MCQs in Huma

ANSWER WHAT YOU ARE SURE OF.

MCQs in Human Physiology

Oliver Holmes DSc, MB, BS, MRCS, LRCP, BA,
Senior Lecturer in Physiology,
University of Glasgow.

Sheila Jennett MD, PhD, MRCP (Glasg.),
Emeritus Professor in Physiology,
University of Glasgow.

CHAPMAN & HALL MEDICAL

London · Glasgow · Weinheim · New York · Tokyo · Melbourne · Madras

**Published by Chapman & Hall, 2–6 Boundary Row,
London SE1 8HN, UK**

Chapman & Hall, 2–6 Boundary Row, London SE1 8HN, UK

Blackie Academic & Professional, Wester Cleddens Road, Bishopbriggs,
Glasgow G64 2NZ, UK

Chapman & Hall GmbH, Pappelallee 3, 69469 Weinheim, Germany

Chapman & Hall USA, 115 Fifth Avenue, New York, NY 10003, USA

Chapman & Hall Japan, ITP-Japan, Kyowa Building, 3F, 2-2-1 Hirakawacho,
Chiyoda-ku, Tokyo 102, Japan

Chapman & Hall Australia, 102 Dodds Street, South Melbourne, 3205,
Victoria, Australia

Chapman & Hall India, R. Seshadri, 32 Second Main Road, CIT East,
Madras 600 035, India

First edition 1996

© 1996 Oliver Holmes and Sheila Jennett

Typeset in 9.5/11pt Times by Mews Photosetting
Printed in Great Britain by Page Bros (Norwich) Ltd

ISBN 0 412 56210 3

A catalogue record for this book is available from the British Library

Library of Congress Catalog Card Number: 95-69152

Contents

Acknowledgements

We owe thanks to many colleagues who have assisted in the assembly of questions over the years, and apologize for any we may have included without attribution to authors no longer known. Professor O.F. Hutter has kindly let us use some of his. We thank Mr Ian Ramsden for drawing the diagrams and Mr Michael Holmes for secretarial assistance.

Introduction

The questions in this book are designed for students of medicine and related life sciences, undergraduate or postgraduate. This type of Yes/No or True/False question is so widespread and so firmly established that its continued use seems likely for some time to come. Even where students of physiology do not anticipate such a test, the questions and their explanatory answers should be an appropriate aid to understanding and revision.

We do not believe that only factual knowledge can be tested in this way, but rather that it is possible to design questions that require the logical thought, calculation and deduction that are the tools of problem-solving.

Most of these questions have been through the mill of repeated use and analysis of answers; many have been modified either as a result of improvements suggested or ambiguities noticed by colleagues or students, or of analytical data such as the discriminative index. Comments on any remaining imperfections will be welcomed.

The questions are arranged in sections, each relating broadly to a topic or system. There is no one obvious starting point or sequence in physiology, since all functions are interrelated, and there is necessarily overlap and repetition among sections. Indexing should allow the location of any particular item. Answers, with explanations, are deferred to the end of each whole section of questions rather than accompanying each one, encouraging the student to refrain from immediate reference to an answer.

In accordance with prevailing practice, five items are grouped under an initial phrase or 'stem' and each item reads on from the stem to make a statement which is either correct or incorrect. The items are designed so that the decision for each statement is independent of the decision about any of the other statements under the same stem. The aim has been to make each statement unequivocally right or wrong, while seeming equally plausible to those with inadequate knowledge.

Advice to students

Each of the five items within a question is designed to be quite separate from the other four, so consider each independently: read the stem and item (a) and decide Yes or No; then read the stem and item (b), and so on.

A candidate who guesses randomly without any basis of knowledge should, in all fairness, be left with a mark of zero. To deal with this, the commonest marking system gives $+1$ for a correct answer, -1 for an incorrect answer and no mark for a blank. Intelligent guessing without sufficient secure information may sometimes be appropriate and useful in an examination – as it can also be in clinical practice, whereas a wild guess is worse than an admission of ignorance. In attempting to answer this type of question, choose Yes or No if you are sure, or if your selection seems reasonably based, but leave the answer blank if choosing Yes or No would be pure guess work.

Note to examiners

In the construction of these questions we have tried to avoid some of the particularly common pitfalls.

1. Statements must not be mutually exclusive. If the answer to one item is 'Yes', this must not imply that the answer to any of the others must be 'No'.

2. Each item in a question should test only one bit of knowledge or deduction. The following is an example of failure to observe this:

A rise in arterial blood pressure:

(a) leads to a decrease in heart rate because of increased baroreceptor activity.

(b) causes cerebral vasoconstriction which reduces cerebral blood flow.

In (a) although both propositions are correct, it is not appropriate to test both the fact (decrease in heart rate) and the mechanism (increased baroreceptor activity): a student who knows that heart rate decreases, but thinks this is due to a reduction in baroreceptor activity, will be puzzled about how to answer, but could gain some credit if the items were separated.

In (b) the fault is similar, but the question is also treacherous because the first part is correct and the second is not.

The items of knowledge tested in this example should have been separated into four independent statements.

1 Body fluids

QUESTIONS

Osmosis, osmotic behaviour of erythrocytes, haemolysis

1.1 Concerning osmosis:

(a) in a dilute solution, the osmotic pressure exerted by a solute is inversely proportional to the molar concentration of that solute.

(b) the total osmotic pressure of the plasma is about one atmosphere.

(c) quantitatively, proteins account for most of the total osmotic pressure of the plasma.

(d) in the process of digestion, when a large molecule is broken down into several smaller molecules, this results in a fall in the osmotic pressure of the intestinal contents.

(e) solutions of sodium chloride and glucose that are of equal molarity exert similar osmotic pressures.

1.2 Concerning the movement of water across cell membranes:

(a) if two solutions are separated by a membrane, the concentration gradient for water is from the solution of higher osmotic pressure towards the solution of lower osmotic pressure.

(b) an erythrocyte immersed in a fluid whose tonicity is twice that of plasma will shrink to less than half its original volume.

(c) when erythrocytes are suspended in a very dilute solution, the hydrostatic pressure difference across the cell membrane rises to about one atmosphere before the cell bursts.

(d) if the hydrostatic pressure applied to a muscle fibre is doubled, the osmotic pressure inside the cell is also approximately doubled.

(e) organic chemicals contribute more to the osmotic pressure of intracellular fluid than to that of extracellular fluid.

1.3 **Concerning the membranes of animal cells and osmosis:**
(a) they consist of a lipid bilayer spanned by protein macromolecules.
(b) the plasma membranes of animal cells can withstand a large pressure difference.
(c) animal cells remain at the same volume irrespective of the osmotic pressure of the solution in which they are bathed.
(d) plasma has an osmolarity of about 300 mosmol per litre.
(e) the osmotic pressure of plasma is about the same as the mean arterial blood pressure.

1.4 **Concerning simple diffusion across cell membranes:**
(a) simple diffusion involves the formation of chemical bonds with structures in the membrane.
(b) if the temperature is reduced from 37°C to 27°C, the rate of diffusion is halved.
(c) the rate of simple diffusion increases with the size of the molecule or ion.
(d) it occurs more rapidly for non-polar than for polar molecules.
(e) the rate of net diffusion of a chemical is inversely proportional to the concentration difference of the chemical across the membrane.

1.5 **Concerning osmotic phenomena:**
(a) movement across the cell membrane of a permeant chemical ceases if the concentration of the chemical on the two sides of the membrane is equal.
(b) if a muscle fibre is immersed in a very dilute solution, the area of its plasma membrane increases by about 2% before the cell bursts.
(c) consider a bag made of a membrane permeable to water but not to sodium or chloride. If the bag were filled with water and immersed in saline, there would be a net entry of water into the bag.
(d) consider a bag made out of a membrane permeable to water, sodium and chloride but not to plasma proteins. If the bag were filled with plasma and immersed in 0.9% saline, there would be a net entry of water into the bag.
(e) if erythrocytes are transferred from a fluid with the composition of plasma to one with the composition of interstitial fluid, the erythrocytes shrink.

1.6 **In a normal adult:**
(a) the osmolarity of intracellular fluid is approximately the same as that of extracellular fluid.
(b) after water is ingested, most of the extra volume is accommodated by the intracellular compartment.
(c) after a 0.9% sodium chloride solution is infused, most of the extra volume is accommodated by the extracellular compartment. (A 0.9% sodium chloride solution is isotonic with plasma).
(d) drinking sea water (3% sodium chloride solution) will lead to shrinkage of cells.
(e) an hour after eating 17 g of solid urea, the cells of the body will have swelled.

1.7 Figure 1.7 represents the volume and osmolarity of intracellular and extracellular fluid in a healthy adult.

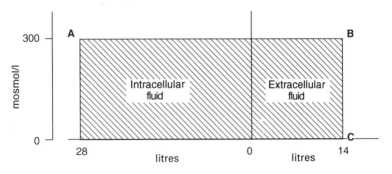

(a) the extracellular fluid contains in total about 300 mosmol of osmolyte.
(b) after the subject drinks and absorbs 1 litre of water, the line AB moves down.
(c) after the subject drinks and absorbs 1 litre of water, the line BC moves to the left.
(d) after infusion of 1 litre of sodium chloride solution at a concentration of 300 mosmol per litre, the line AB will be at about the same level.
(e) after rapid absorption of 17 g sodium chloride, the line AB will have moved up.

1.8 **With further reference to Figure 1.7, concerning the shaded region:**
(a) its area increases if the subject drinks water.
(b) its area increases if the subject drinks isotonic saline.
(c) its area increases if the subject eats salt.
(d) sodium and potassium together contribute about 10% of the total shaded area.
(e) inorganic ions contribute a greater proportion of the shaded area in intracellular fluid than in extracellular fluid.

1.9 **Concerning blood and interstitial fluid:**
(a) the protein content of normal plasma is about 70 g per litre.
(b) the concentration of protein in normal interstitial fluid is similar to that in plasma.
(c) in a muscle capillary, the fluid passing from lumen to interstitial fluid at the arteriolar end contains about half as much albumin as does the plasma.
(d) an amount of albumin equivalent to about half the total plasma albumin passes to the interstitial fluid in 24 hours.
(e) the albumin that passes from plasma to interstitial fluid is returned to the circulation.

1.10   Concerning blood freshly taken from a healthy person:
(a)   the packed cell volume is typically 0.45.
(b)   the protein concentration (in g per litre) in plasma is equal to that in erythrocytes.
(c)   the erythrocytes have a lower specific gravity than the leucocytes.
(d)   the plasma has a lower specific gravity than the erythrocytes.
(e)   when erythrocytes are lysed, the blood loses its colour.

1.11   For blood freshly taken from a healthy person, will the erythrocytes undergo lysis if they are suspended in solutions of:
(a)   sodium chloride at 100 mmol per litre?
(b)   sodium chloride at 100 mosmol per litre?
(c)   sucrose at 300 mosmol per litre?
(d)   sodium chloride at 300 mosmol per litre plus a detergent?
(e)   urea at 300 mosmol per litre plus a detergent?

1.12   0.5 ml of distilled water is added to 1 ml of freshly-taken anticoagulated blood in a test tube. As a result of adding the water, there will be:
(a)   an increase in the volume of individual erythrocytes.
(b)   an increase in the total number of erythrocytes in the test tube.
(c)   an increase in the concentration of haemoglobin within erythrocytes.
(d)   an increase in the amount of haemoglobin (in g) in each erythrocyte.
(e)   a change in shape of erythrocytes towards being nearer to spherical.

1.13   In blood taken from a normal adult person:
(a)   serum differs from plasma in that it lacks fibrinogen.
(b)   in 1 ml of blood there is typically 0.3 ml of plasma.
(c)   in 1 ml of blood the total number of osmotically active particles in erythrocytes is about twice that of the number in the plasma.
(d)   if the extracellular compartment is increased in volume by the addition of more fluid of the same tonicity as plasma, the erythrocytes swell.
(e)   if extra sodium chloride were added the erythrocytes would shrink.

1.14 The cell membranes of erythrocytes in a fresh sample of human blood are permeable to urea but not to sodium chloride. The osmolarity of the plasma for this sample is 300 mosmol/litre. Will the cells swell if they are suspended in the following solutions?
(a) sodium chloride at 150 mmol.
(b) urea at 300 mmol.
(c) sodium chloride at 150 mmol plus urea at 300 mmol.
(d) sodium chloride at 200 mmol plus urea at 200 mmol.
(e) sodium chloride at 100 mmol plus urea at 400 mmol.

1.15 Are the ratios on the right approximately correct for the difference between ionic concentrations outside and inside a cell, e.g. a mammalian nerve cell?

Outside:Inside

(a) K^+ 1:30
(b) Na^+ 10:1
(c) Ca^{2+} 10:1
(d) H^+ 1:1
(e) Cl^- 12:1

1.16 Concerning distribution of the major inorganic ionic species across resting cell membranes:
(a) cell membranes are more permeable to potassium ions than to water.
(b) cell membranes are more permeable to sodium ions than to other inorganic ions.
(c) the electrochemical gradient for bicarbonate favours its movement out of cells.
(d) inorganic anions are in greater total concentration outside than inside cells.
(e) if sodium–potassium pump activity is poisoned, all inorganic ion species will move in or out down their concentration gradients.

1.17 Concerning diffusion and blood:
(a) in a capillary bed, the transfer of oxygen from the erythrocyte to the interstitial fluid is by passive diffusion.
(b) comparing the rates of passive diffusion of two chemicals in a bulk solution, if one chemical has twice the molecular weight of the other it will diffuse at half the rate.
(c) if you can read the written page through 5 ml of a solution to which one drop of blood has been added, the erythrocytes are intact.
(d) the packed cell volume of blood taken from a peripheral vein is an underestimate of the whole body packed cell volume.
(e) when blood is stored, the erythrocytes progressively shrink.

1.18 **With reference to water and body fluids:**
(a) there is a continuous loss of water via the skin.
(b) ingestion of an unusually large quantity of water results in a transient decrease in plasma osmolarity.
(c) interstitial fluid is an ultrafiltrate of plasma.
(d) the concentration of bicarbonate ions in interstitial fluid is less than one-tenth that in plasma.
(e) extracellular fluid has a lower concentration of sodium ions than intracellular fluid.

1.19 **Concerning the body water in an adult person:**
(a) it readily permeates all cell membranes.
(b) it comprises a smaller percentage of the total body mass in a fat person than in a thin person.
(c) it is held constant to within about 100 ml during a day.
(d) it may decrease by 4 litres due to sweating without threatening life.
(e) its volume can be estimated with inulin injected intravenously as a marker.

1.20 **Concerning osmotic pressure:**
(a) a solution of 5 g/litre of haemoglobin (molecular weight 67 000) has a higher osmotic pressure than a solution of 5 g/litre of urea (molecular weight 60).
(b) the total osmotic pressure of the plasma globulins is about 25 mmHg.
If erythrocytes are placed in a hypertonic solution of sodium chloride:
(c) the erythrocytes swell.
(d) haemolysis may occur.
(e) water diffuses out of the erythrocytes.

Fluid compartments, electrolytes

1.21 **Compared with intracellular fluid, extracellular fluid has:**
(a) a greater osmotic strength.
(b) a lower sodium ion concentration.
(c) a lower chloride ion concentration.
(d) a lower potassium ion concentration.
(e) a lower hydrogen ion concentration.

1.22 **With reference to extracellular fluid volume and composition in the human:**
(a) if blood volume is depleted, adjustments involve an increase in aldosterone secretion.
(b) if the body is short of water, the collecting ducts of the nephrons become less permeable to water.
(c) plasma sodium concentration is regulated by varying the fraction of the sodium in the glomerular filtrate which is reabsorbed in the proximal tubules.
(d) increased osmolality leads to an increase in the secretion of anti-diuretic hormone (ADH).
(e) plasma sodium concentration is regulated by varying the proportion of ingested sodium that is absorbed in the gut.

1.23 **With reference to water and solutes:**
(a) diffusion means that molecules move in one direction only from a region of greater to a region of lesser concentration.
(b) the colloid osmotic pressure of the plasma represents about one-tenth of the total plasma osmolality.
(c) in plasma, chloride is in higher concentration than any other anion.
(d) the sum of the concentration of sodium and chloride ions on one side of a membrane permeable to these ions must equal the sum of the two on the other side.
(e) carrier-mediated mechanisms are more susceptible to temperature changes than are diffusional processes.

1.24 **If about 0.5 litre of isotonic saline (sodium chloride solution) were rapidly infused intravenously in a healthy adult, the consequences would include:**
(a) an increase in cardiac stroke volume.
(b) an increase in flow of lymph from peripheral tissues.
(c) an increase in renin secretion by the kidneys.
(d) an increase in cerebral blood flow.
(e) equal distribution of the excess volume between intracellular and extracellular compartments.

1.25 **If an excessive amount of water is drunk:**
(a) only a small fraction of it is absorbed from the gastro-intestinal tract.
(b) the osmolality of interstitial fluid decreases.
(c) receptors in the right atrium may be stimulated.
(d) receptors in the carotid body may be stimulated.
(e) an increase in the glomerular filtration rate is the main means of disposing of the extra water.

1.26 **Concerning plasma albumin:**
(a) less than 10% is degraded each week.
(b) its molecular weight (MW) is greater than that of globulin.
(c) it is responsible for most of the colloid osmotic pressure.
(d) in normal subjects, the albumin:globulin ratio is about 2:1 (weight for weight).
(e) a reduction in plasma albumin concentration is liable to be associated with oedema.

1.27 **With reference to the control of extracellular fluid volume and osmolarity:**
(a) the action of anti-diuretic hormone on the kidney is by increasing the permeability of the distal tubules to water.
(b) renin is secreted by cells situated close to the afferent glomerular arterioles.
(c) anti-diuretic hormone is released in response to the action of hypothalamic releasing factors.
(d) an increase in right atrial pressure leads to a decrease in aldosterone activity.
(e) an excessive secretion of aldosterone results in increased loss of potassium in the urine.

1.28 **Are the values given appropriate for a healthy 70 kg man?**
(a) the body contains about 40 litres of water.
(b) the minimal daily water intake to maintain fluid balance in temperate conditions is approximately 450 ml.
(c) a suitable daily calorie intake for moderate physical activity would be 3500 kcal.
(d) the glomerular filtration rate (GFR) (both kidneys) is approximately 1200 ml/min.
(e) plasma osmolarity is about 300 mosmol/litre.

1.29 **With reference to water in the body:**
(a) the total accounts for approximately 60% of body weight in a lean adult man.
(b) approximately two-thirds of the total volume is intracellular.
(c) the total volume may be estimated using radioactively labelled plasma albumin.
(d) there is inevitably a continuous loss of water via the skin under average temperature conditions.
(e) ingestion of an unusually large quantity of water results in a transient decrease in plasma osmolarity.

1.30 **With reference to potassium in the body:**
(a) the equivalent of most of the daily dietary intake of potassium is secreted into the tubular fluid in the kidneys.
(b) an increase in extracellular potassium concentration endangers cardiac function.
(c) a decrease in extracellular potassium concentration endangers cardiac function.
(d) an increase in extracellular potassium concentration (e.g. to 8 mmol per litre) relaxes vascular smooth muscle.
(e) deficiency of aldosterone secretion results in an increase in extracellular potassium concentration.

1.31 **In a normal human adult:**
(a) the total concentration of electrolytes in plasma is less than that in interstitial fluid.
(b) the total number of osmotically active particles in the intracellular compartment is about the same as in the extracellular compartment.
(c) if pure water were added to the extracellular compartment, the cells of the body would swell.
(d) if the extracellular compartment were increased in volume by the addition of fluid of the same composition as extracellular fluid, the cells of the body would shrink.
(e) if extra sodium chloride were dissolved in the extracellular fluid, there would be a net entry of water into the cells.

1.32 **Concerning the movement of solutes and solvent across the wall of a typical capillary (e.g. in muscle):**
(a) at the arteriolar end of the capillary, the hydrostatic force favouring filtration of fluid is typically 35 mmHg.
(b) in the capillary, the colloid osmotic pressure favouring reabsorption of fluid is typically 25 mmHg.
(c) in a given capillary (assumed to be unbranching), the total flow of blood at the arteriolar end of the capillary is greater than the total flow half way along it.
(d) at the venular end of the capillary, there is usually a net filtration of fluid.
(e) in a given capillary (assumed to be unbranching), the total flow of blood at the venular end of the capillary is greater than the total flow half way along it.

1.33 In blood plasma:
(a) calcium is the cation present in greatest concentration.
(b) bicarbonate is the anion present in greatest concentration.
(c) the total osmotic pressure of the plasma opposes filtration of fluid across the capillary wall.
(d) the colloid osmotic pressure of the plasma falls as blood traverses typical capillaries (e.g. in skeletal muscle).
(e) as blood descends in the vasa recta to the medullary region of the kidney, the colloid osmotic pressure of the plasma rises several fold.

1.34 Concerning blood in the circulation:
(a) as blood passes down the vasa recta of the kidney in the anti-diuretic subject, the erythrocytes shrink to about a quarter of their usual volume.
(b) as blood traverses the systemic capillaries, its packed cell volume increases.
(c) as blood traverses the systemic capillaries, the colloid osmotic pressure decreases.
(d) in capillaries in skeletal muscle, erythrocytes move to and fro across the capillary wall.
(e) leucocytes move to and fro across capillary walls.

1.35 A marker (such as a dye) is selected to measure the plasma volume of a human. It should possess the following properties:
(a) it should be rapidly metabolized.
(b) it should adhere to the membranes of erythrocytes.
(c) it should bind to plasma proteins.
(d) it should readily cross the walls of capillaries.
In order to make the calculation:
(e) the concentration of the marker in whole blood is used.

1.36 Is it possible for a person to survive the reduction of the concentrations of the following substances to one half of their normal value?
(a) water in plasma.
(b) haemoglobin in blood.
(c) sodium ions in plasma.
(d) hydrogen ions in plasma.
(e) bicarbonate in plasma.

1.37 **Is it possible for a person to survive the reduction of the concentrations of the following substances to one half of their normal value?**
(a) chloride in plasma.
(b) potassium ions in plasma.
(c) ionized calcium in plasma.
(d) glucose in plasma.
(e) oxygen in mixed venous blood.

1.38 **Oedema formation in a tissue is promoted by:**
(a) arteriolar constriction with a constant mean arterial blood pressure.
(b) constriction of the vein draining the tissue.
(c) a decrease in the sodium concentration of the plasma.
(d) histamine release by the tissue.
(e) surgical removal of the lymphatics draining the tissue.

1.39 **Oedema in the limbs is likely to be associated with:**
(a) right ventricular failure.
(b) chronic severe liver disease.
(c) allergic reactions.
(d) chronic over-administration of aldosterone.
(e) loss of 20% of the blood volume.

1.40 **Decide if the following values lie within normal limits:**
(a) plasma sodium concentration 140 mmol/litre.
(b) plasma potassium concentration 10 mmol/litre.
(c) plasma bicarbonate concentration 4 mmol/litre.
(d) total plasma osmotic pressure 150 mosmol/litre.
(e) intracellular potassium concentration 8 mmol/litre.

1.41 **Concerning movement of solutes across the capillary wall:**
(a) non-polar molecules diffuse across the endothelial cell membranes more readily than polar molecules.
(b) small polar molecules readily pass through the channels between endothelial cells.
(c) plasma proteins readily pass through the channels between endothelial cells.
(d) pinocytotic vesicles in endothelial cells carry solute molecules between the plasma and the interstitial fluid.
(e) pinocytosis is the mechanism of movement across fenestrations in endothelial cells.

1.42 **If an animal cell is immersed in a solution of sodium chloride at two-thirds the normal osmolarity:**
(a) the cell will initially swell.
(b) membrane transporter mechanisms are activated.
(c) after any initial change in volume, the cell slowly returns towards its initial volume.
(d) if the cell is subsequently returned to saline of normal osmolarity, the cell's volume will fall to below its initial value.
(e) if membrane transporter mechanisms are blocked, all volume changes in response to hypotonicity of the bathing fluid are prevented.

1.43 **With respect to the ways in which substances enter and leave cells:**
(a) potassium ions move in and out through water-filled 'pores'.
(b) glucose enters by dissolving in the cell membrane.
(c) amino acids enter by a carrier-mediated transport mechanism.
(d) all healthy cells have sodium pumps which extrude sodium ions against a concentration gradient.
(e) only water-soluble substances can cross cell walls.

Cell structure and membrane function

1.44 **Concerning the contents of cells:**
(a) the cytosol is the term for the intracellular fluid.
(b) microtubules provide routes for internal transport.
(c) microfilaments can change a cell's shape.
(d) messenger RNA is made in the endoplasmic reticulum.
(e) lysosomes contain enzymes in a package of internal membrane.

1.45 **The cell membrane:**
(a) has hydrophilic heads of lipid molecules pointing only to the side interfacing with the extracellular fluid.
(b) allows movement of water across it, over the whole of its surface.
(c) allows movement of oxygen and carbon dioxide across it over the whole of its surface.
(d) has protein molecules embedded in it.
(e) has glycogen granules embedded in it.

ANSWERS

1.1

(a) No. Osmotic pressure is a colligative property, i.e. the osmotic pressure depends on the number of solute particles in a given volume of solution, not on their chemical nature. In a dilute solution, the osmotic pressure exerted by a solute is directly proportional to the molar concentration of that solute.

(b) No. The total osmotic pressure of the plasma is between 6 and 7 atmospheres. (A solution of 1 osmol per litre exerts an osmotic pressure of 22.4 atmospheres; the osmolarity of plasma is about 0.3 osmol per litre, so its osmotic pressure is $0.3 \times 22.4 = 6.7$ atmospheres.

(c) No. Quantitatively, electrolytes account for most of the total osmotic pressure of the plasma. Proteins account for a tiny fraction, typically 25 mmHg.

(d) No. In the process of digestion, when a large molecule is broken down into several smaller molecules, this results in an increase in concentration of osmotically active particles and hence a rise in the osmotic pressure of the intestinal contents.

(e) No. Each mole of sodium chloride dissociates in solution into 2 osmol. So for solutions of sodium chloride and of glucose of equal molarity, sodium chloride solution exerts twice the osmotic pressure of glucose solution.

1.2

(a) No. If two solutions of different osmotic pressure are separated by a membrane, the concentration of water is greater in the solution of lower osmotic pressure, so the gradient for water is from the solution of lower osmotic pressure towards the solution of higher osmotic pressure. There is liable to be confusion on this point and it arises because osmotic 'pressure' is an unfortunate expression; osmotic 'suck' would be much more intuitively meaningful since a strong solution sucks in water.

(b) No. When an erythrocyte is immersed in a fluid whose tonicity is twice that of plasma, about half the water initially within the erythrocyte will leave due to osmotic forces. However, the haemoglobin inside the erythrocyte makes up a significant proportion of the cell contents and its volume will not change. Hence the erythrocyte will shrink, but not by as much as a half.

(c) No. The plasma membrane of erythrocytes and of other animal cells can withstand only a negligible mechanical distortion before they break.

(d)   No. Aqueous fluids are virtually incompressible, so doubling the hydrostatic pressure has almost no effect on the volume of the intracellular fluid. The amount of solute is unaltered, so the osmotic pressure remains unchanged.

(e)   Yes. Intracellular fluid is rich in proteins and amino acids whereas extracellular fluid contains very little of them.

1.3

(a)   Yes. Most of the membrane consists of a lipid bilayer, but here and there are to be found protein macromolecules that span the lipid bilayer; these protein macromolecules form ion channels, etc.

(b)   No. The plasma membranes of animal cells are very delicate and can withstand only negligible pressure differences.

(c)   No. Cell membranes are in general permeable to water since they can withstand negligible hydrostatic pressure differences. If the osmolarity of the solution in which they are bathed changes, there is a net movement of water across the cell wall until the osmotic gradient is evened out. Net movement of water results in changes in volume.

(d)   Yes.

(e)   No. The osmotic pressure of plasma is around 6 atmospheres (4 500 mm Hg;) the mean arterial blood pressure is typically 90 mm Hg.

1.4

(a)   No. Simple diffusion is a physicochemical phenomenon that does not involve the formation of chemical bonds with structures in the membrane.

(b)   No. The rate of diffusion, unlike many biological processes, is very little affected by a change in temperature from 37°C to 27°C.

(c)   No. The rate of simple diffusion decreases with the size of the molecule or ion.

(d)   Yes. Diffusion occurs more rapidly for non-polar than for polar molecules because non-polar molecules dissolve in the cell membrane.

(e)   No. The rate of net diffusion of a chemical is directly proportional to the concentration difference of the chemical across the membrane.

1.5

(a)   No. To-and-fro movement across the cell membrane of a permeant chemical occurs if the concentration of the chemical on the two sides of the membrane is equal. However, there is no net movement of the chemical.

(b)   Yes. The membrane of any animal cell, including a muscle cell, has very little elasticity; if it is immersed in a very dilute solution, the area of its plasma membrane will only increase by about 2% before the cell bursts.

(c)   No. The saline surrounding the bag sucks water out; there would be a net exit of water out of the bag.

(d)   Yes. The only impermeant particles are the plasma proteins so these are the only particles providing an effective osmotic pressure; they therefore suck water into the bag.

(e)   No. Interstitial fluid, being protein free, has a lower osmotic strength than does plasma. So if erythrocytes are transferred from a fluid with the composition of plasma to one with the composition of interstitial fluid, the erythrocytes swell.

1.6

(a)   Yes.

(b)   Yes. Extra- and intracellular compartments shows similar relative increases in volume in this situation, so about one-third of the ingested water is accommodated in the extracellular compartment.

(c)   Yes.

(d)   Yes. The hypertonicity of the extracellular fluid will suck water out of the cells and cause shrinkage.

(e)   No. Urea crosses the cell wall with ease so does not alter the osmotic relationship between intra- and extracellular fluids.

1.7

(a)   No. The extracellular fluid contains in total about $(300 \times 14) = 4200$ mosmol of osmolyte.

(b)   Yes. Water dilutes the body fluids.

(c)   No. The extracellular volume (and also the intracellular volume) are expanded by the ingestion of water, so line BC moves to the right.

(d)   Yes. Infusion of isosmotic saline does not alter the osmolarity of the body fluids.

(e)   Yes. Absorption of sodium chloride increases the osmolarity of the body fluids.

1.8

(a)   No. The total shaded area represents the total number of osmolytes in the body; this is unaltered by drinking water.

(b)   Yes. Drinking isotonic saline adds to the total number of osmolytes in the body fluids.

(c)   Yes. Eating salt adds to the total number of osmolytes in the body fluids.

(d)   No. Sodium and potassium contribute about half the osmolarity of extracellular and intracellular fluid respectively, so together they contribute about 50% of the total shaded area.

(e)   No. In intracellular fluid, organic ions such as amino acids and peptides contribute far more to osmolarity than in extracellular fluid.

1.9

(a)   Yes.

(b)   No. 1 g per litre is a typical value.

(c)   No. The range is 1–2%.

(d)   Yes.

(e)   Yes. The albumin that passes from plasma to interstitial fluid is returned to the circulation in the lymph.

1.10

(a)   Yes.

(b)   No. In plasma, the protein concentration is typically 70 g per litre; in erythrocytes the protein haemoglobin is at a concentration of typically 320 g per litre.

(c)   No. The erythrocytes have a higher specific gravity than the leucocytes, as witnessed by the fact that after centrifuge the leucocytes form the 'buffy coat' above the erythrocytes.

(d)   Yes. This is why the erythrocytes are thrown to the bottom of the tube.

(e)   No. When erythrocytes are lysed, the blood is a clear red.

1.11

(a)   No. Sodium chloride at 100 mmol per litre has an osmolarity of 200 mosmol per litre; erythrocytes haemolyse when bathed in solutions of about half normal plasma osmolarity or less and the normal osmolarity of plasma is around 300 mosmol per litre.

(b)   Yes. Erythrocytes haemolyse when bathed in solutions of about half normal plasma osmolarity or less, and the normal osmolarity of plasma is around 300 mosmol per litre.

(c)   No. Sucrose does not permeate the erythrocyte membrane and so provides an effective extracellular osmolarity similar to that of the intracellular fluid to counteract the osmotic pressure exerted by intracellular large impermeant chemicals.

(d)   Yes. Detergent dissolves the cell membrane, so no matter what other particles are present, a detergent will cause lysis.

(e)   Yes. As in (d).

1.12

(a) Yes. The added water dilutes the plasma increasing its water concentration. There is a net entry of water into the erythrocytes, which therefore swell.

(b) No. No erythrocytes have been added and individual erythrocytes do not divide. So there is no change in the total number of erythrocytes in the test tube.

(c) No. There is a net entry of water into erythrocytes, so the concentration of haemoglobin within erythrocytes falls.

(d) No. The amount of haemoglobin in each erythrocyte is unaltered.

(e) Yes. As the volume of an erythrocyte increases, there is a change from the normal biconcave disc shape to a more spherical shape.

1.13

(a) Yes. Plasma is the supernatant after centrifuging blood to which an anticoagulant has been added. Serum is the fluid expressed when blood is allowed to clot. The clotting removes fibrinogen.

(b) No. Since a typical value for the packed cell volume is 0.45, in 1 ml of blood there is typically 0.55 ml of plasma.

(c) No. Since the packed cell volume for normal blood is below 0.5, and since the osmolality in intra- and extracellular fluid is the same, the total number of osmotically active particles is rather less in erythrocytes than in plasma in 1 ml of blood.

(d) No. If the extracellular compartment is increased by adding more fluid of the same composition, there is no alteration in osmotic balance across the erythrocyte membrane and so there is no net movement of water; the erythrocyte volume remains constant.

(e) Yes. Addition of sodium chloride to the extracellular fluid increases its osmolality and this sucks water out of the erythrocytes, which therefore shrink.

1.14

(a) No. In solution, each molecule of sodium chloride dissociates into two osmotically active particles. A solution of sodium chloride at a concentration of 150 mmol therefore has an osmolarity of 300 mosmol per litre and the erythrocytes will experience no change in the osmotic strength of their environment. There will be no net movement of water.

(b) Yes. Urea permeates the erythrocyte membrane and so its concentration inside the erythrocyte tends to equalize with the extracellular concentration. There are therefore no extracellular impermeant particles to balance the osmotic pressure exerted by intracellular large impermeant chemicals such as proteins. So erythrocytes immersed in a solution of urea alone, no matter what its concentration, will swell and burst.

(c)   No. For this and parts (d) and (e), we can ignore the effects of urea, since it exerts no effective osmotic pressure across the membrane. Urea will diffuse into the cells until its concentration on the two sides of the membrane is equal. The sodium chloride has an osmolarity of 300 mosmol per litre so the erythrocytes do not swell.

(d)   No. Here the sodium chloride solution has an osmolarity of 400 mosmol per litre, so the erythrocytes will shrink.

(e)   Yes. The sodium chloride has an osmolarity of 200 mosmol per litre which is less than the osmolarity of the intracellular fluid. There is net movement of water into the erythrocytes and they swell.

1.15

(a)   Yes.

(b)   Yes.

(c)   No. The difference is much greater than this: 10^4:1.

(d)   No. Intracellular pH is more acid than extracellular; 0.4:1 is a likely ratio for [H^+].

(e)   Yes.

1.16

(a)   No. The membrane permeability to water is around 10^7 times as great as that for potassium ions.

(b)   No. The membrane conductance for sodium ions is low by comparison with that for potassium ions in resting cells. The result of electrical (outwards) and chemical (inwards) gradients is a small net movement inwards, continually corrected actively by the Na–K pump.

(c)   Yes. Although the outside:inside ratio for bicarbonate is about 3:1, this is more than counteracted by the inside negativity tending to expel it.

(d)   Yes. Both chloride and bicarbonate are in lower concentration outside than inside. Only phosphate is higher inside. The balance of charges inside cells is made up by organic anions.

(e)   Yes. The conductance of the membrane for the different ion species varies greatly, but it is not totally impermeable to any of them; each will tend to equilibrate by diffusion across the membrane. The large organic molecules, however, cannot move out, so there is an increase in particle concentration, and therefore in osmolarity, inside. Such cells therefore swell and eventually burst.

1.17

(a)   Yes.

(b)   No. The rate of passive diffusion of a chemical in a bulk solution is inversely proportional to the cube root of the molecular weight.

So the difference in diffusion rate will be the cube root of 2 which is about 1.1. Thus small differences in molecular weight have relatively little effect on the rate of diffusion.

(c)　No. Intact erythrocytes disperse light passing through them and it is impossible to read the written page through such a suspension. If you can read the written page, it means that the erythrocytes have been haemolysed.

(d)　No. The packed cell volume taken from a peripheral vein is an overestimate of the whole body packed cell volume. There are several reasons for this. One is that many capillaries are so narrow that they contain few or no erythrocytes but they do contain plasma. This blood is not sampled in a venepuncture. Another reason is that in venous blood the mean corpuscular volume is greater than for peripheral arterial blood. This is because most of the carbon dioxide taken up during transit through the systemic capillaries is transformed in the erythrocytes into bicarbonate and this increases the number of osmotically active particles in the erythrocytes.

(e)　No. When blood is stored, sodium leaks into the erythrocytes. The difference in intra- and extracellular concentration of sodium declines. There is therefore a reduction in the extracellular osmolarity balancing the osmotic pressure exerted by intracellular large impermeant chemicals such as proteins. So erythrocytes swell and eventually burst.

1.18

(a)　Yes. The continuous loss of water via the skin is called 'insensible perspiration'.

(b)　Yes.

(c)　Yes. Interstitial fluid is an ultrafiltrate of plasma. The fluid passes through small water-filled channels in the endothelial lining.

(d)　No. The concentration of bicarbonate ions in interstitial fluid is close to its value in plasma.

(e)　No. Extracellular fluid has a higher concentration of sodium ions than intracellular fluid. Sodium is the principal cation in the extracellular fluid; in the intracellular fluid it is potassium.

1.19

(a)　No. The cells of the ascending limb of the loop of Henle in the kidney have membranes impermeable to water. So does the epithelium lining the ureters and bladder.

(b)　Yes. Fatty tissue is almost devoid of water, so a fat person has a smaller proportion of water than a thin person.

(c)　No. The total body water typically varies by about 1 litre during a day.

(d)   Yes. A decrease in body water of 4 litres is mild to moderate; it is not life-threatening. A loss of above 10 litres would be life-threatening.

(e)   No. Inulin does not cross cell membranes readily; it is used to estimate the extracellular fluid volume.

1.20

(a)   No. Osmotic pressure depends on the number of particles per unit volume; 5 g/litre of urea has about 1000 times as many particles as 5 g/litre of Hb.

(b)   No. The osmotic pressure of the plasma proteins is around 25 mm Hg, but most of this is due to albumin.

(c)   No. The cells will lose water by osmosis. They will shrink.

(d)   No. Haemolysis occurs when cells swell in a hypotonic solution.

(e)   Yes.

1.21

(a)   No. In this situation, the cells would shrink.

(b)   No. Extracellular sodium is much the higher.

(c)   No. Extracellular chloride is much the higher.

(d)   Yes. Intracellular potassium is much the higher.

(e)   Yes. Intracellular pH is less than extracellular.

1.22

(a)   Yes. Aldosterone tends to restore blood volume, by reabsorption of sodium, which brings water with it osmotically.

(b)   No. They become more permeable to water (by the action of ADH), which allows greater water reabsorption down the osmotic gradient.

(c)   No. The amount reabsorbed in the proximal tubules is always the same proportion of the filtered load. The variation is in the distal tubules, by the action of aldosterone.

(d)   Yes. Increased extracellular fluid osmolality stimulates hypothalamic osmoreceptors, leading to secretion of ADH, retention of water, and hence correction of osmolality.

(e)   No. All ingested sodium is absorbed in the gut; absorption is active and does not depend on a diffusion gradient. Correction for changes in plasma sodium concentration is by the kidneys, not by controlling absorption.

1.23

(a)   No. Diffusion is the continuous movement of molecules in all directions. Diffusion from a region of greater concentration to one of lesser concentration implies a net movement in that direction.

(b)   No. It is about 1/200.

(c)   Yes. Cl^- concentration is over 100 mmol per litre.

(d)   No. It is the products, not the sums, that must be equal (Donnan equilibrium).

(e)   Yes.

1.24

(a)   Yes. Increased venous return leads to higher ventricular filling pressure, and hence to an increase in stroke volume.

(b)   Yes. Dilution of plasma protein enhances movement of fluid out of capillaries, therefore leads to greater lymph flow.

(c)   No. Renin secretion, hence angiotensin, hence aldosterone would decrease, leading to a decrease in Na^+ reabsorption.

(d)   No. Even though arterial blood pressure may rise, cerebral autoregulatory vasoconstriction keeps blood flow steady.

(e)   No. Most of the fluid remains extracellular.

1.25

(a)   No. Water absorption is independent of intake or need.

(b)   Yes. Any dilution of the blood will lead to transfer of water across capillary walls, by osmosis.

(c)   Yes. An increase in blood volume can lead to stimulation of atrial receptors and hence to stimulation of release of the appropriate hormones.

(d)   No. These are chemoreceptors which are stimulated by low PO_2, high PCO_2 and low pH.

(e)   No. The main means is by altering reabsorption rate in the distal tubules and collecting ducts.

1.26

(a)   No. About 10% is degraded every day.

(b)   No. Molecular weight 69 000 and 156 000 respectively.

(c)   Yes. Its **molar** concentration accounts for the major part of the colloid osmotic pressure.

(d)   Yes.

(e)   Yes. Because of the lowering of colloid osmotic pressure.

1.27

(a)   Yes. This is the action of anti-diuretic hormone (ADH).

(b)   Yes.

(c)   No. ADH is released from the posterior pituitary; the control is via the direct neural pathway from the hypothalamus. Releasing hormones act on the anterior pituitary.

(d)   Yes. Receptors in the atrium initiate a neuroendocrine reflex which leads to less aldosterone secretion, therefore less retention of sodium and water, therefore a reduction in blood volume. Atrial natriuretic factor is also released and has similar renal effects.

(e)   Yes. Aldosterone promotes the secretion of potassium, as well as the retention of sodium, in the kidney.

1.28

(a)   Yes.

(b)   No. Minimal water intake must balance obligatory fluid loss which is approximately 1–1.5 litres:

urine	430–450 ml/24 h
faeces	70–150 ml/24 h
evaporation	400–500 ml/24 h
respiration	200–300 ml/24 h

(c)   Yes.

(d)   No. About one-tenth of the renal blood flow or one-fifth of the plasma flow is filtered. Renal blood flow is in turn about one-fifth of cardiac output, giving a GFR of about 120 ml/min.

(e)   Yes. This is the total osmolarity; not to be confused with colloid osmotic pressure.

1.29

(a)   Yes.

(b)   Yes.

(c)   No. Plasma albumin is not distributed outside the plasma. This 'label' would measure plasma volume only.

(d)   Yes. By 'insensible perspiration' when not sweating.

(e)   Yes. Absorption of excessive water from the gut leads to some degree of haemodilution, transient because it is rapidly corrected by osmotic movement into the extravascular compartment and by decreased secretion of anti-diuretic hormone.

1.30

(a)   Yes. In a state of balance, little is lost by other routes, and virtually all is reabsorbed from the glomerular filtrate.

(b)   Yes. Accelerates repolarization and can lead to cardiac arrest.

(c)   Yes. Weakens contraction.

(d)   Yes. This may contribute to vasodilatation in active muscle and neural tissue.

(e)   Yes. Aldosterone stimulates distal tubular potassium secretion in the kidney.

1.31

(a)   No. The total concentration of electrolytes in plasma is close to that in interstitial fluid (it is, in fact, slightly more because of Donnan effects influencing the distribution of permeant ions across the capillary wall). The total osmotic strength of plasma is greater than that of the interstitial fluid because of the plasma proteins, the interstitial fluid being virtually protein free.

(b)   No. Since the volume of the intracellular compartment is about twice that of the extracellular compartment, the total number of osmotically active particles is about twice as great in the intracellular compartment as in the extracellular compartment.

(c)   Yes. Water would enter the cells due to the pressure gradient and this would cause swelling.

(d)   No. Since there would be no disturbance of osmotic equilibrium across the cell membrane, the cells would stay the same size.

(e)   No. There would be a net exit of water, because of the increased osmolality of the extracellular fluid.

1.32

(a)   Yes.

(b)   Yes.

(c)   Yes. Some of the fluid entering the capillary at the arteriolar end leaves the plasma to pass across the capillary wall. So the total flow of blood at the arteriolar end of the capillary is greater than the total flow half way along it.

(d)   No. At the venular end of the capillary, there is usually a net reabsorption of fluid back into the plasma.

(e)   Yes. Towards the venular end of the capillary, fluid enters the capillary from the interstitial fluid. So the total flow of blood at the venular end of the capillary is greater than the total flow half way along it.

1.33

(a)   No. In plasma, sodium is the cation present in greatest concentration, typically 140 mmol.

(b)   No. In plasma, chloride is the anion present in greatest concentration, typically 100 mmol.

(c)   No. Only the particles that cannot cross the capillary wall (i.e. plasma proteins) oppose filtration. The colloid osmotic pressure of the plasma is the osmotic force opposing filtration of fluid across the capillary wall.

(d)   No. As blood traverses capillaries, there is a net loss of protein-free fluid from the plasma, so the concentration of protein in the plasma rises; the colloid osmotic pressure of the plasma rises.

(e)   Yes. As blood descends in the vasa recta to the medullary region of the kidney, the hypertonicity of the interstitial fluid 'sucks' fluid out of the blood. As plasma protein cannot follow, its concentration rises and the colloid osmotic pressure of the plasma rises several fold.

1.34

(a)   Yes. The tonicity of the interstitium of the renal medulla and the plasma in the loops of the vasa recta is about four times that of normal plasma and so the erythrocytes are exposed to a solution that is about four times the usual tonicity.

(b)   Yes. The erythrocytes swell due to uptake of CO_2 and release of bicarbonate, which increases the total concentration of osmotically-active particles in the erythrocyte. Even though much of this intracellular bicarbonate moves back into the plasma, each bicarbonate ion moving out is in exchange for a chloride ion moving in; this mechanism has no influence on the number of osmotically-active particles in the plasma.

(c)   No. The colloid osmotic pressure increases by a small amount due to the net loss of fluid from the plasma to the interstitial fluid.

(d)   No. The erythrocytes are constrained to remain in the circulating blood.

(e)   Yes. Leucocytes can wander freely between the blood and the interstitial fluid.

1.35

(a)   No. Metabolism of the marker would remove it from the system.

(b)   No. In order to be of use in estimating plasma volume, the marker must remain in the plasma.

(c)   Yes. Binding to plasma proteins helps to keep it in the plasma compartments.

(d)   No. If the marker readily crosses the walls of capillaries, it does not stay in the plasma.

(e)   No. The concentration of the marker in plasma is used.

1.36

(a)   No. A reduction in water concentration of about 25% is fatal.

(b)   Yes. The haemoglobin concentration is normally around 150 g haemoglobin per litre of blood. It is not uncommon for an anaemic person to have a haemoglobin concentration of 50 g haemoglobin per litre of blood. Oxygen carrying capacity in such a person is one-third that of normal, but oxygen supply to the tissues may be maintained by an increase in cardiac output and increasing the proportion of oxygen lost by each litre of blood as it passes through the systemic capillaries.

(c)   No. Sodium ions are the principal cation osmolyte in the blood and a reduction in concentration of about 25% is fatal.

(d)   Yes. A two-fold change of hydrogen ion concentration in plasma (corresponding to a change in pH of 0.2 units) is compatible with life.

(e)   Yes. Bicarbonate concentrations vary widely, beyond two-fold changes, in compensated acid-base disturbances.

1.37

(a)   No. Chloride ions are the principal anion osmolyte in the blood and a reduction in concentration of about 25% is fatal.

(b)   Yes. The normal concentration of potassium ions in the plasma is about 4 mmol per litre and a reduction to 2 mmol per litre although life-threatening, is a value not uncommonly found in patients.

(c)   Yes. Such a reduction in calcium would produce profound clinical effects such as hypocalcaemic tetany, but halving of the calcium concentration is compatible with life.

(d)   Yes. A fall in blood glucose from its normal 5 mmol per litre to half this value occurs in hypoglycaemic episodes occurring, for instance, in a diabetic who receives an insulin injection and then omits to eat a meal.

(e)   Yes. A halving of oxygen content of mixed venous blood occurs in a healthy person who exercises moderately vigorously.

1.38

(a)   No. Arteriolar constriction with a constant mean arterial blood pressure reduces the mean capillary hydrostatic pressure and reduces the tendency for formation of tissue fluid.

(b)   Yes. Constriction of the vein draining the tissue increases the mean capillary hydrostatic pressure and increases the tendency for formation of tissue fluid.

(c)   No. A decrease in the sodium concentration of the plasma is without effect on the balance of forces across the capillary wall.

(d)   Yes. Histamine release by the tissue causes an increase in permeability of the walls of capillaries and hence the formation of oedema.

(e)   Yes. Surgical removal of the lymphatics draining the tissue removes the route for drainage of excess tissue fluid and so favours the formation of oedema.

1.39

(a)   Yes. In right ventricular failure, the central venous pressure rises and this predisposes to oedema in the limbs.

(b)   Yes. In chronic severe liver disease, there is a reduced concentration of plasma albumin, which is produced by the liver. Consequent on this low plasma albumin, the colloid osmotic pressure of the plasma is low and oedema forms.

(c)   Yes. In allergic reactions the permeability of the capillaries is increased and an excess of tissue fluid forms.

(d)   Yes. Aldosterone causes fluid retention and this predisposes to oedema formation.

(e)   No. A haemorrhage of this magnitude constitutes a loss of body fluid and oedema is not a feature of hypovolaemia.

1.40

(a)   Yes.

(b)   No. The plasma potassium concentration is typically 4 mmol per litre; 10 mmol per litre would be fatal.

(c)   No. The plasma bicarbonate concentration is typically 24 mmol per litre.

(d)   No. The total plasma osmotic pressure is typically 300 mosmol per litre.

(e)   No. The intracellular potassium concentration is typically 150 mmol per litre.

1.41

(a)   Yes. Non-polar molecules dissolve in the lipid part of the cell membrane and so diffuse across the endothelial cell membranes more readily than polar molecules, which do not dissolve in lipids.

(b)   Yes. Passage through the channels between endothelial cells is by diffusion; small polar molecules pass readily.

(c)   No. Plasma proteins are too large to pass readily through the channels between endothelial cells.

(d)   Yes. Pinocytotic vesicles act as tiny ferry boats.

(e)   No. The movement of chemicals across fenestrations in endothelial cells is passive diffusion directly from plasma to interstitial fluid without traversing the endothelial cell.

1.42

(a)   Yes. The concentration of water in the extracellular fluid initially exceeds that of the intracellular fluid so water enters and the cell swells.

(b)   Yes. Swelling stretches the membrane and stretch activates transporter mechanisms.

(c)   Yes. The membrane transporter mechanisms move osmolytes out of the cell, thereby returning the cell volume towards normal.

(d)   Yes. As a result of activation of the transporter mechanisms, the intracellular compartment has lost osmolyte, so subsequent transfer to the previously isosmotic solution results in a fall in volume to below the initial value; this subsequently slowly returns to normal.

(e)   No. The passive responses remain; when the cell is transferred to the hypotonic solution, its volume increases and this increase is maintained for much longer than if transporter mechanisms were active.

1.43
(a)   Yes.
(b)   No. Glucose is not lipid-soluble.
(c)   Yes.
(d)   Yes.
(e)   No. Lipid-soluble substances enter by dissolving in the membrane.

1.44
(a)   Yes.
(b)   Yes.
(c)   Yes.
(d)   No. mRNA is made in the nucleus, then moves out.
(e)   Yes.

1.45
(a)   No. There are two rows of molecules, with heads on the inner and outer sides of the membrane.
(b)   No. The lipid itself is waterproof; water enters and leaves through sub-microscopic pores in the membrane.
(c)   Yes. The respiratory gases are lipid-soluble.
(d)   Yes. There may be thousands in the membrane of a single cell. They include enzyme molecules which act as 'pumps', and receptor molecules providing binding sites for hormones or transmitters.
(e)   No. Glycogen stores are intracellular.

2 Alimentary tract

QUESTIONS

Mouth, oesophagus, stomach

2.1 Concerning the intake of food:
(a) mastication of food is entirely a voluntary action.
(b) swallowing can occur reflexly.
(c) nerve pathways serving swallowing go to and from the hypothalamus.
(d) peristalsis in the oesophagus is under the control of the vagus nerves.
(e) the lower oesophageal sphincter relaxes when the stomach is full.

2.2 Concerning saliva:
(a) it has the same osmolarity as plasma.
(b) it contains digestive enzymes.
(c) the increase in flow of saliva associated with eating appetizing food starts about 1 min after food is taken into the mouth.
(d) the average salivary flow is typically 100 ml per 24 h.
(e) the mucus content is increased by parasympathetic stimulation.

2.3 Salivary amylase:
(a) is a protein.
(b) is secreted mainly by the parotid glands.
(c) is secreted in response to parasympathetic stimulation.
(d) is most active at pH 1–2.
(e) is necessary for any digestion of carbohydrate to occur.

2.4 Concerning saliva and the salivary glands:
(a) saliva has a pH in the range 1 to 2.
(b) stimulation of the parasympathetic nerve supply to the parotid gland causes vasoconstriction within the gland.
(c) the concentration of sodium ions in saliva is lower than in plasma.
(d) salivary amylase acts mainly in the stomach.
(e) saliva contains substances with antibacterial action.

2.5   With reference to gastric function:
(a)   an average meal has moved on from the stomach after half an hour.
(b)   contractility is augmented by sympathetic stimulation.
(c)   when the quantity of ingested material increases, the intragastric pressure increases.
(d)   the longitudinal muscle coat has a basic electrical rhythm.
(e)   histamine inhibits the production of gastric acid.

2.6   On the left is a list of gastric secretions. Are the items on the right appropriately associated with each secretion?
(a)   Hydrochloric acid   Increase in bicarbonate in gastric venous blood.
(b)   Hydrochloric acid   Necessary to life.
(c)   Pepsinogen   Is inactive above pH 6.
(d)   Intrinsic factor   Another name for vitamin B12.
(e)   Gastrin   Secretion stimulated by vagal activity.

2.7   Concerning gastric secretion in a normal adult:
(a)   the lowest pH that can be attained in the stomach is about 4.5.
(b)   the histamine receptors in the stomach can be pharmacologically stimulated without significant stimulation of histamine receptors in the lungs.
(c)   pentagastrin injection can cause maximal secretion of acid by the stomach.
(d)   excessive acid secretion is prevented by an effect originating in antral receptors.
(e)   gastrin comes mainly from cells in the fundus of the stomach.

2.8   Concerning gastro-intestinal secretions:
(a)   gastro-intestinal hormones are steroids.
(b)   secretin is secreted from the pancreas.
(c)   the pancreatic secretion that is stimulated by secretin has a high concentration of bicarbonate ions.
(d)   the maximal flow of pancreatic juice in response to cholecystokinin and secretin given together is greater than the maximum produced by either hormone alone.
(e)   the pancreas secretes more than 1 litre of juice per 24 hours.

2.9   In the stomach:
(a)   secretion of enzymes is by parietal (oxyntic) cells.
(b)   secretion of acid is from parietal (oxyntic) cells.
(c)   gastrin is secreted by the same cells that secrete acid.
(d)   the main digestive function is the breakdown of carbohydrates.
(e)   the products of carbohydrate digestion are absorbed.

2.10 Functions of the stomach include:
(a) storage of food during digestion.
(b) secretion into the lumen of intrinsic haemopoietic factor.
(c) the secretion into the blood of secretin.
(d) the secretion into the blood of gastrin.
(e) the maintenance of iron in the Fe^{2+} state.

2.11 Histamine injection results in:
(a) an increase in the rate of secretion of gastric juice.
(b) an increase in the concentration of hydrogen ions in the gastric juice.
(c) an increase in blood flow in the gastric mucosa.
(d) an increase in the osmolarity of the gastric juice.
(e) an extracellular alkalosis.

2.12 Gastric emptying is delayed by:
(a) vagotomy.
(b) muscular exercise.
(c) cholecystokinin.
(d) fat in the duodenum.
(e) secretin.

2.13 Consider a subject who is digesting a normal meal. He or she swallows a tube and 100 ml of a solution at pH 3 is infused into the duodenum. As a result of the infusion, there is:
(a) an increase in gastric secretion of acid.
(b) an increase in the rate of gastric emptying.
(c) an increase in the rate of pancreatic secretion.
(d) an increase in the rate of bile secretion.
(e) relaxation of the gall bladder.

Duodenum, bile, pancreatic function

2.14 In the normal human:
(a) cholecystokinin is the most important hormone concerned in the neutralization in the small bowel of acid from the stomach.
(b) in the gall bladder, chloride ions are secreted into the bile.
(c) the emulsification of dietary lipid by bile salts assists intestinal absorption of lipid.
(d) at least 95% of bile pigments secreted by the liver are reabsorbed in the gut.
(e) most of the water absorbed in the intestinal tract is directly derived from dietary intake.

2.15 Concerning bile:
(a)   water is absorbed from bile in the gall bladder.
(b)   a high ratio of bile salts to cholesterol favours the formation of gall stones.
(c)   the cholesterol normally present in bile is derived mainly from the breakdown of steroid hormones.
(d)   the volume of bile entering the duodenum is about 500 ml per 24 hours.
(e)   about 10% of the bile salts entering the duodenum are lost in the faeces.

2.16 Concerning bile and bile salts:
(a)   the secretion of bile by the liver is intermittent.
(b)   bile contains significant amounts of digestive enzymes.
(c)   bile salts accompany fatty acids in their absorption through the wall of the jejunum.
(d)   the synthesis of bile salts by the liver is inhibited by an increasing concentration of bile salts in portal venous blood.
(e)   The secretion of bile salts by the liver is inhibited by an increasing concentration of bile salts in portal venous blood.

2.17 In a normal subject:
(a)   the gall bladder has a capacity, when full, of about 50 ml.
(b)   the gall bladder concentrates hepatic bile by a factor of 100.
(c)   the flow of hepatic bile is about 50 ml per 24 hours.
(d)   the secretions from the Brunner's glands of the duodenum protect its mucosa against stomach acid.
(e)   the liver holds a store of vitamin B12 sufficient for the needs of the body for at least several months.

2.18 Bile acids:
(a)   are derived from the breakdown products of haemoglobin.
(b)   are secreted into the bile in the gall bladder.
(c)   are concentrated in the gall bladder.
(d)   are water soluble.
(e)   break down fats to fatty acids.

2.19 Compared with hepatic duct bile, gall bladder bile contains a higher concentration of:
(a)   water.
(b)   bile salts.
(c)   bicarbonate.
(d)   hydrogen ions.
(e)   bile pigments.

2.20 Concerning pancreatic juice:
(a) the enzyme component of pancreatic juice is secreted largely by acinar cells.
(b) the bicarbonate component of pancreatic juice is secreted largely by cells that form the walls of the ducts.
(c) as the flow rate of pancreatic juice increases, the bicarbonate concentration of the juice increases.
(d) as the flow rate of pancreatic juice increases, the chloride concentration of the juice increases.
(e) the sodium concentration of pancreatic juice is typically 10 mmol.

2.21 Concerning pancreatic juice:
(a) the flow of pancreatic juice is typically 100 ml per day.
(b) gastrin is an important stimulant of secretion of bicarbonate by the pancreas.
(c) secretin inhibits the secretion of pancreatic juice.
(d) cholecystokinin (CCK) stimulates the secretion of pancreatic enzymes.
(e) there are pancreatic enzymes for the breakdown of all the major nutrients – proteins, fats and starches.

2.22 Concerning pancreatic secretion:
(a) the pancreatic juice secreted in response to vagal stimulation is rich in enzymes.
(b) secretin can produce a greater flow of pancreatic juice than the maximal flow in response to vagal stimulation.
(c) atropine blocks the secretogogue effects of vagal stimulation.
(d) atropine blocks the secretogogue effects of secretin.
(e) secretin causes the production of a pancreatic secretion which is more alkaline than that secreted in response to cholecystokinin (CCK).

2.23 Concerning the pancreas:
(a) it is an exocrine organ.
(b) it is an endocrine organ.
(c) some of its secretory activity is influenced by hormones from elsewhere.
(d) it receives innervation from the autonomic nervous system.
(e) increase in secretion is accompanied by vasoconstriction of pancreatic arterioles.

Small intestine

2.24 Concerning the autonomic nerve supply to the small intestine:
(a) the parasympathetic nerve supply is through the vagus nerves.
(b) the parasympathetic nerve fibres running from the central nervous system relay at synapses before entering the gut wall.
(c) increased parasympathetic activity results in relaxation of the ileocolic sphincter.
(d) the sympathetic nerve supply leaves the central nervous system in the thoracolumbar region of the spinal cord.
(e) the sympathetic neuro-effector endings in the gut liberate acetylcholine.

2.25 Concerning intestinal absorption:
(a) a volume of fluid in excess of 10 litres per day is absorbed from the gut.
(b) protein is absorbed only in the form of dipeptides.
(c) absorption of the products of protein digestion depends on active transport mechanisms.
(d) vitamin B12 is largely absorbed in the stomach.
(e) products of fat digestion can reach the systemic blood before reaching the liver.

2.26 Concerning fat absorption:
(a) in a healthy person, 5% is the upper limit of ingested fat that appears in the faeces.
Malabsorption of lipids is likely to occur as a result of:
(b) hepatocellular damage.
(c) obstructive jaundice.
(d) failure of pancreatic secretion.
(e) removal of the gastric antrum in a partial gastrectomy.

2.27 The ileum is the principal site for the absorption of:
(a) glucose.
(b) the products of fat digestion.
(c) bile salts.
(d) vitamin K.
(e) iron.

2.28 Vitamin B12:
(a) contains iron.
(b) can be absorbed readily without the participation of gastro-intestinal secretions.
(c) is absorbed mainly in the distal ileum.
(d) is degraded by digestive enzymes.
(e) deficiency leads to macrocytic anaemia.

2.29   Concerning intestinal motility:
(a)   motility in general is inhibited by sympathetic activity.
(b)   a region of relaxation moves ahead of peristaltic constriction.
(c)   peristalsis is dependent on vagal (parasympathetic) innervation.
(d)   the basic electric rhythm (BER) is a function of the intrinsic nerve plexuses.
(e)   every wave of the BER is accompanied by a wave of contraction.

2.30   In the lining of the small intestine:
(a)   enterocytes on the surface of villi secrete digestive enzymes.
(b)   enterocytes on the surface of the villi survive for only a few days.
(c)   glucose absorption can occur without there being a diffusion gradient.
(d)   active pumping of sodium ions occurs across the luminal surface.
(e)   enterokinase secretion is necessary for the activation of pancreatic proteases.

2.31   Concerning the movements of water in the intestine:
(a)   water is secreted from the lining of the crypts between the villi of the small intestine.
(b)   water is absorbed through the enterocytes covering the villi of the small intestine.
(c)   more water is absorbed in the large intestine than in the small intestine.
(d)   on an average intake, about a litre of water is absorbed daily in the large intestine.
(e)   typically about 500 ml water daily remains to be lost in the faeces.

Large intestine

2.32   In the colon:
(a)   the secretions lack significant digestive enzymes.
(b)   sympathetic stimulation results in enhanced motility.
(c)   stimulation of the nervi erigentes (parasympathetic supply) results in increased mucus secretion.
(d)   more than half the water that enters the colon is absorbed from the contents.
(e)   bacterial synthesis of vitamin K is of vital importance.

2.33 **Concerning large bowel function:**
(a) constipation results in the absorption of toxic substances from the bowel.
(b) defaecation is a spinal reflex that can be voluntarily overridden.
(c) distension of the stomach with food initiates contractions of the colon.
(d) the parasympathetic nerve supply is excitatory to the musculature of the colon (excluding sphincters).
(e) the sympathetic nerve supply is excitatory to the internal (involuntary) anal sphincter.

Vomiting

2.34 **Concerning vomiting:**
(a) vomiting as a component of travel sickness is primarily the result of irritation of gastro-intestinal receptors.
(b) the drug apomorphine can be given to inhibit vomiting.
(c) the central nervous centre for the vomiting reflex is in the cerebral cortex.
(d) vomiting involves the same muscles as a strong expiratory effort against a closed glottis.
(e) the efferent pathways of the vomiting reflex involve both autonomic and somatic components.

2.35 **Figure 2.35 represents the pH of the digestive juices aspirated from the alimentary tract as a function of position along the alimentary tract during digestion of a meal.**

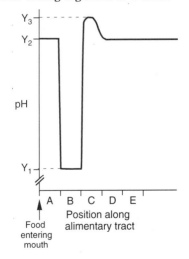

(a)   a typical value for Y2 is 7.0.
(b)   a typical value for Y1 is 4.0.
(c)   a typical value for Y3 is 10.0.
(d)   the fall in pH from segment A to segment B is due to stomach acid.
(e)   the rise in pH from segment B to segment C is due to active reabsorption of hydrogen ions.

2.36   With further reference to Figure 2.35:
(a)   segment C represents the duodenum.
(b)   vomiting as a result of a blockage between segments B and C results in metabolic acidosis.
(c)   vomiting as a result of an obstruction between segments C and D may result in metabolic acidosis.
(d)   the digestive enzymes active in segment A are inactivated by the acidity in B.
(e)   the digestive enzymes active in segment B are inactivated by the alkalinity of segment C.

ANSWERS

2.1
(a)   No. Mastication can occur reflexively, as well as voluntarily. Material put into the mouth can elicit the reflex, via the brain stem, when all higher brain function has ceased.
(b)   Yes. Swallowing can be initiated voluntarily, but also reflexively in response to stimulation of the oropharynx when liquids or solids reach the back of the mouth.
(c)   No. The pathways for swallowing go to and from the medulla; it can therefore occur as long as medullary function is intact, or it can be disturbed by medullary damage.
(d)   Yes. Unlike peristalsis further down the gut which can occur in isolation from any extrinsic nerve supply, peristalsis in the oesophagus requires the vagus nerves.
(e)   No. The lower oesophageal sphincter closes when the stomach is full (except as part of the complex coordinated act of vomiting which may be triggered by over-distension).

2.2
(a)   Yes.
(b)   Yes. Saliva contains amylase, an enzyme that splits carbohydrates, and also lipase.
(c)   No. Saliva starts to flow in anticipation of appetizing food, before the food enters the mouth.

(d)   No. The flow of saliva is typically about 1 litre per 24 h.

(e)   No. Parasympathetic stimulation yields a watery saliva rich in digestive enzymes.

2.3

(a)   Yes. This is true of all enzymes.

(b)   Yes. The other salivary glands (sublingual, submandibular) produce primarily a mucous secretion.

(c)   Yes.

(d)   No. It is most active when the pH is around 7, which is the pH of saliva.

(e)   No. Carbohydrate digestion can proceed without the participation of salivary amylase by the action of intestinal secretions.

2.4

(a)   No. Saliva is approximately neutral.

(b)   No. Stimulation of the parasympathetic nerve supply to the parotid gland causes vasodilatation; this increases the blood supply to the acinar cells whose secretion is stimulated by the parasympathetic activity.

(c)   Yes. Sodium ions are reabsorbed from the secretion as it passes from the acini along the ducts, and potassium ions are secreted into the saliva.

(d)   No. Salivary amylase acts mainly in the mouth, although it can continue in the centre of a bolus of food before exposure to low pH in the stomach.

(e)   Yes.

2.5

(a)   No. Three hours is about right, although there is variation with the nature and size of the meal.

(b)   No. Vagal activity enhances, sympathetic depresses.

(c)   No. There is 'receptive relaxation' as food enters, so that pressure is unchanged.

(d)   Yes. This produces waves of contraction, every 20 seconds.

(e)   No. Histamine stimulates acid secretion.

2.6

(a)   Yes. This is the 'alkaline tide': extrusion of H^+ into the lumen is associated with a rise in HCO_3^- concentration in cells: this moves out into plasma.

(b)   No. Digestion is assisted by gastric acidity, but no vitally necessary process is impossible without it.

(c)   Yes. Pepsin is split off only when pH falls (acidity increases) below about 5.

(d)   No. Intrinsic factor is a necessary adjunct to the vitamin B12 that comes from the diet. Without intrinsic factor, B12 is not absorbed and pernicious anaemia ensues.

(e)   Yes. In the cephalic phase, vagal stimulation accounts for pepsinogen and acid secretion, directly by stimulation of secretory cells and indirectly by causing release of gastrin.

2.7

(a)   No. The correct value is between 1 and 2.

(b)   Yes. The gastric receptors are H_2 receptors. The standard histamine blockers such as anthisan block pulmonary histamine receptors (H_1) but not the receptors in the stomach.

(c)   Yes. This is the standard means of eliciting a maximal secretion of acid and thus assessing the 'parietal cell mass'.

(d)   Yes. This is a negative feedback mechanism – gastrin stimulates acid secretion in the body of the stomach, and increasing acidity of the chyme inhibits gastrin secretion in the antrum.

(e)   No. Gastrin is secreted by G cells located in the antrum.

2.8

(a)   No. They are polypeptides.

(b)   No. Secretin is secreted by the duodenal mucosa.

(c)   Yes.

(d)   Yes.

(e)   Yes. About 1.5 litres in 24 hours.

2.9

(a)   No. Secretion of enzymes is by 'chief' cells, which contain zymogen granules.

(b)   Yes.

(c)   No. Gastrin is secreted by G cells.

(d)   No. The main digestive function of the stomach is the breakdown of protein.

(e)   No. The small intestine is the principal site of absorption of the products of carbohydrate digestion. The stomach has little absorptive function.

2.10

(a)   Yes. The stomach stores and churns food thus allowing digestion to proceed.

(b)   Yes.

(c)   No. Secretin is secreted in the duodenum and first part of the jejunum.

(d)   Yes. Gastrin is secreted by the antral G cells.

(e)   Yes. The acidity of the gastric contents contributes to maintaining iron in the ferrous state.

2.11

(a)   Yes. Histamine stimulates the parietal cells of the stomach to secrete a profuse, acid-rich juice.

(b)   Yes. As for (a).

(c)   Yes. An increase in local blood flow occurs in association with an increase in acid secretion.

(d)   No. Gastric juice is always approximately isosmotic with plasma.

(e)   Yes. Secretion of acid into the stomach is accompanied by alkalinization of the extracellular fluid.

2.12

(a)   Yes. The vagus provides an excitatory innervation for gastric motility, so gastric emptying is delayed by vagotomy.

(b)   Yes. Sympathetic activity and catecholamine secretion in response to exercise reduce gastric motility.

(c)   No. Cholecystokinin causes constriction of the gall bladder and has no significant effect on the stomach.

(d)   Yes. This is an important component of the reflex slowing of the entry of chyme into the duodenum, thus allowing time for digestion of the fat content.

(e)   Yes. Secretin is the hormone mediating the slowing of the propulsion of chyme from the stomach. In this way, the duodenum controls the rate at which it receives material to neutralize and digest.

2.13

(a)   No. Duodenal contents at a pH of 4.5 or less results in the release of secretin, which inhibits gastric secretion of acid.

(b)   No. Acid in the duodenum leads to a slowing of gastric emptying. Secretin acts in the stomach to induce inhibition of gastric motility.

(c)   Yes. See (d) below.

(d)   Yes. These are also effects of secretin. The alkaline secretions of the pancreas and liver neutralize acid in the duodenum.

(e)   No. The gall bladder contracts. This is due to secretin augmenting the action of cholecystokinin which promotes contraction of the gall bladder.

2.14

(a)   No. Secretin is the important hormone.

(b)   No. Chloride ions are reabsorbed from the bile into the interstitial fluid.

(c)   Yes. The emulsification of dietary lipid is a preliminary to micelle formation, which in turn leads to diffusion of lipids into mucosal cells.

(d)   No. This would be true of bile salts but not of bile pigments, only a tiny proportion of which are reabsorbed.

(e)   No. Dietary intake is usually around 1.5 litres per day. Secretions into the gastro-intestinal tract total at least 10 times this amount.

2.15

(a)   Yes. But bile remains isosmotic with plasma partly because of micelle formation.

(b)   No. The reverse is true since bile salts render cholesterol soluble.

(c)   Yes. This is also the route for excretion when plasma cholesterol is raised.

(d)   Yes.

(e)   No. A figure of 10% indicates malabsorption; the figure for a healthy human is about 1%.

2.16

(a)   No. The secretion of bile by the liver is continuous, but bile is discharged into the duodenum only during digestion.

(b)   No.

(c)   No. Bile salts remain in the lumen and contribute to the emulsification of more fats, until fat absorption is complete; they are then reabsorbed in the ileum – about 75% actively as bile salts, and most of the rest passively as the primary cholic and chenic acids after bacterial deconjugation.

(d)   Yes. The higher the concentration of bile salts in the portal blood, the lower the rate of their synthesis in the liver; the secretion of bile is stimulated, however, and the same bile salts are thus recirculated.

(e)   No. The opposite is true: a rise in plasma concentration of bile salts stimulates secretion of bile salts and flow of bile: the so-called chola-gogue action. This positive feedback mechanism ensures escalating enterohepatic circulation of bile salts during digestion of a meal. It is stopped when the sphincter of Oddi closes and the gall bladder relaxes, as secretion of cholecystokinin (CCK) by the duodenum declines.

2.17

(a)   Yes.

(b)   No. The concentration by the gall bladder is about five-fold.

(c)   No. The flow of hepatic bile is about 500 ml per 24 hours (so, from (b), bile flow from the gall bladder is about 100 ml per 24 hours).

(d)   Yes. Brunner's glands, found only in the duodenal submucosa, protect the mucosa against stomach acids by the secretion of alkali and mucus.

(e)   Yes. This is the reason that after a gastrectomy evidence of vitamin B12 deficiency does not appear for a year or so.

2.18
(a) No. This would be true for bile pigments.
(b) No. They are secreted into the bile canaliculi in the liver.
(c) Yes. Because sodium and water are absorbed.
(d) Yes.
(e) No. This is the function of lipases; bile salts assist the breakdown by taking part in emulsification and micelle formation.

2.19
(a) No. Bile is concentrated in the gall bladder.
(b) Yes. They are concentrated because of the reabsorption of water from the bile in the gall bladder.
(c) No. The gall bladder reabsorbs bicarbonate from the bile disproportionately to the absorption of water.
(d) Yes. See (c).
(e) Yes. They are concentrated because of the reabsorption of water from the bile in the gall bladder.

2.20
(a) Yes.
(b) Yes. Sodium ions are actively secreted by the walls of the duct; bicarbonate follows, derived from CO_2 with the assistance of carbonic anhydrase.
(c) Yes. Secretion of bicarbonate occurs in the first (intralobular) duct tributaries, and reabsorption in the next (extralobular) ducts. When flow is faster, there is less time for reabsorption.
(d) No. As the flow rate of pancreatic juice increases, the chloride concentration of the juice decreases, balancing an increase in bicarbonate.
(e) No. Sodium ion concentration in acinar secretion is similar to that in plasma; sodium ions are moved into the fluid in the intralobular ducts, and are variably reabsorbed further along. The sodium concentration of pancreatic juice is typically 160 mmol per litre.

2.21
(a) No. The flow of pancreatic juice is 500–1000 ml per day.
(b) No. Gastrin stimulates the secretion of acid in the stomach.
(c) No. Secretin stimulates the secretion of pancreatic juice rich in bicarbonate.
(d) Yes. (This same hormone used to be called pancreozymin or CCK-PZ).
(e) Yes. The enzymes secreted by the pancreas are important in the digestion of all the major classes of foodstuffs.

2.22

(a)   Yes. Small volume, enzyme-rich fluid is secreted in the 'cephalic phase'.
(b)   Yes. Copious water and electrolyte-rich secretion is the response to secretin.
(c)   Yes. Atropine blocks the muscarinic effects of acetylcholine, which is the mechanism for vagal stimulation of secretion.
(d)   No. Secretin acts directly on the pancreas.
(e)   Yes. CCK elicits enzyme containing secretion (although it does also enhance the HCO_3^- secretion in response to secretin).

2.23

(a)   Yes. It secretes alkaline digestive juices into the duodenum.
(b)   Yes. The islets of Langerhans, in the pancreas, secrete the hormones insulin and glucagon into the blood.
(c)   Yes. Its exocrine activity is stimulated by cholecystokinin-pancreo-zymin, from the duodenum.
(d)   Yes. Both exocrine and endocrine secretions are influenced by the autonomic nervous system.
(e)   No. As in all organs, increase in secretion is accompanied by vasodilatation.

2.24

(a)   Yes.
(b)   No. The postganglionic fibre originates at a synapse within the wall in the myenteric plexus.
(c)   Yes.
(d)   Yes. And it relays in the coeliac or superior mesenteric ganglia.
(e)   No. They are noradrenergic.

2.25

(a)   Yes. Most of this is from gut secretions.
(b)   No. About half the ingested protein is absorbed as amino acids.
(c)   Yes.
(d)   No. Most absorption of vitamin B12 occurs in the ileum.
(e)   Yes. Much of the lipid absorption is into lymphatics, which bypass the liver to drain into the great veins in the thorax and thence into the circulating blood.

2.26

(a)   Yes.
(b)   Yes. This causes inadequate bile salt secretion and hence deficient fat absorption.
(c)   Yes. As (b).

(d)   Yes. Inadequate lipase secretion results in deficient fat digestion.

(e)   No. The stomach does not contribute significantly to fat digestion and absorption.

2.27

(a)   No. Glucose is absorbed mostly in the proximal small gut.

(b)   No. The jejunum is the principal site for the absorption of the products of fat digestion.

(c)   Yes.

(d)   No. Most vitamin K is absorbed in the large bowel after bacteria synthesize it in the lumen of that region.

(e)   No. Most iron is absorbed in the jejunum.

2.28

(a)   No. It contains cobalt.

(b)   No. It must be complexed with intrinsic factor excreted by the parietal cells of the stomach before it can be absorbed.

(c)   Yes. The B12 intrinsic factor complex is absorbed by specific receptors in the distal ileum.

(d)   No. Neither B12 nor the B12 intrinsic complex is readily degraded by gastro-intestinal secretions. Intrinsic factor itself, uncomplexed with B12, is readily digested.

(e)   Yes.

2.29

(a)   Yes.

(b)   Yes. This increases the capacity of the part of the gut immediately ahead of peristaltic constriction.

(c)   No. Peristalsis occurs independently of the extrinsic nerve supply, although it can be influenced by it. It is coordinated by the intrinsic system of ganglion cells and fibres in the submucosal and myenteric plexuses.

(d)   No. The BER is a function of the smooth muscle itself, a fluctuation of membrane potential, spreading from pacemaker cells in the wall of the duodenum.

(e)   No. Whether or not action potentials and contraction are superimposed on the depolarizing phase of the BER depends on other excitatory and inhibitory neural or chemical influences.

2.30

(a)   Yes. A high proportion of the final stages of digestive breakdown occurs close to the microvilli (at the 'brush border').

(b)   Yes. Enterocytes are continually lost from the tips of villi and replaced by migration from the depths of the crypts, where cell division maintains the supply.

(c)   Yes. Glucose is absorbed by co-transport with Na ions, dependent on sodium pump activity, although it will also be passively absorbed when there is a diffusion gradient from chyme through cells to blood. (Similar mechanisms apply to amino acids.)

(d)   No. Active pumping of Na out of these cells occurs across the basolateral membrane (as also, for example, in the proximal convoluted tubules of the kidney); this maintains a gradient for Na entry across the luminal surface.

(e)   Yes. This occurs in the jejunum.

2.31

(a)   Yes.

(b)   Yes. Together with secretion in the crypts, this creates a local recirculation of water. The overall ratio of absorption to secretion increases down the length of the small intestine.

(c)   No. Although water absorption is a prime function of the large bowel, the small bowel absorbs much more.

(d)   Yes. Comparing (c): although colonic absorption may seem a substantial fraction of intake by mouth, the small bowel has already absorbed many more litres of water, from gastro-intestinal secretions as well as from the rest of the intake.

(e)   No. Normally only about 100 ml water is lost in the faeces daily.

2.32

(a)   Yes. Secretion is essentially mucous.

(b)   No. Sympathetic stimulation decreases colonic motility.

(c)   Yes. This is one mechanism of emotional diarrhoea.

(d)   Yes. Water is absorbed consequent on active sodium reabsorption.

(e)   Yes. Dietary intake is normally insufficient.

2.33

(a)   No. There is no evidence that the adverse effects of constipation are due to factors other than abdominal discomfort and distension.

(b)   Yes. Distension of the rectum stimulates receptors; via sacral segments of the spinal cord, parasympathetic (nervi erigentes) efferents cause contraction of rectal and relaxation of internal sphincteric smooth muscle. This is superimposed on a weaker local reflex.

(c)   Yes. This is the gastrocolic reflex. Distension of the stomach is frequently accompanied by an urge to defaecate.

(d)   Yes. See (b).

(e)   Yes.

2.34

(a)   No. Vestibular receptors are primarily involved.

(b)   No. It promotes vomiting.

(c)   No. The vomiting centre is in the medulla.

(d)   Yes.

(e)   Yes. For example, the autonomic nervous system is responsible for stomach relaxation and the somatic nervous system for contraction of the abdominal musculature.

2.35

(a)   Yes.

(b)   No. A typical value for Y1 is 1.0.

(c)   No. A typical value for Y3 is 8.0.

(d)   Yes.

(e)   No. The rise in pH from segment B to segment C is due to alkaline secretions from the liver and pancreas. These juices neutralise the acid in the chyme.

2.36

(a)   Yes.

(b)   No. Vomiting as a result of a blockage between segments B and C results in loss of acid from the body and hence a metabolic alkalosis.

(c)   Yes. Vomiting as a result of a blockage between segments C and D results in loss of acid and alkali from the body; in some cases the loss of alkali exceeds that of acid and so there is a metabolic acidosis.

(d)   Yes. The activity of digestive enzymes is very sensitive to pH. So salivary enzymes are active at the pH of the mouth (typically pH = 7.0) and are inactivated by acidity. Within the food mass, the salivary enzymes act until gastric acid has penetrated.

(e)   Yes. As for (d), Gastric enzymes (protein-splitting) are inactivated by the alkalinity of the duodenum.

3 Metabolism, liver function

Metabolism (except exercise – see	
Section 10)	3.1–3.10
Liver function (except bile secretion	
see Section 2)	3.11–3.15

QUESTIONS

Metabolism

3.1 Carbohydrates:
(a) start to be digested in the stomach.
(b) are ultimately broken down at the brush border of intestinal mucosal cells.
(c) pass into the blood as monosaccharides.
(d) after digestion, can be absorbed only down a diffusion gradient (i.e. only when the intestinal luminal concentration is higher than plasma concentration).
(e) have about the same calorific value weight for weight as fat.

3.2 The disaccharide, sucrose:
(a) is composed entirely of glucose subunits.
(b) is absorbed unchanged in the alimentary tract.
(c) readily crosses the walls of capillaries.
(d) when injected intravenously becomes rapidly distributed throughout the body water.
(e) about 50% of ingested sucrose is excreted unchanged in the faeces.

3.3 Glucose in the plasma of a healthy person:
(a) remains elevated for about two hours after ingesting 50 g glucose.
(b) is entirely removed from all plasma flowing through the glomerular capillaries.
(c) is replenished, if its concentration decreases, from breakdown of liver glycogen.
(d) is the essential energy source for the central nervous system.
(e) is bound to albumin.

3.4 **With reference to the endocrine control of carbohydrate metabolism:**
(a) cortisol inhibits tissue glucose utilization.
(b) uptake of glucose into brain cells depends on an adequate amount of insulin.
(c) insulin promotes synthesis of glycogen in muscle.
(d) glucagon secretion exceeds insulin secretion during fasting.
(e) adrenaline promotes glycogenolysis.

3.5 **Concerning metabolism:**
(a) a man who has been eating nothing but carbohydrate for 24 hours has a respiratory quotient (RQ) at rest of less than 0.8.
(b) 1 mol of glucose enables production of more high-energy phosphate compounds if metabolism is aerobic than if it is anaerobic.
(c) in a healthy person at rest, the liver contains most of the body's glycogen.
(d) the release of glucose from the liver is increased by glucagon.
(e) the calorific value of 1 g of fat is greater than that of 1 g of protein.

3.6 **The following statements apply to the energy stores and sources of an average well-nourished but not obese 70 kg man:**
(a) fat makes up about 15% of the total body weight.
(b) the normal daily energy requirement can be supplied by 0.3–0.4 kg of stored fat.
(c) fat is stored extracellularly.
(d) the complete oxidative breakdown of 1 g of glucose yields approximately 17 kJ (4 kcal).
(e) the complete oxidative breakdown of 1 g of protein yields approximately 37 kJ (9 kcal).

3.7 **Protein synthesis in most tissues is promoted by:**
(a) growth hormone.
(b) insulin.
(c) cortisol.
(d) androgens.
(e) glucagon.

3.8 **With reference to the turnover of lipids:**
(a) insulin promotes entry of fatty acids into fat cells.
(b) the brain can use fatty acids as a fuel if glucose is in short supply.
(c) fatty acids normally make a much smaller contribution to whole-body nutrient utilization than glucose.
(d) the metabolic rate during prolonged exercise is mainly fuelled by fatty acids.
(e) adrenaline promotes the release of free fatty acids from adipose tissue.

3.9   **If a healthy person goes without food for a week:**
(a)   blood glucose is unlikely to fall below 2.5 mmol per litre (half normal).
(b)   insulin secretion decreases.
(c)   ketone formation increases in the liver.
(d)   the liver forms glucose from amino acids.
(e)   brain metabolizes free fatty acids.

3.10   **If a normal person is deprived of food for three weeks but has as much water as he or she wishes, at the end of this time there will be:**
(a)   a high blood glucose concentration.
(b)   an increase in the rate of breakdown of proteins.
(c)   an increase in plasma concentration of glucagon.
(d)   an increase in plasma concentration of ketone bodies.
(e)   an increase in lipolysis.

Liver function (for bile secretion see Section 2)

3.11   **Functions of the liver include:**
(a)   synthesis of plasma albumin.
(b)   detoxication of drugs.
(c)   storage of vitamin B12.
(d)   secretion of digestive enzymes.
(f)   synthesis of erythropoietin.

3.12   **Functions that can be carried out ONLY in the liver include:**
(a)   synthesis of prothrombin.
(b)   breakdown of red blood cells.
(c)   conversion of glucose to glycogen.
(d)   excretion of cholesterol.
(e)   secretion of bile salts.

3.13   **With reference to hepatic blood flow:**
(a)   about one-third of the blood flowing to the liver is arterial blood (hepatic artery).
(b)   the total flow from the liver accounts for about one-quarter of the venous return to the heart (at rest and in the postabsorptive state).
(c)   the flow rate decreases during exercise.
(d)   portal venous and arterial blood mix in the capillaries (sinusoids).
(e)   portal venous blood contains all the absorbed products of digestion.

3.14   Urobilinogen:
(a)   is responsible for the yellow colour of normal urine.
(b)   is at a higher concentration in the hepatic portal venous blood than in the general systemic circulation.
(c)   is carried in the blood attached to the plasma albumin.
(d)   is derived from bilirubin.
(e)   is at a higher concentration than normal in the blood in cases of mild hepatocellular damage.

3.15   The following are features of chronic severe liver disease:
(a)   portal hypertension.
(b)   ascites.
(c)   a tendency to haemorrhage.
(d)   a low concentration of plasma proteins.
(e)   a raised core temperature.

ANSWERS

3.1
(a)   No. Carbohydrate digestion starts in the mouth: salivary amylase (ptyalin) acts on starch: this amylase activity is inhibited by gastric acidity.
(b)   Yes. Final breakdown occurs at the brush border of the enterocytes, where the appropriate enzymes are located.
(c)   Yes. Monosaccharides are the final product of digestion, and these are absorbed.
(d)   No. An active carrier mechanism is involved; inhibition of sodium pump activity interferes with absorption; different sugars have different absorption rates. Glucose is absorbed down a diffusion gradient when there is one, but this is not necessary for absorption.
(e)   No. Fats have more than twice the energy value (39 kJ compared with 17 kJ, or about 9:4 kcal, per g).

3.2
(a)   No. The sucrose molecule comprises one glucose and one fructose subunit.
(b)   No. Sucrose cannot be absorbed as such in the alimentary tract; it is split and the component monosaccharides are absorbed.
(c)   Yes. Sucrose is a small molecule and readily crosses the walls of capillaries.
(d)   No. Sucrose does not readily cross cell membranes so, when injected intravenously, it becomes distributed only throughout the extracellular compartment.
(e)   No. Almost all ingested sucrose is digested and absorbed.

3.3
(a)   No. It is normally back to normal within one-and-a-half hours.
(b)   No. It is 'completely filtered', but only one-fifth of the plasma is filtered off.
(c)   Yes. This is the first source.
(d)   Yes. Brain normally uses only glucose; in starvation it can use keto-acids only if there is also some glucose.
(e)   No. Glucose in the plasma is in free solution.

3.4
(a)   Yes. Hence cortisol tends to raise blood glucose.
(b)   No. Glucose enters without the help of insulin – otherwise, how would brain obtain its crucial supply when blood glucose falls and therefore the insulin level also falls?
(c)   Yes. Insulin assists glucose to enter muscle cells and promotes storage as glycogen.
(d)   Yes. A rise in glucagon and a fall in insulin promotes restoration of blood glucose from gluconeogenesis in the liver.
(e)   Yes. This occurs in 'fight or flight'.

3.5
(a)   No. The RQ would be close to 1, because oxidation of hexoses yields one mole of CO_2 for every mole of O_2.
(b)   Yes. The ratio of aerobic to anaerobic yield is about 16:1.
(c)   No. About 80% of the glycogen is in muscle, and about 20% in the liver.
(d)   Yes. Glucagon stimulates glycogenolysis and release of glucose into the blood.
(e)   Yes. Weight for weight, fat provides twice as much energy as protein.

3.6
(a)   Yes.
(b)   Yes. 0.3–0.4 kg of fat would yield 2700–3600 kcal.
(c)   No. Fat is stored in large cells, each containing a single fat droplet.
(d)   Yes.
(e)   No. The figure for protein is similar to that for carbohydrate: about 17 kJ per g. It is metabolism of fat which yields approximately 37 kJ per g.

3.7
(a)   Yes.
(b)   Yes. Insulin promotes muscle and liver uptake of amino acids, as well as of glucose, and hence provides for increased protein synthesis.

(c)   No. Cortisol promotes protein breakdown.

(d)   Yes. These are some of the notorious anabolic steroids which promote 'body-building' and athletic performance.

(e)   No. In this, as in other respects, glucagon has the opposite action to insulin. In starvation, it assists mobilization of amino acids from muscle protein breakdown for gluconeogenesis in the liver.

3.8

(a)   Yes. Insulin thus promotes storage of fats, as well as that of carbohydrates and proteins.

(b)   No. The central nervous system can use keto-acids – not fatty acids – along with glucose in starvation.

(c)   No. Fatty acids make the greater contribution overall to nutrient utilization, except after a high carbohydrate meal.

(d)   Yes.

(e)   Yes.

3.9

(a)   Yes. Blood glucose is maintained at this level, even in more prolonged fasting, by liver gluconeogenesis using amino acids derived in turn from muscle protein breakdown after liver glycogen is depleted within the first day.

(b)   Yes. Insulin secretion is regulated by the level of blood glucose, so it decreases and this prevents uptake of glucose in muscle but not in brain.

(c)   Yes.

(d)   Yes. Liver gluconeogenesis is promoted by a decrease in insulin and an increase in glucagon.

(e)   No. Brain requires glucose and takes what is available (see (b)); it is also able to utilize keto-acids, after a few days, along with glucose.

3.10

(a)   No. In starvation the blood glucose concentration falls.

(b)   Yes. Protein breakdown is a source of energy when glycogen stores have been depleted.

(c)   Yes. In starvation, glucagon is released into the blood to combat the fall in blood glucose concentration.

(d)   Yes. Metabolism of fatty acids when the concentration of insulin is low leads to the formation of ketone bodies.

(e)   Yes. A starved person can derive energy by metabolism of fats.

3.11

(a)   Yes.

(b)   Yes.

(c)   Yes.
(d)   No.
(e)   No. The kidneys synthesize erythropoietin.

3.12

(a)   Yes. Prothrombin is formed only in the liver, and its formation requires vitamin K.
(b)   No. Red blood cells disintegrate after about four months, and phagocytes in the mononuclear phagocytic system (formerly called the 'reticulo-endothelial system'), take them up.
(c)   No. The conversion of glucose to glycogen occurs not only in the liver but also in other tissues, such as muscle.
(d)   Yes. Cholesterol is excreted in the bile.
(e)   Yes. Liver produces and secretes bile salts from bile acids, conjugated with glycine or taurine.

3.13

(a)   Yes. Hepatic artery flow is estimated to be about one-half that of portal vein flow, but the latter varies with intestinal activity.
(b)   Yes.
(c)   Yes. Flow decreases during exercise, probably by means of increased sympathetic outflow causing hepatic vasoconstriction; a fall in portal flow is secondary to a decrease in flow to the gut.
(d)   Yes. Hepatic arterioles and portal venules both open into the sinusoids so that the liver cells are supplied with oxygen and also with the nutrients absorbed from the gut.
(e)   No. All types of foodstuff are represented in the portal vein, and it carries all of the protein and carbohydrate; but lymphatics carry some of the fat.

3.14

(a)   No. Urobilinogen is colourless. The yellow colour of normal urine is due to the pigment urochrome.
(b)   Yes. Urobilinogen is absorbed from the gut mainly in the colon and then travels in the portal venous blood to the liver where it is mostly taken up and re-excreted (another enterohepatic circulation: compare bile salts).
(c)   No. Urobilinogen is water soluble and so is carried in the blood in solution.
(d)   Yes. Urobilinogen is formed by the action of bacteria in the intestine on bilirubin.
(e)   Yes. Because uptake and re-excretion of urobilinogen from the blood by the liver is impaired.

3.15

(a)   Yes. In chronic severe liver disease, the structural changes in the liver impede the flow of blood delivered to it by the portal vein. So one consequence is back pressure – portal hypertension.

(b)   Yes. Associated with the raised portal vein pressure, there is excessive loss of fluid from the vessels of the abdominal viscera into the peritoneal cavity and consequently ascites.

(c)   Yes. One of the functions of the liver is to synthesize prothrombin. When this function is impaired, there is a tendency to haemorrhage. Impaired absorption of the fat-soluble vitamin K contributes to this.

(d)   Yes. The liver synthesizes plasma proteins, so when this function is impaired, their concentration is reduced. A low albumin concentration creates a tendency to oedema.

(e)   No. Much of the heat generated in basal metabolism comes from the liver and, with impairment of hepatic function, the core temperature tends to be low rather than high.

4 Respiration

QUESTIONS

In this section (and elsewhere relevant), **P** is used as the accepted symbol for **partial pressure** of a gas in the gas phase, or **tension** when referring to gas in solution that is in equilibrium with that partial pressure.

Breathing and gas exchange

Lung volumes and mechanics of breathing

4.1 The functional residual capacity (FRC) in the lungs of a young healthy adult of average size:
- (a) is about 1 litre.
- (b) becomes smaller if airflow resistance increases.
- (c) can be estimated using a helium dilution method.
- (d) has the effect of damping fluctuations of alveolar gas concentrations during the breathing cycle.
- (e) is the volume at which some airways normally begin to close during expiration.

4.2 In a healthy subject sitting upright at rest:
- (a) tidal volume is one-tenth or less of the total lung volume.
- (b) the lungs inflate and deflate around a mean volume that is about one-quarter of their full capacity.
- (c) if the person breathes right out, small airways start to close in the lower parts of the lungs sooner than in the upper parts.
- (d) if he or she breathes right out to residual volume (RV), the first air subsequently inhaled will enter the apical regions of the lungs.
- (e) if a resistance is added to airflow, the tidal exchange will shift to a higher lung volume.

$VC = TV + Insp. R + Exp. R$

4.3 An adult subject breathing air was found to have the following lung volumes:

Vital capacity	3.5 litres
Forced expiratory volume in 1 sec (FEV₁)	2.8 litres
Functional residual capacity (FRC)	1.8 litres
Residual volume (RV)	0.8 litre

(a) airflow resistance is normal.
(b) the subject must be abnormal.
(c) the expiratory reserve volume is 1 litre.
(d) all of these measurements could have been made using only a spirometer.
(e) there would be approximately 250 ml of oxygen in this subject's lungs at the end of a tidal expiration.

4.4 Figure 4.4 represents the change in volume when an isolated lung is inflated; A–B represents a typical curve for a lung that is normal and air-filled.

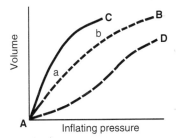

(a) the lower part of the curve, A–a shows the difficulty of initial expansion against surface tension forces.
(b) the upper part, b–B represents the volume at which the lung is most compliant.
(c) during deflation, the same pathway would be followed in reverse (B–b–a–A).
(d) the curve A–C could represent expansion of the same lung when filled with saline instead of air.
(e) the curve A–D could represent a lung with more surfactant activity.

4.5   Compliance of the lungs *in vivo*:
(a)   depends partly on airway conductance when measured during continuous breathing.
(b)   is defined as the change in volume per unit change in expanding (inflating) pressure.
(c)   is greatest, for the whole lung, between residual volume and functional residual capacity.
(d)   is decreased if surfactant is depleted.
(e)   within the tidal range, is greater at the apex than at the base of the lungs in the upright posture.

4.6   Concerning mechanical factors in breathing:
(a)   in the tidal range, there is more muscular work involved in breathing in than in breathing out.
(b)   forced expiration is more difficult than forced inspiration.
(c)   recoil of the chest wall assists inspiration.
(d)   the 'negative pressure' holding the lungs inflated is less effective (less negative) at the bases than at the apices.
(e)   respiratory muscles use about one-tenth of the whole body oxygen consumption in normal people at rest.

4.7   Figure 4.7 represents measurements made continuously during a single normal tidal breath, in and out, in a human subject at rest:

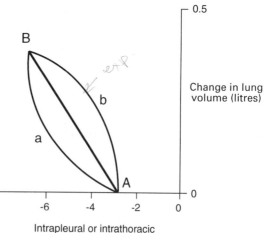

(a)   the curve B–a–A represents expiration.
(b)   zero on the vertical scale represents functional residual capacity.

(c) the volume change shown here could be increased by a factor of 16 in very strenuous exercise.

(d) the slope of the straight line drawn from A to B measures the compliance of the lungs.

(e) the 'loop' shown would be 'fatter' if the person had increased resistance to airflow.

4.8   The muscular work done during inspiration:

(a) is made less by the effect of surfactant.

(b) is greater if the elastic recoil of the lungs is greater.

(c) is greater if inspiration starts at a high lung volume than if it is in the normal tidal range.

(d) could be lessened by bronchial dilatation.

(e) is partly spent in overcoming surface tension forces.

Ventilation

4.9   In relation to oxygen consumption and its measurement in an average-sized man:

(a) if the subject is at rest and hyperventilates, the oxygen percentage in the expired air will decrease.

(b) during moderate muscular exercise, ventilation increases linearly as oxygen consumption increases.

(c) using the spirometer method, the oxygen consumption is measured from the rate of emptying of the spirometer bell.

(d) the average resting oxygen consumption is about 0.25 litres per minute.

(e) consumption of 1 litre of oxygen is equivalent to an energy expenditure of approximately 4.8 kcal (20 kJ).

4.10   In the alveolar region of the lungs:

(a) the barrier to diffusion of gases is about 10 μm thick.

(b) surfactant-secreting cells form a continuous cytoplasmic layer lining the alveoli.

(c) alveoli are larger in the upper and smaller in the lower zones of the lungs.

(d) if any fluid escapes from capillaries, it goes into the alveoli.

(e) macrophages in the alveoli are carried to the respiratory bronchioles by the activity of cilia.

4.11   Decreased arterial oxygen tension is a consequence of:
✓ (a)   hypoventilation.
✗ (b)   low haemoglobin concentration.
✗ (c)   carbon monoxide poisoning.
✓ (d)   living at high altitude.
✓ (e)   ventilation-perfusion mismatch in the lungs.

4.12   In a healthy person, the following values were found for end-tidal (end-expired) gas, and can be taken to represent alveolar partial pressures:

PO$_2$:   115 mmHg (15 kPa)
PCO$_2$:   25 mmHg (3.5 kPa) *(normal 40 (5.2))*

(a)   the subject was overbreathing (hyperventilating).
(b)   the oxygen percentage in the inspired gas must have been higher than in room air.
✓ (c)   the arterial PCO$_2$ would be close to 25 mmHg.
(d)   the arterial PO$_2$ would be 90–100 mmHg (12–13.5 kPa).
(e)   there must be a respiratory alkalosis.

4.13   Figure 4.13 shows simultaneous recordings of CO$_2$ concentration in gas sampled from the nostril and inspired tidal volume in a healthy person.

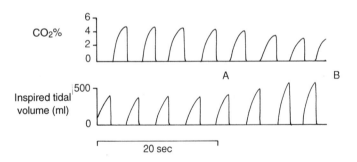

(a)   the inspired gas contained about 5% CO$_2$.
✓ (b)   the subject showed a typical resting breathing pattern at the start.
✗ (c)   the subject started to hypoventilate towards the end.
(d)   arterial oxygen tension would be lower at B than at A.
(e)   over the period from A to B, the rate of excretion of CO$_2$ from the body must have been greater than the initial rate.

4.14 Figure 4.14 shows the effect on alveolar PCO_2 of alterations in alveolar ventilation. The solid curve refers to a typical healthy subject at rest who deliberately changes his ventilation (assuming a constant rate of metabolic CO_2 production); his normal undisturbed alveolar ventilation and PCO_2 are shown at point a:

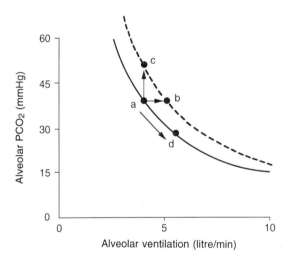

(a) the arrow a to b could represent what happens when this same subject increases his metabolic activity.

(b) the arrow a to d represents what happens during hyperventilation.

(c) the arrow a to c shows the ventilatory response to rising PCO_2.

(d) CO_2 production in the condition represented at point a is a little over 200 ml per min.

(e) the broken curve could refer to a different subject of larger size.

4.15   Figure 4.15 shows a spirometer tracing from a healthy human adult at rest. The spirometer was filled with oxygen and there was a carbon dioxide absorber in the circuit. The subject was switched to breathe from the spirometer at the end of a normal expiration (at functional residual capacity).

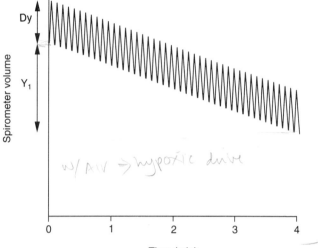

Time (min)

  (a)   the steady fall in the trace is due to oxygen usage by the subject.
  (b)   the excursion Dy is the tidal volume.
  (c)   the value of Y_1 is typically 5 litres.
  (d)   if during the trace the carbon dioxide absorber stopped working, the trace would start to fall more steeply.
  (e)   if the subject had not rested prior to the recording, the steepness of the slope would decrease with time.

4.16   **With further reference to Figure 4.15:**
  (a)   if the apparatus were filled with air rather than oxygen, the amplitude of the rapid excursions would decrease with time.
  (b)   if the apparatus were filled with air rather than oxygen, the frequency of the rapid excursions would decrease with time.
  (c)   if the apparatus were filled with air rather than oxygen, the steepness of the slope would increase.
  (d)   if the spirometer initially contained 6 litres of **oxygen** the subject could be left to breathe from it until the spirometer contained only sufficient gas to match the tidal volume.
  (e)   if the spirometer initially contained 6 litres of **air**, the subject would be in danger from hypoxia if the volume of gas in the spirometer at the end of expiration were allowed to decrease below 5 litres.

Control of breathing

4.17 **With reference to the control of breathing:**
(a) the increase in ventilation in exercise is proportional to a rise in arterial PCO_2.
(b) the peripheral (arterial) chemoreceptors are stimulated by any form of diminished oxygen content in the arterial blood. ↓ O_2 tension
(c) afferent fibres in the vagus nerves carry information on the state of inflation of the lungs.
(d) breathing can continue when the brain stem is the only functioning part of the brain.
(e) breathing can be influenced voluntarily via direct pathways from the cerebral cortex to spinal motoneurones.

4.18 **A healthy person at rest is given pure oxygen to breathe for five minutes:**
(a) in the first minute the ventilation will be considerably depressed.
(b) in the fifth minute the ventilation will be virtually the same as it was breathing air.
(c) the arterial PCO_2 will decrease considerably.
(d) the arterial PO_2 will rise to over 80 kPa (600 mmHg).
(e) the subject would be able to hold his breath at the end of the five minutes for significantly longer than when he was breathing air.

4.19 **Concerning breathing, in a healthy person:**
(a) speech involves modified expiration.
(b) inhalation of 100% oxygen results in apnoea (cessation of breathing).
(c) inhalation of a gas mixture containing 5% CO_2 stimulates breathing.
(d) the respiratory centres lie in the diencephalon.
(e) after hyperventilating, the breath can be held for longer than after normal breathing.

4.20 **The neurones whose activity causes inspiratory muscle activity:**
(a) are situated in the medulla.
(b) are stimulated by their own extracellular acidity.
(c) show an increase in frequency of action potentials during inspiration when there is an increase in chemoreceptor stimulation.
(d) cease firing instantly at the end of inspiration.
(e) project directly on to spinal motoneurones.

4.21   The central (medullary) chemoreceptors:
(a)   are stimulated by a rise in the acidity of the cerebral interstitial fluid.
(b)   are stimulated when arterial carbon dioxide tension increases.
(c)   are stimulated when arterial oxygen tension decreases.
(d)   are stimulated when arterial pH decreases because of metabolic acidaemia (e.g. lactic acid).
(e)   are entirely responsible for the increase in ventilation in response to rebreathing expired air.   NO – peripheral.

4.22   Stimulation of the carotid bodies
(a)   occurs when there is a low arterial oxygen tension.
(b)   occurs when there is a raised arterial carbon dioxide tension.
(c)   causes an increase in ventilation.
(d)   causes a decrease in arterial blood pressure.
(e)   is prevented by breathing a high percentage of oxygen.

Gas transport in the blood

4.23   Concerning the carriage of gases by the blood:
(a)   a rise in PCO_2 increases the oxygen carrying capacity of the blood.
(b)   at a fixed PO_2 of 40 mmHg, a rise in PCO_2 would increase the oxygen content of the blood.
(c)   a rise in PCO_2 assists in off-loading of oxygen in the tissues.
(d)   for blood with a given content of CO_2, a rise in PO_2 increases the PCO_2 of the blood.
(e)   a rise in PO_2 assists in off-loading of CO_2 in the pulmonary capillaries.

4.24   2,3-DPG (diphosphoglycerate):
(a)   decreases the affinity of haemoglobin for oxygen.
(b)   increases in concentration in the erythrocytes in chronic hypoxia.
(c)   is a product of glycolysis.
(d)   increases in concentration in stored blood.
(e)   binds to deoxygenated haemoglobin.

4.25   As blood passes through the lungs, the CO_2 that is released into the alveolar gas:
(a)   has been carried in the blood mainly as bicarbonate.
(b)   has been carried in the blood partly in physical solution.
(c)   has been carried in the blood partly by attachment to haemoglobin.
(d)   is released with the assistance of carbonic anhydrase.
(e)   is actively transported across the capillary–alveolar barrier.

4.26 **As blood passes through the lungs, the CO$_2$ that is released into the alveolar gas:**

(a) matches, in mol per minute, in a steady state, the rate of metabolic production of carbon dioxide by the tissues.

(b) is greater, in mol per minute, than the amount of oxygen taken into the blood, at a respiratory quotient (RQ) of 0.8.

(c) in ml per minute, might increase by a factor of 10 during exercise.

(d) diffuses down a partial pressure gradient of about 45 mmHg at rest.

(e) causes the alveolar carbon dioxide partial pressure to rise during expiration.

4.27 **With reference to carbon dioxide:**

(a) more is taken up at any given PCO$_2$ by desaturated than by fully oxygenated blood.

(b) most of the blood 'CO$_2$ content' is in the form of bicarbonate in the plasma.

(c) it readily diffuses in and out of red blood cells.

(d) it forms carbonic acid more readily in plasma than in red blood cells.

(e) its uptake by blood passing through the tissues is enhanced by carbonic anhydrase inhibitors.

4.28 **Figure 4.28 shows the oxygen dissociation curve for normal fresh arterial blood as the full line; the dashed line shows a different oxygen dissociation curve.**

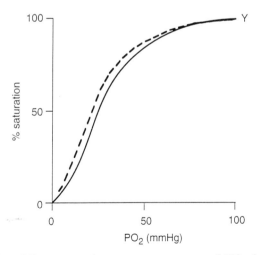

(a) the value of Y corresponds to an oxygen content of 100 ml oxygen per litre of blood.

(b)   The P_{50} is greater for the dashed line than for the full line.
(c)   the full line would represent blood with a lower affinity for oxygen than the dashed line.
(d)   the dashed line would represent blood equilibrated with the PCO_2 of mixed venous blood.
(e)   the dashed line would represent fetal blood.

4.29   In each case, the figure shows the oxyhaemoglobin dissociation curve for normal fresh arterial blood as the full line and the dashed line shows a different oxygen dissociation curve. Is this dashed dissociation curve appropriate for the situation given?:

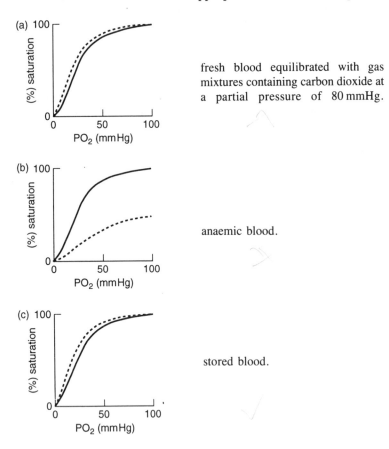

(a)

fresh blood equilibrated with gas mixtures containing carbon dioxide at a partial pressure of 80 mmHg.

(b)

anaemic blood.

(c)

stored blood.

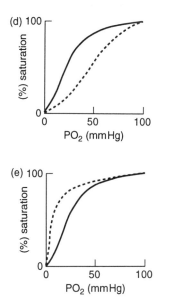

(d) 100

(%) saturation

0

0   50   100

PO$_2$ (mmHg)

blood from a subject with carbon monoxide poisoning.

(e) 100

(%) saturation

0

0   50   100

PO$_2$ (mmHg)

a solution of myoglobin.

Pulmonary circulation

4.30   In the pulmonary circulation:
(a)   the vascular resistance decreases at birth.
(b)   hypoxia is a vasodilator.   *vasoconstrictor*
(c)   the arterioles are thinner walled than systemic arterioles of similar diameter.
(d)   the vascular resistance is about 10 times lower than the total peripheral (systemic) resistance.
(e)   if cardiac output doubles, e.g. in exercise, pulmonary artery pressure also doubles.

4.31   Concerning the pulmonary circulation, in the upright posture:
(a)   the pulmonary artery pressure at the apices is close to zero.
(b)   vessels are more distended at the bases of the lungs than at the apices.
(c)   pulmonary artery and pulmonary vein pressure increase by the same amount from heart level to the base of the lungs.
(d)   the blood flow per unit lung volume is greater at the bases than at the apices.
(e)   there is a greater tendency for fluid to escape from pulmonary capillaries at the apices than at the bases.

4.32   **Movement of fluid out of pulmonary capillaries:**
(a)   is increased if surfactant is deficient.
(b)   normally occurs to some extent all the time.
(c)   implies movement of fluid into the alveoli.
(d)   is increased in rate by any increase in pulmonary capillary pressure.
(e)   is increased in rate by any increase in pulmonary blood flow.

Ventilation-perfusion ratios in the lungs

4.33   **Consider the blood leaving a lobe of the lung for which the ventilation-perfusion ratio is initially 1.**
If the ventilation-perfusion ratio then increases to 2, in the blood leaving this lobe:
(a)   the oxygen content will rise by about 5%.
(b)   the PO_2 will rise by at least 20 mmHg.
(c)   the PCO_2 will be approximately halved.
(d)   the CO_2 content will be reduced by less than 10%.
If, instead, the ventilation-perfusion ratio were to decrease from 1 to 0.5:
(e)   the oxygen content of the blood leaving this lobe would fall by about 5%.

4.34   **Concerning ventilation-perfusion matching/mismatching:**
(a)   in the upright posture alveolar ventilation per unit lung volume is greater at the apices than at the bases.
(b)   in the upright posture, the ventilation-perfusion ratio is greater at the apices than at the bases.
(c)   in the supine posture, the ventilation-perfusion ratio is lowest in the back of the lungs.
(d)   blockage of pulmonary capillaries by scattered emboli causes an increase in alveolar dead space.
(e)   collapse of alveoli causes an increase in venous admixture.

4.35   **Concerning ventilation/perfusion ratios (V_A/Q) in different regions of the lungs:**
(a)   an 'infinite' ratio implies alveolar dead space.
(b)   a ratio of zero implies venous admixture.
(c)   a high ratio causes a higher than average PO_2 in the blood leaving that region.
(d)   a low ratio causes pulmonary capillary blood to leave without reaching the PO_2 in the alveoli of that region.
(e)   an excess of areas with low ratios would necessarily cause a rise in arterial PCO_2.

Calculation questions

4.36 An individual has 135 g Hb per litre of blood and his Hb is 100% saturated at a PO_2 of 100 mmHg (13.3 kPa). When he is breathing air, his cardiac output is 6 litres per min, and his oxygen usage is 300 ml per min. (Assume Hb carries 1.34 mlO_2 per g, and that 3 ml of O_2 dissolves in 1 litre of blood at a PO_2 of 100 mmHg (13.3 kPa).) In this person:

(a)   the arteriovenous difference for oxygen is 50 ml per litre.

(b)   the mixed venous oxygen content is 150 ml per litre.

(c)   if he increases his oxygen usage four-fold, to 1.2 litres per min, and doubles his cardiac output, the tissues must be extracting twice as much oxygen from each litre of blood.

(d)   if he changes from breathing air to breathing oxygen, so that the alveolar PO_2 becomes 600 mmHg (80 kPa), the arterial oxygen content will be increased by 15 ml per litre.

(e)   when the alveolar PO_2 becomes 600 mmHg (80 kPa), the arterial PO_2 will rise above 120 mmHg (16 kPa).

4.37 A subject under anaesthesia, with healthy lungs, is mechanically ventilated at 8 litres per min. The anatomical dead space is estimated to be 150 ml. The stroke volume of the respirator (tidal volume) is set at 0.8 litres. The inspired gas contains 50% oxygen. CO_2 production is 195 ml per min and O_2 usage is 240 ml per min. Alveolar CO_2 is 3%:

(a)   the alveolar ventilation is 6.5 litres per min.

(b)   the patient is being hyperventilated.

(c)   at this alveolar CO_2 concentration, the patient is likely to have cerebral vasodilatation.

(d)   given that his pulmonary gas exchange is normal, his arterial oxygen tension (PO_2) should be over 300 mmHg (40 kPa).

(e)   the respiratory quotient (RQ) is greater than 1.2.

ANSWERS

4.1

(a)   No. The FRC is at least twice this volume.

(b)   No. When resistance to flow increases, the tidal excursion moves to a higher lung volume, so FRC is increased.

(c)   Yes. Helium is not taken up appreciably into the blood; a known concentration is rebreathed from a known volume in a spirometer until there is a constant concentration in the mixed gas; thence total volume of lungs + spirometer can be estimated from the final concentration of He.

(d)   Yes. Because tidal volume is small relative to the volume remaining in the lungs continuously, there is very little fluctuation in CO_2 and O_2 concentrations in alveoli, and therefore in the blood leaving the lungs.

(e)   No. Airways begin to close only as residual volume is approached in healthy young people.

4.2

(a)   Yes. A typical total lung capacity might be 6 litres, and tidal volume 400–500 ml.

(b)   No. The mean volume around which tidal excursion takes place is at about mid-lung volume.

(c)   Yes. In healthy young subjects, during forced expiration, airways in lower regions start to close just before RV is reached. Gravity causes intrapleural pressure to be less around the upper than around the lower parts of the lungs; the upper airways are therefore held open longer, as expiration proceeds.

(d)   Yes. At residual volume, airways in upper parts are held more open than those in lower parts; so the first air will enter the apices.

(e)   Yes. A complex mechanical feedback results in an appropriate compensation: when air is shifted in and out at a higher lung volume, there is more help during expiration from the elastic recoil.

4.3

(a)   Yes. The FEV_1 is 80% of the VC; this is a normal value, indicating that airflow resistance is normal.

(b)   No. These could be perfectly normal values for a small woman: they are all in the correct proportions.

(c)   Yes. The ERV is found by subtracting RV from FRC.

(d)   No. It is not possible to measure RV by spirometer: a dilution method is required – a spirometer may be one component of the apparatus used.

(e)   Yes. FRC is the volume concerned. At the end of expiration, the lungs are full of alveolar gas, which has about 14% oxygen; $0.14 \times 1.8 = 0.25$ litres.

4.4

(a)   No. A–a shows easier expansion than b–B. Surface tension is most strongly opposed by surfactant at low lung volume.

(b)   No. The part b–B shows a decreasing change in volume for a given change in pressure – the lung is becoming less compliant as it becomes full.

(c)   No. There would be hysteresis: that is, the path in the other direction (from full to residual volume) would be different (it would lie above and to the left of B–b–a–A).

(d)   Yes. Filling the lung with liquid abolishes the surface tension factor, expansion is easier, compliance is greater, a given change in pressure causes a larger change in volume.

(e)   No. A greater surfactant activity would make the lung more compliant. Curve A–D suggests a lack of normal surfactant activity.

4.5

(a)   Yes. Resistance to airflow during the breathing cycle affects the area of the pressure volume loop, and the slope of the line joining its ends.

(b)   Yes. This is the definition.

(c)   No. The system is most compliant in the normal tidal volume range, above functional residual capacity.

(d)   Yes. Compliance is increased by surfactant, decreased by surface tension.

(e)   No. Alveoli at the apex, being already more stretched at end-expiratory volume due to gravity, are less easily expanded than lower alveoli.

4.6

(a)   Yes. During inspiration, the elastic recoil of the lungs and surface tension necessitate muscular work; they assist expiration and at rest can account for all the work needed to overcome airflow resistance and chest compression.

(b)   Yes. During forced expiration the intrathoracic pressure becomes positive, and tends to close small airways, increasing the resistance to airflow.

(c)   Yes. The position of rest is above the tidal range.

(d)   Yes. There is more 'pull away' of the lungs from the chest wall at the top, so the pressure here is more negative.

(e)   No. They use only a tiny fraction: about 1 ml per min per litre per min which is of the order of 5–10 ml per min, or less than one-twenty-fifth of the whole body oxygen consumption.

4.7

(a)   No. Curve B–b–A, to the right, shows expiration.

(b)   Yes. This is a normal tidal breath, so inspiration starts from the functional residual capacity.

(c)   No. The volume change shown is 400 ml. $16 \times 0.4 = 6.4$ litres, which is a possible vital capacity but not a possible tidal volume in exercise. Oxygen consumption can increase by 16 times, and minute volume by a comparable factor; tidal volume does not usually become more than half the vital capacity.

(d)   Yes. Compliance is change in volume/change in pressure.

(e)   Yes. Resistance to airflow is one of the factors that makes it necessary to exert a greater pressure change to cause any given volume change during inflation and deflation, than would be needed if the lungs were simply elastic structures. The greater the resistance, the further would the curves be from the straight line of compliance.

4.8

(a)   Yes. Surfactant diminishes the effect of surface tension in the alveoli and therefore limits the work required to expand them.

(b)   Yes. Work in expanding the lungs is done in part against the elastic recoil, the force tending always to deflate the lungs.

(c)   Yes. The compliance of the lungs – the ease with which they can be expanded – becomes less at volumes above the normal tidal range.

(d)   Yes. Bronchial dilatation leads to a decrease in resistance to airflow, against which work has to be done during inspiration (and expiration).

(e)   Yes. Despite the modifying effect of surfactant, there is a surface tension force that must be overcome in any increase in lung volume.

4.9

(a)   No. Hyperventilation only very slightly increases the oxygen consumption. So a smaller fraction of the oxygen is removed from the much larger volume of inspired gas. So the 0_2% in expired gas increases.

(b)   Yes. In a healthy person, ventilation keeps up with oxygen consumption in exercise, so ventilation increases linearly with oxygen consumption. The increase is about 20 litres per min per additional litre of oxygen uptake per minute.

(c)   Yes. In this method, the subject rebreathes oxygen and the CO_2 is absorbed. Therefore the rate of decrease of volume is a direct measure of the O_2 consumed.

(d)   Yes. But varies, of course, according to body size.

(e)   Yes. This conversion factor is used to calculate the metabolic rate from measurement of O_2 usage.

4.10

(a)   No. The barrier to diffusion is a whole order of magnitude thinner: $0.5–1\mu m$.

(b)   No. The surfactant (type II alveolar epithelial) cells are relatively rounded structures. It is the alveolar epithelial type I cells that form an attenuated layer lining the alveoli, with tight junctions between the cytoplasm of neighbouring similar cells. The surfactant is secreted from the Type II cells into the alveolus, and spreads over the surface of the Type I cell epithelium.

(c)   Yes. One of the effects of gravity is to expand the uppermost and relatively 'squash' the lowermost air spaces (but note that the larger expanded alveoli are ventilated less than smaller ones, because they are less readily expanded).

(d)   No. The net loss of fluid from capillaries in the lungs is drained, as elsewhere in the body, via lymphatics. Fluid seeps through connective tissue between alveoli to reach the lymphatics, which extend to the end of the bronchial tree. Only when a considerable fluid pressure builds up in the interstitial tissue does oedema extend into and thicken the thin alveolar–capillary interface and ultimately break through the alveolar epithelium into the air spaces.

(e)   No. There are no cilia between alveoli and respiratory bronchioles. Macrophages must migrate to reach the 'staircase' of cilia that starts at the proximal end of respiratory bronchioles.

4.11

(a)   Yes. A decrease in alveolar ventilation below the level required to keep PCO_2 normal will necessarily also cause a fall in O_2 if the inspired gas is normal air.

(b)   No. Low haemoglobin concentration results in there being less oxygen carried per ml of blood, but the PO_2 will be normal if the lungs are normal, and the ventilation is adequate.

(c)   No. Like low Hb, CO poisoning causes the 'anaemic' type of hypoxia: CO occupies oxygen-carrying sites in Hb, thus putting it out of action for O_2 transport. The PO_2 is normal if the lungs are functioning normally. Dissolved O_2 is normal. There can be a severe or lethal lack of oxygen with a normal PO_2.

(d)   Yes. At high altitude the total barometric pressure is low, so 20% oxygen in inspired air represents progressively less than 160 mmHg partial pressure at increasing height above sea level. As inspired PO_2 decreases, alveolar PO_2 decreases, likewise arterial PO_2.

(e)   Yes. A greater than normal divergence of ventilation-perfusion ratios in the lungs results in some mixed venous blood being relatively poorly oxygenated in its passage through under-ventilated regions of the lungs. The smaller amount of blood flowing past over-ventilated regions does not make up for this, and arterial hypoxaemia is the result.

4.12

(a)   Yes. If PCO_2 is lower than normal, there is, by definition, a state of hyperventilation. The normal PCO_2 is around 40 mmHg (5.2 kPa).

(b)   No. This is the expected increase in alveolar oxygen partial pressure when alveolar CO_2 pressure is this much decreased.

(c)   Yes. In normal people, the arterial PCO_2 is within 3 mmHg
       (0.4 kPa) of the alveolar PCO_2.
(d)   No. In normal people, the alveolar-arterial PO_2 difference will
       be not more than 10 mmHg (1.4 kPa); the rise in arterial PO_2
       during hyperventilation does not, however, appreciably increase
       the Hb saturation or content of O_2 per litre of arterial blood.
(e)   Yes. A decrease of PCO_2 depletes plasma bicarbonate and must
       cause an alkalaemia in accordance with the interrelation among pH,
       bicarbonate and PCO_2, as defined in the Henderson-Hasselbalch
       equation. Even if the hyperventilation has continued for a long time,
       and pH has been restored to near normal by other compensatory
       mechanisms, there is still, by definition, a respiratory alkalosis when
       PCO_2 is low.

4.13
(a)   No. The end-tidal (end-expired) gas is about 5% CO_2; the inspired
       gas is air, with no significant CO_2 content.
(b)   Yes. The tidal volume (400 ml) and frequency of breathing (12 per
       min) give a minute volume of 4.8 litres. This is within the normal
       range for a smallish person.
(c)   No. The subject hyperventilated between A and B, reducing the end-
       tidal CO_2.
(d)   No. It would be higher, because of hyperventilation.
(e)   Yes. Hyperventilation implies a greater rate of excretion of CO_2,
       resulting in a lower alveolar and arterial concentration.

4.14
(a)   Yes. The ventilation increases as metabolic activity increases so that
       arterial PCO_2 is kept normal.
(b)   Yes. The point d would reflect a new steady state at higher ventila-
       tion but the same CO_2 output as before.
(c)   No. This could not be so because the ventilation is unchanged. This
       arrow could represent an increase in metabolic CO_2 production or
       addition of CO_2 to the inspired gas in a patient on constant con-
       trolled ventilation.)
(d)   Yes. The alveolar ventilation shown is about 4 per min, the PCO_2
       about 38 mmHg, corresponding to 5% CO_2 in alveolar gas; 5% of
       4 litres per min = 200 ml per min.
(e)   Yes. A larger subject would have a greater ventilation at any given
       PCO_2; his CO_2 output at rest would be greater. His resting condi-
       tion would be represented at b. (The curve could equally refer to
       the same subject as the solid curve, but at an increased metabolic
       rate.)

4.15

(a)   Yes.

(b)   Yes.

(c)   No. The value of Y_1 is typically 1 litre – representing oxygen consumption at a rate of 250 ml per minute.

(d)   No. If the carbon dioxide absorber stopped working, the trace would level out because accumulation of carbon dioxide would counteract absorption of oxygen. The tidal volume would also increase due to hypercapnic stimulation of respiration.

(e)   Yes. If the subject had not rested prior to the recording, initially the oxygen usage would be above resting, but as the recording progressed, oxygen usage would fall towards basal and the steepness of the slope would decrease with time.

4.16

(a)   No. If the apparatus were filled with air rather than oxygen, there would be progressive hypoxic drive to respiration and the tidal volume would increase.

(b)   No. For the same reason as (a), the frequency of respiration would rise.

(c)   No. Oxygen usage would be little affected and the slope would be unchanged.

(d)   Yes. The subject's lungs at functional residual capacity (FRC) initially contained about 2.5 litres, of which approximately 80% was nitrogen; this 2 litres of N_2 remains in the lung-spirometer system. Assuming a 0.5 litre tidal volume, when the lung-spirometer volume is 3 litres there is just sufficient gas to match the tidal volume. Of this, two-thirds will be nitrogen, one-third oxygen; the inspired oxygen percentage is therefore still greater than in normal air.

(e)   Yes. Leaving a subject rebreathing in a spirometer circuit filled with air and with a CO_2 absorber in place is very dangerous; hypoxia without hypercapnia may cause little discomfort and the subject could become confused and lose consciousness without raising any alarm. Again, assuming FRC = 2.5 litres, the initial lungs + spirometer volume of 2.5 + 6 = 8.5 litres contained approximately 80% nitrogen, and this 6.8 litres of N_2 remains in the lung-spirometer system. When the lungs + spirometer volume has decreased to 2.5 + 5 = 7.5 litres, the N_2 fraction is therefore 6.8/7.5, which is just over 90%. Oxygen can be no more than 10%. Any decrease below this would be dangerous.

4.17

(a)   No. In healthy people, arterial PCO_2 remains at its resting value in moderate exercise and decreases at high work rates.

(b)   No. They are stimulated only by the types of hypoxia that reduce the arterial oxygen tension.

(c)   Yes. Afferents from stretch receptors take part in the control of the pattern of breathing.

(d)   Yes. Although higher centres normally influence breathing, it can continue when only the brain-stem is intact and functioning (as in the 'persistent vegetative state' when the cerebral cortex no longer functions).

(e)   Yes. Voluntary pathways 'bypass' the medullary centres and activate spinal motoneurones.

4.18

(a)   No. There is a small transient depression, but as this leads to a rise in PCO_2, it is promptly corrected and ventilation would be as before within a minute.

(b)   Yes. See (a).

(c)   No. This would mean that ventilation had been stimulated since PCO_2 depends on the balance between metabolic CO_2 production and alveolar ventilation, not on the inspired O_2 concentration.

(d)   Yes. After five minutes virtually all the nitrogen would be washed out of the alveolar gas, so the partial pressures of O_2, CO_2 and water vapour must add up to 1 atmosphere.

(e)   Yes. The break point in breath-holding depends on the combined stimulus of increasing PCO_2 and decreasing PO_2. After breathing oxygen, the rate rise of PCO_2 is unchanged, but the hypoxic enhancement of the stimulus is absent.

4.19

(a)   Yes.

(b)   No. Oxygen may depress breathing very slightly and very briefly. Although oxygen suppresses tonic impulses from the peripheral (arterial) chemoreceptors, central sensitivity to CO_2 promptly corrects the depression and maintains normal breathing.

(c)   Yes. CO_2 stimulates both central and peripheral chemoreceptors.

(d)   No. Respiratory neurones are in the brain-stem (medulla oblongata and pons).

(e)   Yes. Hyperventilation washes CO_2 out of the body fluids, so if the subject subsequently holds the breath, it takes longer for the accumulating CO_2 to reach a stimulating level. Meanwhile, however, the oxygen has fallen lower than in a normal breath-hold; this contributes to the stimulus, so that CO_2 may not rise quite so high before the breakpoint.

4.20

(a)   Yes. They lie in the 'ventral respiratory group' of neurones in the medulla.

(b)   No. It is the chemosensitive region under the ventral surface of the medulla that is stimulated by acidity; the stimulus is neurally transmitted to the inspiratory neurones.

(c)   Yes. Any reflex stimulus, from peripheral (arterial) or central (medullary) chemoreceptors causes the 'ramp' of discharge during inspiration to become steeper; this in turn generates a stronger inspiratory effort and a greater tidal volume.

(d)   No. There is a brief continuation, with a steep decline in activity during early expiration: the inspiratory muscles therefore do not 'let go' suddenly, but allow a smooth transition into expiration.

(e)   Yes.

4.21

(a)   Yes. Decrease in the pH of their immediate environment stimulates them; this can occur as a result of a rise in carbon dioxide in the blood supplying the medulla or, because they are situated close to the medullary surface, as a result of a rise in acidity for any reason of the cerebrospinal fluid that bathes that surface.

(b)   Yes. Because carbon dioxide freely diffuses through the blood–brain barrier. See (a).

(c)   No. Whole body hypoxia stimulates breathing only by acting at the peripheral (arterial) chemoreceptors. Brain hypoxia depresses breathing, and this competes with the chemoreflex stimulation.

(d)   No. The central chemoreceptors are not readily accessible to increasing H^+ in the blood because of the blood–brain barrier; stimulation of ventilation in these circumstances is via the peripheral chemoreceptors.

(e)   No. When rebreathing expired air, as in a small enclosed space, both decreasing oxygen and rising carbon dioxide stimulate breathing via the peripheral (arterial) chemoreceptors.

4.22

(a)   Yes. Decrease in oxygen tension alone (without an increase in carbon dioxide tension) becomes a significant stimulus only when it falls below about 60 mmHg; below this the response is progressively steeper.

(b)   Yes. An increase in PCO_2 or in acidity for any reason stimulates the carotid bodies; such a stimulus enhances the effect of any concomitant decrease in PO_2; thus even small changes in the direction of asphyxia can be strong stimuli.

(c)   Yes.

(d)   No. There is reflex peripheral vasoconstriction. Whether or not the blood pressure rises depends on the balance between this and the direct vasodilatory effect of hypoxia. In the absence of intact innervated carotid bodies, hypoxia causes a fall in blood pressure.

(e)   Yes. Because hyperoxia silences the carotid bodies, the response of ventilation to rising carbon dioxide combined with high oxygen reflects only the sensitivity of the central chemosensitive mechanism, and may be used to assess this.

4.23

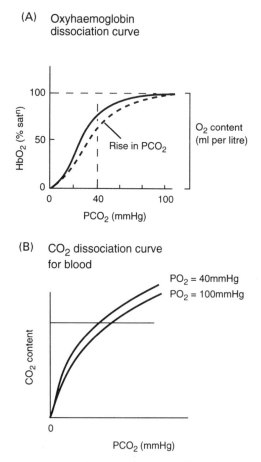

(A) Oxyhaemoglobin dissociation curve

(B) CO_2 dissociation curve for blood

(a)   No. The oxygen carrying capacity of the blood is the amount of oxygen per litre of blood when the haemoglobin is fully saturated. A rise in PCO_2 shifts the oxyhaemoglobin dissociation curve to the right. The oxygen carrying capacity of the blood, which depends only on the haemoglobin concentration, is not altered. (Figure A4.23(A)).

(b) No. See Figure A4.23(A); the vertical line at $PO_2 = 40\,mmHg$ shows that as the PCO_2 rises, the oxygen content falls (the 'Bohr effect').

(c) Yes. Because of the effect in (b) a rise in PCO_2 forces oxygen out of the blood.

(d) Yes. See Figure A4.23(B). The horizontal line represents blood with a given CO_2 content. Raising the PO_2 increases the PCO_2 of the blood.

(e) Yes. Because of the effect in (d), a rise in PO_2 forces CO_2 out of the blood.

4.24

(a) Yes. The normal oxyhaemoglobin dissociation curve depends on the presence of 2,3-DPG; without it, the curve is to the left of its normal position, i.e. there is greater saturation at a given partial pressure of oxygen.

(b) Yes. This has an adverse effect on oxygen uptake in the lungs at low PO_2 but conversely assists release in the tissue. The effect is greater where off-loading is over the steeper part of the dissociation curve.

(c) Yes. 2,3-DPG is formed from 3-phosphoglyceraldehyde, which is a product of anaerobic glycolysis. 2,3-DPG also itself promotes glycolysis by acting as a 'shunt' in a glycolytic pathway in erythrocytes.

(d) No. The concentration decreases in stored blood, which impairs off-loading of oxygen in the tissues when it is used for transfusion; unless cardiac output can increase to decrease the arterio-venous difference for oxygen, the tissue PO_2 must decrease if sufficient oxygen is to be extracted.

(e) Yes. 2,3-DPG binds to deoxygenated haemoglobin: this is one mechanism whereby it effectively decreases the affinity of haemoglobin for oxygen (the other is by maintaining a low internal pH relative to plasma, contributing to the Bohr effect).

4.25

(a) Yes. The major component of exchange from tissues to blood, and from blood to lungs, is in the form of bicarbonate.

(b) Yes.

(c) Yes. As carbamino-haemoglobin.

(d) Yes. Carbonic anhydrase accelerates the reaction in both directions, so takes part in both uptake and release.

(e) No. Transfer is purely passive.

4.26

(a) Yes. Because ventilation is regulated in such a way as to maintain this balance.

(b)   No. Carbon dioxide output is the numerator, and oxygen uptake the denominator, of this ratio; CO_2 output is the smaller value at RQ 0.8.

(c)   Yes. Say, from 200 to 2000 ml per minute – or more in the physically fitter.

(d)   No. The partial pressure difference between mixed venous blood, at rest, and alveolar gas is only 5–10 mmHg – from 45–50 mmHg in blood to 37–42 mmHg in alveolar gas.

(e)   Yes. Mixed venous blood continues to deliver CO_2 during expiration while there is no dilution of alveolar gas with fresh air until the next inspiration. But the fluctuation in alveolar gas PCO_2 is only by a few mmHg.

4.27

(a)   Yes. This is because more carbamino-Hb is formed when Hb is not saturated with oxygen and because Hb becomes a progressively better buffer as more oxygen is removed from it, taking up H^+ and thus promoting bicarbonate formation.

(b)   Yes. In this context CO_2 content means the amount of CO_2 that can be chemically released from the blood. In normal blood, the CO_2 content is around 500 ml per litre of blood, of which around 90% is in the form of bicarbonate.

(c)   Yes. As for all cells.

(d)   No. Carbonic anhydrase is present in red blood cells but not in plasma, so the reaction (either uptake or release of CO_2) is faster in the cells.

(e)   No. Carbonic anhydrase accelerates the uptake of carbon dioxide, by conversion to bicarbonate in the red blood cells. Inhibition of this enzyme makes the process slower. The rate of uptake must still match the rate of production, so the result is a rise in tissue PCO_2 and acidity: the higher partial pressure maintains the rate of uptake in the face of a slower reaction.

4.28

(a)   No. The value of Y corresponds to an oxygen content of 200 ml oxygen per litre of blood.

(b)   No. The P_{50} is the partial pressure of oxygen at which the blood is 50% saturated with oxygen. The dashed line therefore has a lower P_{50} than the full line.

(c)   Yes. At a given PO_2 the blood giving the dashed curve holds more oxygen than that giving the full curve; this indicates a greater affinity.

(d)   No. In mixed venous blood, the PCO_2 is greater than in arterial blood and the dissociation curve is shifted to the right.

(e)   Yes. Fetal blood has a greater affinity for oxygen than adult blood and this enhances transfer of oxygen from maternal to fetal blood.

4.29

(a)   No. An increase in PCO_2 causes the curve to shift to the right, not to the left.

(b)   No. In anaemia, the haemoglobin concentration is reduced, but the haemoglobin that is present takes up oxygen normally. The dissociation curve with the y-axis representing percentage saturation, as here, is normal; it is the oxygen-carrying capacity of the blood that is reduced.

(c)   Yes. In stored blood, the concentration of 2,3-DPG falls and, as a consequence, the oxygen dissociation curve is shifted to the left.

(d)   No. With carbon monoxide poisoning, the affinity of haemoglobin for oxygen is reduced and the dissociation curve for haemoglobin still available for oxygen transport is changed; it is no longer sigmoid and it is shifted to the left.

(e)   Yes. As shown in the figure, myoglobin has a higher affinity for oxygen than does haemoglobin.

4.30

(a)   Yes. When the lungs inflate at the first breath, the pulmonary vascular bed is expanded and the negative pleural pressure and surface tension in air-filled alveoli tend to hold all intrapulmonary vessels open.

(b)   No. In the lungs, hypoxia has a vasoconstrictive action.

(c)   Yes. There is virtually no smooth muscle in the walls of the smallest arterioles.

(d)   Yes. Because the flow is the same (cardiac output) the resistances are in inverse proportion to the systemic and pulmonary driving pressures. (Say, 100 mmHg mean systemic, and 15 mmHg mean pulmonary artery pressure minus 5 mmHg left atrial pressure = 10 mmHg pressure difference. This gives a factor of 10.)

(e)   No. This would be so if there were no change in pulmonary vascular resistance. But in the lungs, as flow increases, resistance decreases, by both distension and recruitment of vessels. (Unlike the systemic circulation, any increase in intravascular pressure leads to distension, not to autoregulatory constriction.)

4.31

(a)   Yes. The vertical distance from heart to apices represents the height of a column of blood that can only just be supported by the mean pulmonary artery pressure: in other words, blood pressure fluctuates around zero in the branches of the pulmonary arteries at the apices.

(b)   Yes. Because the intravascular pressure is greater at the bases in the upright posture. The increase in diameter by distension diminishes the vascular resistance.

(c)   Yes. The increase in pressure is due to the weight of a column of blood of that height, in whatever type of vessel.

(d)   Yes. The blood flow is greater at the bases.

(e)   No. The intravascular pressure is greater at the bases than at the apices, so the force tending to move fluid out of capillaries is greater.

4.32

(a)   Yes. Surface tension forces tend to create a 'suction', drawing fluid out of capillaries. Surfactant counteracts this.

(b)   Yes. There is some net loss of fluid and a steady small lymph flow.

(c)   No. Fluid escapes into the interstitial corners between alveoli; it only bursts through into alveoli when the pressure has risen and increased lymph flow cannot keep up with it.

(d)   Yes. As in any vascular bed.

(e)   No. It is the intravascular pressure that is the driving force, not flow.

4.33

(a)   No. With a ventilation-perfusion ratio of 1, PO_2 is about 100 mmHg and the haemoglobin is saturated with oxygen; doubling the ventilation relative to blood flow would raise PO_2 to about 12 mmHg and the increase in oxygen content due to dissolved oxygen would be negligible (less than 1 ml per litre, or 0.5%).

(b)   Yes. The arterial PO_2, typically 100 mmHg with a ventilation-perfusion of 1, rises to about 125 mmHg with a ventilation-perfusion of 2.

(c)   Yes. Doubling the ventilation with no change in blood flow will approximately halve the alveolar, and hence the pulmonary vein, PCO_2.

(d)   No. Because of the shape of the CO_2 dissociation curve, halving of the CO_2 tension will result in a fall in CO_2 content of less than 50%, but much more than 10%.

(e)   Yes. The fall in PO_2 will be from 100 mmHg to about 80 mmHg, at which level saturation is still close to 95%. (Note that the asymmetry of the answers to (a) and (e) arises from the shape of the dissociation curve.)

4.34

(a)   No. Alveolar ventilation at the apices is less than at the bases.

(b)   Yes. The ratio of ventilation to blood flow is greater at the apices: both ventilation and blood flow are less than at the bases, but the difference from base to apex is greater for blood flow than for ventilation.

(c)   Yes. Because the differences in ratios up and down the lungs are due to gravity, blood flow is greatest, and ventilation-perfusion ratio lowest, in the most dependent parts of the lungs.

(d)   Yes. Blockage of capillaries, with zero blood flow, represents 'infinite' ventilation-perfusion; the affected alveoli are ventilated, but there is no gas exchange, which is by definition dead space.

(e)   Yes. When alveoli are not ventilated due to collapse or filling with fluid, the affected areas receive mixed venous blood but there is no gas exchange. The unchanged ('shunted') blood is added to the oxygenated blood from normal parts of the lung; this is venous admixture.

4.35

(a)   Yes. Alveolar dead space means that the alveoli in question receive tidal air, but no blood flow. A finite value for ventilation, divided by zero perfusion, gives an infinite ratio.

(b)   Yes. Venous admixture means that some venous blood (from the pulmonary artery) has passed alveoli that are not ventilated and so is mixing, unchanged, with blood leaving other normally function-ing regions of the lungs. Zero ventilation, divided by a finite value for blood flow, gives a ratio of zero.

(c)   Yes. The alveoli in the region concerned are relatively over-ventilated and therefore have higher than average oxygen, and lower than average carbon dioxide partial pressures; the blood leaving them reflects these values.

(d)   No. Unless there is also defective diffusion, blood leaving a region will have virtually the same partial pressures of oxygen and carbon dioxide as those in the alveoli of that region. The ventilation-perfusion ratios do not affect equilibration.

(e)   No. An excess of areas with low ventilation-perfusion ratios will necessarily cause arterial hypoxaemia, but not hypercapnia. This is because any tendency for PCO_2 to rise, together with a fall in PO_2, stimulates ventilation; all regions will thereby have their alveolar PCO_2 decreased and PO_2 increased; oxygen, however, will still be low in low-ratio regions, and where it is high in high-ratio regions this cannot force any more oxygen into the already saturated haemo-globin. For carbon dioxide, however, the situation is different: low alveolar concentration in high-ratio regions can compensate for high concentration in low-ratio regions. If the hypoxaemia is severe, venti-lation is further stimulated and may bring CO_2 below normal. So the arterial blood is likely to have a normal or low carbon dioxide tension.

4.36

(a) Yes. From the Fick principle, cardiac output = oxygen consumption divided by the arterio-venous difference for oxygen content.

(b) No. Arterio-venous difference is 50 ml per litre; arterial oxygen content is (1.34×135) ml per litre in Hb and 3 ml per litre in solution giving 184 ml per litre. So mixed venous is lower than 150 ml per litre (133.9 ml).

(c) Yes. This follows from the equation relating the three variables (see (a)).

(d) Yes. Oxygen in solution is simply proportional to the PO_2. So it has increased six-fold, from 3 ml to 18 ml per litre.

(e) Yes. In normal lungs, the blood virtually equilibrates with the alveolar gas, so arterial PO_2 will approach 600 mmHg.

4.37

(a) Yes. Ventilation   = 8 litres per min
tidal volume   = 0.8 litres
so frequency   = 10 per min
and dead space ventilation   = 10×150 ml per min
  = 1.5 litres per min.
Alveolar ventilation   = total minus dead space ventilation
  = 8 − 1.5
  = 6.5 litres per min.

(b) Yes. Alveolar CO_2 = 3%.
If barometric pressure = 706 mmHg, alveolar PCO_2 = 22.8 mmHg. This very low PCO_2 implies hyperventilation, by definition.

(c) No. Low PCO_2 causes cerebral vasoconstriction.

(d) Yes. The inspired PO_2 will be about 380 mmHg (50 kPa). Alveolar PO_2 is roughly this minus alveolar PCO_2, which has been calculated as less than 23 mmHg (3 kPa). So the range is right for alveolar PO_2, and if pulmonary gas exchange is normal, arterial PO_2 will be not more than 10 mmHg (1.5 kPa) lower.

(e) No. To answer this you need only know that RQ is expressed as CO_2 output ÷ O_2 uptake. 195/240 is clearly less than 1.

5 Breathing in abnormal environments and respiratory pathophysiology

Altitude	5.1–5.3
Diving	5.4–5.6
Respiratory pathophysiology	5.7–5.16

QUESTIONS

Altitude

5.1 Persistent, but tolerable, hypoxia at high altitude is likely to result in:

✓(a) increase in pulmonary ventilation.
✓(b) low arterial PCO_2.
✓(c) increase in cardiac output.
✗(d) increase in acidity of the urine.
✗(e) decreased blood viscosity.

5.2 Side-effects of tolerable acute altitude hypoxia (or of the compensatory changes it leads to) include:

✓(a) increased pulmonary vascular resistance.
✗(b) decrease in metabolic rate.
✓(c) increase in cerebrospinal fluid (CSF) pH.
✗(d) increased bicarbonate reabsorption in the kidneys.
✓(e) increased heart rate.

5.3 Compensations for the low partial pressure of oxygen in inspired air at high altitude include the changes listed on the left. Are the mechanisms on the right appropriate in each case?

✗(a) increased ventilation — carotid sinus receptor stimulation.
✓(b) increased cardiac output — increase in sympathetic activity.
✓(c) increased red blood cell count — increase in erythropoietin secretion.
✓(d) shift of oxyhaemoglobin dissociation curve to the right — increase in 2, 3-diphosphoglycerate (DPG) in erythrocytes.
✗(e) hypocapnia — decreased tissue metabolism.

Diving

5.4 **With reference to hyperbaric conditions:**
(a) during a breath-hold dive the volume of the lungs decreases.
(b) diving, breathing air from a cylinder, at a depth of about 30 ft, the inspired oxygen partial pressure is about 300 mmHg (40 kPa).
(c) oxygen can be safely breathed for several hours at a depth of 100 ft.
(d) there is a danger of CO_2 narcosis when breathing air at a pressure of 3 atmospheres.
(e) after exposure to high ambient pressure, fat people require more prolonged decompression than thin people.

5.5 **At 2 atmospheres ambient pressure (e.g. about 30 ft under water), in a healthy adult breathing air from a cylinder:**
(a) the arterial oxygen tension is over twice normal.
(b) the arterial PCO_2 is about twice the normal value.
(c) the alveolar $CO_2\%$ is about half normal.
(d) the arterial nitrogen tension is higher than normal.
(e) the volume of the lungs is about half normal.

5.6 **At 2 atmospheres ambient pressure (e.g. about 30 ft under water) a healthy adult breathing air from a cylinder:**
(a) given that he maintains a normal PCO_2, would have an arterial oxygen tension of about 260 mmHg (33.5 kPa).
(b) if he remained long enough for equilibration, would have twice as much nitrogen dissolved in the body fluids as he would normally have at sea level.
(c) has twice the amount of oxygen per unit volume of arterial blood than he would normally have at sea level.
(d) is at risk from oxygen poisoning.
(e) to maintain the same carbon dioxide output as at sea level, breathes at about half his normal tidal volume.

Respiratory pathophysiology

5.7 **An increase in pulmonary ventilation (minute volume) would be expected:**
(a) when a patient in respiratory failure (with hypoxia and hypercapnia) is given oxygen.
(b) when a normal subject breathes a mixture of 5% CO_2 and 95% oxygen.
(c) when multiple small pulmonary emboli occur (i.e. when pulmonary blood flow is obstructed in some areas).
(d) in diabetic ketosis (acidaemia).
(e) when there is persistent vomiting of gastric juice.

5.8 **Concerning inhalation of oxygen:**

✓ (a) when a healthy person breathes pure oxygen, the small amount normally dissolved in arterial blood increases by a factor of six to seven.

✗ (b) high concentrations of oxygen in inspired gas decrease any tendency to alveolar collapse.   Mercone

✗ (c) breathing 100% oxygen will bring the arterial PO_2 to normal in a patient who has a 50% right-to-left shunt.

(d) breathing 100% oxygen at 2 atmospheres pressure could provide a normal arterial oxygen content in a patient with life-threatening anaemia, with a haemoglobin concentration of 40 g per litre.

✓ (e) the best concentration of oxygen to give a hypoxic patient in ventilatory failure is less than 30%.

5.9 **If a person on artificial ventilation is over-ventilated:**

✓ (a) the arterial PO_2 will rise.

✓ (b) the arterial PCO_2 will fall.

✓ (c) the urine will become alkaline.

✗ (d) the cerebral arterioles will dilate.

✗ (e) the pulmonary arterioles will constrict.

5.10 **The arterial oxygen tension is low in:**

✗ (a) poisoning with a sublethal dose of cyanide.

(b) pulmonary fibrosis.

(c) bronchial obstruction.

(d) anaemia.

(e) hyperventilation in panic attacks.

5.11 **The arterial PO_2 is decreased:**

✗ (a) by inhalation of a sublethal dose of carbon monoxide.

✓ (b) by shunting of blood from the right to the left side of the heart.

(c) by shunting of blood from the aorta to the pulmonary artery (patent ductus).

(d) an hour after a loss of 20% of the blood volume.

(e) in an average healthy subject exercising vigorously.

5.12 **A subject has a low arterial PO_2 (60 mmHg) with a normal or low arterial PCO_2. Could the following account for this condition?**

✓ (a) breathing air at a low barometric pressure, e.g. at altitude.

✗ (b) asphyxia, e.g. due to a plastic bag over the head.

✗ (c) partial obstruction of the trachea.

(d) partial obstruction of the bronchi supplying one lobe of a lung.

(e) right to left shunt of blood in the heart or lungs.

5.13   The data refer to two subjects of the same sex and with similar body build. One subject is healthy; the other is not.

	Normal	Patient
Total lung capacity	6 litres	4 litres
Functional residual capacity (FRC)	2.4 litres	1.9 litres
FEV1/forced vital capacity (FVC)	80%	90%
Residual volume (RV)	1.5 litres	1.1 litres

Are the values for the patient compatible with the following?
(a)   an attack of asthma.
(b)   partial paralysis of the respiratory muscles.
(c)   pulmonary fibrosis.
(d)   thickening of the pleura.
(e)   emphysema.

5.14   Consider the following abnormality of gas exchange in the lungs. One lung is abnormal: 2 litres of blood per minute leave it, with an abnormally low PO_2 of 46 mmHg. The other lung is normal: 2 litres of blood per minute leave it, at a PO_2 of 100 mmHg (13 kPa). The standard 'physiological' oxygen dissociation curve for whole blood is shown in Figure 5.14 to assist you. Are the following statements true?

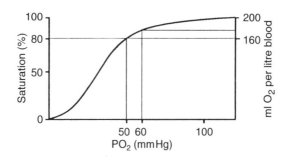

(a)   the mixture of blood from both lungs (4 litres per min) will have a PO_2 of approximately 60 mmHg.
(b)   if the concentration of haemoglobin is normal, the amount of oxygen in the arterial blood will be approximately 180 ml per litre.
(c)   the abnormality could be a high ventilation-perfusion ratio in the whole of the abnormal lung.
(d)   the abnormality could be some barrier to diffusion in the abnormal lung.
(e)   The concentration of dissolved oxygen in blood leaving the abnormal lung would be a little less than 1.5 ml per litre.

5.15 **The values below represent measurements made on an abnormal subject, at rest, breathing air.**

Blood volume	5.5 litres
Right atrial pressure	20 mmHg
Arterial blood pressure	100/60 mmHg
Arterial PCO_2	60 mmHg (8 kPa)
Arterial blood pH	7.34
Weight	70 kg

Are the following statements correct?
(a) he is suffering from hypovolaemic shock.
(b) there is a respiratory acidosis.
(c) there is some degree of failure of the heart as a pump.
(d) the arterial PO_2 must be lower than normal.
(e) bicarbonate reabsorption in the kidneys is likely to be proceeding at a lower rate than normal.

5.16 **Consider the following values, obtained from an average-sized patient at rest.**

Systolic pressure
  in the pulmonary artery: 40 mmHg
  in the aorta: 140 mmHg.
Oxygen content in blood
  from the pulmonary artery: 140 ml per litre
  from the aorta: 200 ml per litre.
Arterial PO_2:   60 mmHg.
Whole body oxygen consumption: 0.30 litre per min.

These values indicate:
(a) the aortic systolic blood pressure is normal.
(b) the pulmonary artery systolic pressure is normal.
(c) there must be a higher than normal haemoglobin concentration.
(d) the cardiac output is 6 litres per min.
(e) the oxygen consumption is low.

ANSWERS

5.1
(a) Yes. This results from stimulation of the peripheral (arterial) chemo-receptors.
(b) Yes. The hyperventilation reduces PCO_2 and increases PO_2. For a given, low, inspired PO_2, the ventilatory response thus allows a

higher alveolar and arterial PO_2 and improves the oxygen content of the blood.

(c)   Yes. An increase in blood flow to all body tissues helps to compensate for the decreased oxygen content of the blood.

(d)   No. The hyperventilation and resulting low PCO_2 causes a respiratory alkalosis. The renal compensation for this is a decrease in acidity of the urine.

(e)   No. Increase in erythropoiesis in the bone marrow, stimulated by erythropoietin from the kidneys, raises the haemoglobin concentration of the blood, allowing greater oxygen content at the low PO_2. The down-side is an increase in viscosity, raising resistance to blood flow.

5.2

(a)   Yes. Hypoxia causes pulmonary vasoconstriction.

(b)   No. Reduced resting metabolic rate (and therefore oxygen consumption) occurs only if hypoxia is lethally severe.

(c)   Yes. Hypocapnia follows from the stimulation of ventilation by hypoxia; since CO_2 is readily diffusible, there is an increase in pH of all body fluids, including CSF. This shift tends to damp the ventilatory stimulus.

(d)   No. Hypocapnia causes alkalaemia: a decreased rate of bicarbonate reabsorption is the compensatory response.

(e)   Yes.

5.3

(a)   No. Carotid body, not sinus.

(b)   Yes.

(c)   Yes.

(d)   Yes. A shift to the right due to an increase in 2,3-DPG allows more ready off-loading of oxygen in the tissues and enables maintenance of a higher tissue PO_2. A shift to the left due to hypocapnia competes with this, however.

(e)   No. There is hypocapnia because ventilation is stimulated. Only in hypoxia so severe as to be fatal is the tissue oxygen consumption diminished.

5.4

(a)   Yes.

(b)   Yes. Inspired oxygen has the same percentage value, but is at about 2 atmospheres pressure, so the partial pressure is about twice that at sea level.

(c)   No. This is an ambient pressure of about 4 atmospheres. Oxygen toxicity would occur.

(d)   No. PCO_2 is regulated by the usual mechanisms for the control of ventilation, but there is a danger of nitrogen narcosis.

(e)   Yes. If exposure lasts long enough for equilibration of tissues with the raised nitrogen partial pressure, there will be a greater amount dissolved when there is a greater amount of fat. Therefore it takes longer to wash out the nitrogen and decompression must be prolonged if bubble formation is to be avoided.

5.5

(a)   Yes. Inspired oxygen is twice normal; because alveolar PCO_2 does not change, and its percentage therefore halves, the alveolar oxygen percentage is higher than at 1 atmosphere. So the alveolar and arterial partial pressures are more than twice normal.

(b)   No. Arterial PCO_2 is kept constant by the physiological control of ventilation, which maintains a normal alveolar partial pressure of CO_2.

(c)   Yes. See (b). The percentage CO_2 will be halved because the total pressure is doubled while the CO_2 partial pressure is unchanged.

(d)   Yes. The arterial PN_2 results from equilibration of blood with alveolar PN_2 and so will be more than twice normal.

(e)   No. Both the water outside the chest and the gas in the lungs inside are at 2 atmospheres pressure as long as breathing continues. Deflation occurs only during a breath-hold dive. It is important for divers to breathe out as they come up towards the surface to counter the expansion of the lungs during decompression.

5.6

(a)   Yes. Alveolar and hence arterial PO_2 is calculated approximately by subtracting arterial PCO_2 from the PO_2 in the humidified inspired gas: $300 - 40 = 260 \, \text{mmHg}$.

(b)   Yes. There is a PN_2 in the blood and in all body fluids in normal circumstances because of equilibration between blood in the lungs with alveolar PN_2. Because nitrogen is so insoluble, this represents a minute amount of dissolved nitrogen. When the amount is increased at higher than normal pressures, it becomes important because firstly, high PN_2 in the central nervous system can cause nitrogen narcosis and, secondly, if pressure is subsequently reduced too rapidly, nitrogen comes out of solution in the tissues before it has had time to be washed out in the lungs, causing the 'bends'.

(c)   No. Because haemoglobin is virtually fully saturated at the normal oxygen partial pressure at sea level, a rise in PO_2 above normal can only increase the dissolved oxygen; this will double; but it is still a small proportion of the total oxygen content.

(d)   No. The increase in alveolar and arterial oxygen partial pressure to about 250 mmHg, breathing air, is not a threat. (However, if they were to breathe 100% oxygen at 2 atmospheres some individuals would develop oxygen toxicity.)

(e)   No. To breathe out the same amount of CO_2, he must exhale the same volume of alveolar gas as at sea level: the percentage CO_2 is halved, but 2.5% of a volume of alveolar gas now contains the same molecular amount as 5% at sea level.

5.7

(a)   No. Ventilation may be further depressed by removal of the hypoxic drive.

(b)   Yes. Increase in PCO_2, in high oxygen, stimulates the central (medullary) chemoreceptors (although the high oxygen suppresses peripheral chemoreceptor sensitivity).

(c)   Yes. There is stimulation of receptors in the lungs, which leads to an increase in ventilation via afferent fibres in the vagus nerves.

(d)   Yes. Acidaemia stimulates ventilation via the peripheral (arterial) chemoreceptors. The consequent reduction in carbon dioxide tension tends to correct the acidaemia.

(e)   No. Vomiting loses acid and results in alkalaemia; if anything, ventilation will be depressed.

5.8

(a)   Yes. The amount dissolved is directly proportional to the PO_2, and this is increased by a factor of at least six in alveolar gas and therefore in arterial blood. (When all nitrogen has been washed out, alveolar gas, at barometric pressure $= 760$ mmHg, contains only CO_2 (40 mmHg), water vapour (47 mmHg) and oxygen (693 mmHg).)

(b)   No. Oxygen increases the likelihood of alveolar collapse, especially in conditions of limited chest movement, e.g. post-operatively. This is because, unlike nitrogen, it can all be absorbed into the blood.

(c)   No. 50% of the blood going through the lungs would have its PO_2 increased to 600 mmHg or more, and content raised by about 15 ml per litre. The 50% shunted would not be exposed to the oxygen, and would be mixed venous blood, say at most 75% saturated. Assuming normal haemoglobin concentration, mixing these two gives an average oxygen content of $(150 + 215) \div 2 = 365/2 = 182.5$ ml per litre. The mixture would therefore have a saturation of 90% and PO_2 60–70 mmHg.

(d)   No. The oxygen content would be usefully increased – but neither this nor PO_2 would be as high as normal. At a PO_2 of 1400 mmHg at most, the dissolved oxygen would be $14 \times 3 = 42$ ml per litre of blood; the 40 g of haemoglobin would carry 50 ml of oxygen per litre, so the total content would be around 90 ml per litre – less than half the normal 200 ml per litre.

(e) Yes. The inspired oxygen fraction must be increased cautiously in such patients because full correction of arterial PO_2 may further depress ventilation by cancelling their hypoxic drive. The PCO_2 is already above normal, these patients have become insensitive to it as a stimulus to breathing, and a further rise depresses cerebral function.

5.9

(a) Yes. See (b).

(b) Yes. These are the changes that characterize over-ventilation of the lungs.

(c) Yes. The hyperventilation leads to respiratory alkalosis; the renal compensation for this is a decrease in bicarbonate reabsorption and hence excretion of alkaline urine.

(d) No. A low PCO_2 causes cerebral arterioles to constrict.

(e) No. In the pulmonary vascular bed it is low PO_2 and high PCO_2 that cause constriction.

5.10

(a) No. Cyanide poisons cellular enzymes that are necessary for the utilization of oxygen. The arterial oxygen tension is not depressed.

(b) Yes. As pulmonary fibrosis develops, there is progressive limitation of diffusion of oxygen, though not of carbon dioxide (which diffuses more readily because of its greater solubility). The arterial hypoxaemia stimulates ventilation, so that PCO_2 may be low until or unless the lungs fail as a pump and hypoventilation ensues.

(c) Yes. In bronchial obstruction, aeration of the lobe(s) supplied by the obstructed bronchi ceases leading to a low oxygen content and hence a low arterial PO_2.

(d) No. In anaemia, the oxygen carrying capacity of the blood is depressed but the arterial PO_2 is normal or may even be raised.

(e) No. Hyperventilation results in an elevation of the arterial PO_2.

5.11

(a) No. The arterial oxygen tension is not reduced by inhalation of a sublethal dose of carbon monoxide; the oxygen content of the blood is reduced because of the high affinity of carbon monoxide for haemoglobin.

(b) Yes. Since the right side of the heart contains deoxygenated blood, shunting of blood from the right to the left side results in venous admixture and hence a decrease in arterial PO_2. This occurs in some congenital abnormalities.

(c)   No. Since the aorta contains oxygenated blood, addition of this to pulmonary artery blood sends it for a second time through the lungs. The cardiac output is higher than normally required, but the arterial PO_2 is normal.

(d)   No. An hour after a loss of 20% of the blood volume there will be some haemodilution but the arterial PO_2 will not be reduced; it may be increased due to stimulation of ventilation.

(e)   No. In an average subject exercising vigorously, ventilation and diffusion are adequate to maintain full oxygenation of the blood despite increased deoxygenation of venous blood and increased pulmonary blood flow. In some highly trained athletes, who attain very high cardiac output, there may be a fall in arterial PO_2 at peak exercise.

5.12

(a)   Yes. When breathing air at a low barometric pressure, breathing is stimulated by the hypoxia. The low inspired PO_2 causes a low arterial PO_2 and the hyperventilation causes the low arterial PCO_2.

(b)   No. Asphyxia leads to a fall in arterial PO_2 with a rise in arterial PCO_2.

(c)   No. Partial obstruction of the trachea, if severe enough to decrease ventilation despite greater effort, could cause hypoventilation with both a fall in arterial PO_2 and a rise in arterial PCO_2.

(d)   Yes. Partial obstruction of the bronchi supplying one lobe of a lung results in under-ventilation of that lobe, and hence a fall in oxygen content and a rise in CO_2 content of blood leaving that lobe. This blood mixes with blood from the unobstructed lobes of the lung, so that the PO_2 of the mixed pulmonary vein blood falls below normal. Reaching the systemic arterial chemoreceptors, this stimulates ventilation; as a result, the alveolar PCO_2 is lowered in the unobstructed lobes, the blood leaving them has a CO_2 content reduced below normal, and this compensates for the extra CO_2 in blood from the obstructed lobe. The over-ventilation of the healthy lobes cannot, however, correct the lowered arterial PO_2, because of the nature of the oxyhaemoglobin dissociation curve (see questions on ventilation–perfusion ratios).

(e)   Yes. With a modest right to left shunt of blood, the increase in ventilation can maintain a normal CO_2 content of blood but cannot do the same for oxygen – as for (d).

5.13

(a)   No. With asthma, the FEV_1/forced vital capacity would be reduced.

(b)   No. Partial paralysis of the respiratory muscles would result in reduced force of expiration, and the FEV1/forced vital capacity would be reduced.

(c)   Yes. See (d).

(d)   Yes. With pulmonary fibrosis or thickening of the pleura, the total lung capacity is reduced, but movements within the range allowed by the pleural thickening are normal. This is a 'restrictive' abnormality.

(e)   No. With emphysema, the FEV_1/FVC is low while the FRC and RV are high (an 'obstructive' abnormality).

5.14

(a)   Yes. Half is 80%, and half 100%, saturated so the mixture is 90% saturated, which is equivalent to an oxygen tension of 60 mmHg.

(b)   Yes. 90% of 200 ml per litre.

(c)   No. Low ventilation–perfusion ratio in the abnormal lung could account for this venous admixture.

(d)   Yes. Diffusion limitation could account for this venous admixture.

(e)   Yes. At an oxygen tension of 50 mmHg, the dissolved oxygen will be half that at 100 mmHg:
$0.03 \times 50 = 1.5$ ml per litre.

5.15

(a)   No. The blood volume is normal for a 70 kg subject.

(b)   Yes. The arterial PCO_2 is raised, which is, by definition, a respiratory acidosis.

(c)   Yes. The right atrial pressure is raised.

(d)   Yes. If the PCO_2 is higher than normal, the arterial PO_2 is inevitably lower than normal, when the inspired gas is air.

(e)   No. In respiratory acidosis, due to CO_2 retention, the plasma bicarbonate is raised, and there is increased reabsorption of bicarbonate in the kidneys.

5.16

(a)   Yes. 140 mmHg is at the high end of the normal range.

(b)   No. Pulmonary artery pressure is normally about 25 mmHg systolic.

(c)   Yes. If there are 200 ml of oxygen per litre of blood this would imply a Hb concentration of 150 g per litre if it were fully saturated, and more than 150 g per litre in this instance as it is not fully saturated at a PO_2 of 60 mmHg. (This could be a chronically hypoxic patient, in whom there is a high haematocrit, and high Hb concentration; the high pulmonary artery pressure is consistent with this.)

(d) No. From the Fick equation, cardiac output

= O_2 consumption/arterio-venous O_2 difference
= (0.30)/(200 − 140) litre per min, per ml per litre
= 5 litres per min.

(e) No. This is higher than the average resting oxygen consumption of 250 ml per min.

6 Blood

QUESTIONS

Normal blood

6.1 In a human adult, red blood cells:
(a) arc formcd continuously in the bonc marrow.
(b) at the end of their life-span, disintegrate, mainly in the spleen.
(c) are produced at a slower rate under the influence of hypoxia.
(d) are discharged from the marrow into the bloodstream as reticulocytes, retaining fragments of the stem cell nucleus for a day or two.
(e) by their breakdown, lead to the formation of bile pigments.

6.2 In a human adult, the neutrophils (polymorphonuclear neutrophil leucocytes)
(a) are actively phagocytic in the bloodstream.
(b) migrate in and out of the bloodstream.
(c) are in the blood in a concentration of 3 to 6 $\times$ 10^9 per litre.
(d) are formed mainly in the spleen and lymph nodes.
(e) decrease in number during many common infective illnesses.

6.3 The haemoglobin in blood:
(a) is completely deoxygenated in the blood drawn from an arm vein.
(b) is the major source of bile pigments.
(c) is responsible for the colour of the blood.
(d) can be estimated by adding dilute hydrochloric acid and comparing the solution with a standard.
(e) contains iron in the ferrous state.

6.4 In the circulating blood of a healthy human adult:
(a) some of the red cells are nucleated.
(b) more than half of the white cells are neutrophil granulocytes.
(c) the red cells utilize glucose as their only metabolic fuel.
(d) the volume of a red cell can increase by 50% without a significant increase in surface area.
(e) the life-span of the red cells is typically 10 days.

6.5 **On a smear of blood taken from a healthy person:**
(a) the ratio of erythrocytes to leucocytes is about 10 000:1.
(b) every leucocyte has a nucleus.
(c) the largest cells seen are megakaryocytes.
(d) the erythrocytes look larger than the leucocytes.
(e) there are more platelets than erythrocytes.

6.6 **Concerning the composition of normal human blood:**
(a) more than 90% of the weight of the erythrocyte is water.
(b) more than 90% of the dry weight of the erythrocyte is haemoglobin.
(c) more than 90% of the weight of plasma is water.
(d) stored red cells need to be provided with an energy source such as glucose.
(e) stored red cells without an energy source tend to shrink.

6.7 **In a fresh sample of human blood, do the following values fall within the normal range?**
(a) plasma sodium: 140 mmol.
(b) plasma potassium: 8 mmol.
(c) haemoglobin concentration: 50 g per litre.
(d) erythrocyte count: 5×10^{12} per litre.
(e) leucocyte count: 6×10^9 per litre.

6.8 **Concerning the blood:**
(a) the number of erythrocytes per litre of blood is greater in the neonate than in the adult.
(b) circulating erythrocytes divide to produce daughter erythrocytes.
(c) 1 g of haemoglobin combines with 20 ml O_2.
(d) in normal arterial blood, one molecule of haemoglobin carries one molecule of oxygen.
(e) as erythrocytes become old, their resistance to haemolysis increases.

6.9 **Concerning iron:**
(a) most of the iron that is ingested is absorbed.
(b) it is more readily absorbed in the gastrointestinal tract in the Fe^{3+} than in the Fe^{2+} state.
(c) the major fraction of the iron in the body is in haemoglobin.
(d) the incorporation of iron into the haemoglobin molecule occurs principally in the peripheral circulation.
(e) iron is a constituent of myoglobin.

6.10 **Concerning iron metabolism in a normal adult human:**
(a) intestinal absorption of iron occurs largely in about the first 40 cm of the small intestine.
(b) the iron content of the body is controlled by renal excretory mechanisms.
(c) iron is present in the plasma bound to transferrin.
(d) iron deficiency anaemia is commonly associated with deficient secretion of gastric acid.
(e) iron released from the breakdown of haemoglobin is largely excreted in the bile.

6.11 **Bilirubin released into the circulation from the mononuclear phagocytic system (the reticulo-endothelial):**
(a) is bound by plasma proteins.
(b) is conjugated with glucuronic acid in plasma.
(c) contains ferric ions.
(d) is readily filtered in the renal glomeruli.
(e) can be reincorporated into haemoglobin.

6.12 **In a resting person, as blood passes through the systemic capillaries:**
(a) the reduction in oxygen content of the blood is on average around 25%.
(b) the increase in carbon dioxide content of the blood is on average around 25%.
(c) the net transfer of fluid from plasma to interstitial fluid is about 25% of the plasma volume.
(d) the blood becomes more alkaline.
(e) the concentration of chloride in the plasma increases.

6.13 **In a resting person, as blood passes through the systemic capillaries, there is:**
(a) an increase in the red cell count.
(b) an increase in plasma protein concentration.
(c) an increase in the mean corpuscular volume (MCV) of the erythrocytes.
(d) an increase in the mean corpuscular haemoglobin of the erythrocytes.
(e) an increase in the mean corpuscular haemoglobin concentration of the erythrocytes.

6.14 **As blood passes through systemic capillaries:**
(a) its pH rises.
(b) bicarbonate ions pass from the red cells to the plasma.
(c) the concentration of chloride ions in the red cells falls.
(d) its oxygen dissociation curve shifts to the right.
(e) the velocity of blood flow is less than in the aorta.

6.15   **With reference to the blood:**

(a)   a blood film stained with Leishman's stain may be used to count the number of white cells per litre of blood.

(b)   in a normal blood film, the number of platelets seen, relative to numbers of other cells, is the same as the number in the original sample of blood.

(c)   reticulocytes are old red blood corpuscles ready for destruction.

(d)   the production of erythropoietin is stimulated by low oxygen tension.

(e)   platelets are the cell membranes of disintegrated erythrocytes.

6.16   **Blood from a healthy subject yielded the following values:**
  Red blood corpuscles (RBC)   5.5 × 10¹² per litre
  Haemoglobin concentration   16 g per decilitre
  Are the following statements true?

(a)   the values are typical of a man rather than a woman.

(b)   from these values, the mean cell volume (MCV) can be calculated.

(c)   from these values, the mean cell haemoglobin (MCH) can be calculated.

(d)   from these values, the mean cell haemoglobin concentration (MCHC) can be calculated.

(e)   if the same investigations were carried out in a patient's blood, it would be possible to discover whether the patient has a microcytosis.

6.17   **A blood sample taken from a young man showed the following values:**
  Packed cell volume (PCV)   0.45 litres per litre
  Haemoglobin concentration   152 g per litre
  Erythrocyte count   5.0 × 10¹² per litre
  Are the following statements true for this subject?

(a)   the red cell count is within normal limits.

(b)   the mean volume of this subject's erythrocytes is 90 femtolitres (1 litre $= 10^{-15}$ femtolitres).

(c)   this blood contains about 55% plasma.

(d)   the concentration of haemoglobin within the red blood corpuscles is more than twice the concentration in whole blood.

(e)   if the same investigations were carried out on a patient's blood it would be possible to determine whether the patient has a microcytic anaemia.

6.18 **Concerning haemoglobin in the blood:**
(a) poisoning with carbon monoxide results in a reduction in the concentration of haemoglobin in the blood.
(b) haemoglobin is an important blood buffer.
(c) haemoglobin catalyses the hydration of carbon dioxide.
(d) when haemoglobin is saturated with oxygen, each molecule of haemoglobin carries one molecule of oxygen.
(e) haemoglobin is attached to AB blood group antigens.

Abnormalities

6.19 **Concerning the blood:**
(a) anaemia is defined as an abnormally low haemoglobin concentration.
(b) an anaemic person looks pink.
(c) cyanosis is a blueness of the skin, conjunctiva and mucosal surfaces.
(d) cyanosis is caused by partial deoxygenation of the haemoglobin in the blood.
(e) cyanosis indicates deoxygenation equivalent to a concentration of 50 g or more of deoxygenated haemoglobin per litre of blood.

6.20 **In an anaemic patient, are the following changes in the blood always present?**
(a) low haemoglobin concentration.
(b) low mean corpuscular volume.
(c) low mean corpuscular haemoglobin concentration (MCHC).
(d) low oxygen-carrying capacity.
(e) low arterial PO_2.

6.21 **The following measurements were made on a resting man:**
Haemoglobin concentration **150 g per litre of blood**
Oxygen content of arterial blood **150 ml per litre of blood**
Are the following statements true?
(a) he is anaemic.
(b) his arterial blood is about 75% saturated with oxygen.
(c) his skin may appear blue.
(d) his mixed venous blood is likely to contain about 130 ml O_2 per litre blood.
(e) his arterial oxygen tension is likely to be 40–50 mmHg.

6.22   **Blood from a patient yielded the following data:**
Red blood corpuscles (RBC) 10×10^{12} per litre
Haemoglobin concentration   220 g per litre
Haematocrit (packed cell volume)   0.6 litre per litre
Are the following statements true for this patient?
(a)   the red blood cell count is within the normal range.
(b)   the haemoglobin concentration is within the normal range.
(c)   the viscosity of the blood is higher than normal.
(d)   the mean corpuscular volume (MCV) is 80 femtolitres
         (fl = 10^{-15} litres).
(e)   The mean corpuscular haemoglobin (MCH) is 22 picograms
         (pg = 10^{-12}g).

6.23   **Can the abnormality on the left be diagnosed from ONLY the**
         investigation on the right?
(a)   microcytosis   red cell count.
(b)   anaemia   mean corpuscular volume (MCV).
(c)   hypochromia   mean corpuscular haemoglobin.
                                 concentration (MCHC).
(d)   leucocytosis   white cell count.
(e)   erythrocytes abnormally   packed cell volume (haematocrit).
         fragile

Haemostasis

6.24   **Platelets:**
(a)   are produced in the bone marrow.
(b)   are destroyed in the spleen.
(c)   are important in plugging deficiencies in the walls of damaged blood
         vessels.
(d)   rupture when the blood makes contact with rough surfaces.
(e)   release prothrombin.

6.25   **Concerning blood clotting:**
(a)   heparin prevents clotting because of the negative charge carried by
         the heparin molecules.
(b)   the reversal of the effect of heparin by protamine is because protamine
         is positively charged.
(c)   platelets are essential for blood clotting.
(d)   addition of vitamin K to blood in a tube causes the blood to clot.
(e)   administration of a calcium binding agent intravenously is a clinical
         method used to prevent the clotting of blood.

6.26 **Concerning coagulation of blood:**
(a) cooling of freshly taken blood to 0°C slows coagulation.
(b) whipping freshly taken blood prevents it from coagulating.
(c) freshly taken blood will coagulate more quickly if kept in a clean glass vessel than in a vaseline-coated vessel.
(d) adding citrate to freshly taken blood prevents coagulation.
(e) adding dicoumarol to freshly taken blood prevents coagulation.

Blood groups

6.27 **Concerning the ABO blood groups:**
(a) a person of group O is a universal recipient.
(b) a person of group B usually has anti-A agglutinins in his plasma.
(c) in an incompatible blood transfusion reaction, donor cells are lysed by recipient antibodies.
(d) a severe transfusion reaction is likely to be followed by jaundice.
(e) antibodies to the A and B agglutinogens are complete cold antibodies.

6.28 **Concerning the rhesus (Rh) blood grouping:**
(a) every baby of a Rh positive father and Rh negative mother is at risk.
(b) the second Rh positive child of a Rh-negative mother is at greater risk than the first.
(c) transfusion of group A Rh positive blood for the first time to a nulliparous young woman whose blood group is A Rh negative, is likely to cause a severe reaction.
(d) the antibodies that cross the placenta from maternal to fetal circulation are incomplete antibodies.
(e) an appropriate treatment for a newborn infant suffering from erythroblastosis neonatorum is transfusion with maternal blood.

ANSWERS

6.1
(a) Yes.
(b) Yes.
(c) No. Hypoxia stimulates release of erythropoetin from the kidneys, which in turn stimulates red cell production.
(d) Yes.
(e) Yes.

6.2
(a) No. They are phagocytic when they migrate outside the bloodstream.
(b) Yes.

(c)   Yes.
(d)   No. They arise from stem cells in the bone marrow.
(e)   No. The polymorphonuclear leucocyte count increases in many types of infection.

6.3
(a)   No. There can never be complete removal of oxygen by the tissues in life, even very active tissues; arm vein blood is a mixture from skin and muscle, and its desaturation will depend on muscular activity, skin temperature and vasodilatation or otherwise.
(b)   Yes. Bilirubin is formed from haem in the reticulo-endothelial system; it is then secreted in the bile; the iron removed from haem is retained for red blood corpuscle formation.
(c)   Yes.
(d)   Yes. This is the essence of the Sahli method.
(e)   Yes. If the Fe is oxidized to the ferric form, methaemoglobin is formed.

6.4
(a)   No.
(b)   Yes.
(c)   Yes. Red blood cells have no mitochondria, cannot use oxygen, and use glucose for anaerobic glycolysis.
(d)   Yes, by changing from a flattened towards a spherical shape.
(e)   No. Red cells live about 10 times as long as this.

6.5
(a)   No. 1000:1.
(b)   Yes.
(c)   Yes.
(d)   No. Leucocytes look larger than erythrocytes.
(e)   No.

6.6
(a)   No. Mean cell haemoglobin concentration is around 320 g per litre; assuming that there is a negligible increase in volume when haemoglobin is dissolved in an aqueous solution, the litre of solution contains at most 1000 g water and 320 g of haemoglobin, so water is not more than $1000/1320 = 76\%$ of the weight.
(b)   Yes.
(c)   Yes. Protein accounts for about 6% and electrolytes for about 0.9%, so the water content is around 93%.
(d)   Yes. Glucose is necessary for the anaerobic erythrocyte metabolism to continue.

(e)   No. Stored red cells tend to swell due to the loss of function of the sodium pump which requires metabolic energy.

6.7

(a)   Yes.
(b)   No. This is a dangerously high concentration.
(c)   No. The normal range is 140–150 g per litre.
(d)   Yes.
(e)   Yes.

6.8

(a)   Yes. The neonate has an erythrocyte count which is about 20% higher than the adult.
(b)   No. Circulating erythrocytes have no nuclei and cannot divide to produce daughter erythrocytes.
(c)   No. 1 g of haemoglobin combines with 1.33 ml O_2.
(d)   No. One molecule of haemoglobin has 4 haem groups and can carry 4 molecules of oxygen.
(e)   No. As erythrocytes become old, their resistance to haemolysis decreases.

6.9

(a)   No. Only a small proportion of the iron that is ingested is absorbed. That which is absorbed into mucosal cells is partly passed into the blood, but partly remains in the cells and is shed into the gut with them as they die off.
(b)   No. Iron is more readily absorbed in the Fe^{2+} than in the Fe^{3+} state.
(c)   Yes. About 2.5 g (nearly 70%) is in haemoglobin.
(d)   No. The incorporation of iron into the haemoglobin molecule occurs in the bone marrow as a component of haemopoiesis.
(e)   Yes. About 5% of total body iron.

6.10

(a)   Yes.
(b)   No. Excretion of iron is not regulated. Absorption intake is regulated according to requirement (by the mechanism of 'mucosal block').
(c)   Yes. Only a very small amount is normally present in plasma; as well as that bound to transferrin, there are traces of ferritin.
(d)   Yes. Inorganic iron is more readily absorbed in the ferrous than in the ferric form, and hydrochloric acid in the stomach favours the conversion of the ferric to the ferrous state.
(e)   No. This would be true of the porphyrin moiety of the haemoglobin molecule. The iron is retained in the body. It is stored as ferritin and haemosiderin in hepatocytes and mononuclear phagocytes, which transport it to the bone marrow.

6.11
(a)   Yes.
(b)   No. This occurs in the liver.
(c)   No. It contains no iron.
(d)   No. Because it is bound to plasma protein.
(e)   No. This product of haemoglobin breakdown cannot be recycled by the body.

6.12
(a)   Yes. The oxygen content falls from around 200 ml to 150 ml per litre of blood.
(b)   No. The carbon dioxide content rises from about 500 ml to 550 ml of carbon dioxide per litre of blood, a change of around 10%. (Note that the change in the amount per litre is similar to the change in oxygen, although only the same when whole body respiratory quotient = 1.)
(c)   No. The net transfer of fluid from plasma to interstitial fluid is about 1% of the plasma volume.
(d)   No. The blood becomes more acid because of uptake of CO_2 and its hydration.
(e)   Yes. As a result of the chloride shift (Cl^- leaving red cells as HCO_3^- is formed within them) the concentration of chloride in the plasma increases.

6.13
(a)   Yes. The net movement of fluid from plasma to interstitial fluid across the capillary wall results in an increase in the red cell count.
(b)   Yes. The net movement of virtually protein-free fluid from plasma to interstitial fluid across the capillary wall results in an increase in plasma protein concentration.
(c)   Yes. As carbon dioxide is hydrated, bicarbonate ions are released in the erythrocytes and so the number of osmotically-active particles in the erythrocytes rises; this sucks in water and increases the mean corpuscular volume. (Outward movement of bicarbonate ions occurs, but is matched by an equal inward movement of chloride ions, so this does not affect the change in MCV.)
(d)   No. The amount of haemoglobin in each erythrocyte is unaltered.
(e)   No. By the mechanism described in (c), there is a reduction in the mean corpuscular haemoglobin concentration.

6.14
(a)   No. pH falls as CO_2 is added.
(b)   Yes. CO_2 diffuses into plasma and red blood cells (RBC): bicarbonate is formed faster in RBC because of carbonic anhydrase; bicarbonate moves out of RBC.

(c)   No. Chloride ions pass into cells, electrically balancing the outward movement of bicarbonate.

(d)   Yes. The rise in CO_2 concentration shifts the curve to the right (Bohr effect).

(e)   Yes. Although the volume of blood per minute flowing through the whole systemic capillary bed must be the same as that in the aorta, flow is slower in capillaries, because the total cross-section is greater.

6.15

(a)   No. This allows only the relative number of different cell types to be counted.

(b)   No. Some platelets are lost or destroyed in the preparation of the film.

(c)   No. Reticulocytes are precursors of mature red cells.

(d)   Yes. This provides a compensatory mechanism for the production of more cells to carry more O_2.

(e)   No. Platelets are formed from megakaryocytes in the bone marrow.

6.16

(a)   Yes. This is at the upper end of the range for healthy men. The average for healthy women is about 10 g per litre (1 g per decilitre) lower than for men.

(b)   No. The packed cell volume (PCV) would also be required. MCV is calculated from the total volume of cells in a litre of blood, divided by the number of cells per litre of blood.

(c)   Yes. The average amount of haemoglobin per cell (MCH) is the amount per litre of blood, divided by the number of cells per litre of blood.

(d)   No. The MCHC is the MCH divided by the mean cell volume, which is PCV/number of cells.

(e)   No. To know whether or not the cells are of normal size, it is necessary to know the PCV as well as the number of cells per litre.

6.17

(a)   Yes.

(b)   Yes. Mean corpuscular volume (MCV) is the PCV divided by the erythrocyte count.

(c)   Yes. The cells occupy 0.45 litre per litre so that plasma occupies 0.55; this is 55%.

(d)   Yes. Mean corpuscular Hb concentration is Hb concentration divided by PCV which gives a value of about 330 g per litre (33 g per decilitre).

(e)   Yes. Microcytosis is indicated by a low mean corpuscular volume, which is normally not less than about 80 femtolitres. Anaemia is indicated by a haemoglobin concentration of 120 g per litre or less.

6.18

(a) No. Carbon monoxide binds tightly to haemoglobin displacing oxygen; carbon monoxide does not influence the concentration of haemoglobin in the blood.

(b) Yes. It is quantitatively the most important non-bicarbonate buffer in blood.

(c) No. Haemoglobin is not an enzyme. The hydration of carbon dioxide is catalysed inside red blood cells, but the relevant enzyme is carbonic anhydrase.

(d) No. Each molecule of haemoglobin, when saturated, carries four molecules of oxygen.

(e) No. The blood group antigens are attached to the erythrocyte membrane, not to haemoglobin.

6.19

(a) Yes. This is the definition of anaemia.

(b) No. An anaemic person looks pale due to a deficiency of haemoglobin in the blood.

(c) Yes.

(d) Yes. Deoxygenated blood is blue and is responsible for the blue colour of the cyanotic subject.

(e) Yes. With less than this 'concentration of deoxygenated haemoglobin' blueness cannot be appreciated by eye. In fact, of course, none of the haemoglobin will be fully deoxygenated – it will all be partially deoxygenated. (If there is 150 g of haemoglobin per litre, and it is only two-thirds saturated ($\sim 66\%$), it is as though there were 50 g deoxygenated and 100 g oxygenated; if there is also anaemia, with haemoglobin of, say, 100 g, at 66% saturation, it is as though there were 33 g per litre deoxygenated: insufficient to look blue.)

6.20

(a) Yes. This is the definition of anaemia, if it is less than 2 standard deviations of the mean for the healthy population (Hb below 120 g per litre for women, 140 g per litre for men).

(b) No. Anaemia can, for example, be macrocytic (pernicious anaemia).

(c) No. There could be a normal MCHC, with a low erythrocyte count.

(d) Yes. The oxygen-carrying capacity is proportional to the haemoglobin concentration.

(e) No. The arterial PO_2 depends on gas exchange in the lungs: it is normal, and the haemoglobin will be saturated if the lungs are normal; it is the oxygen content of the blood, in ml per litre, that is always low.

6.21

(a)   No. This is a normal haemoglobin concentration.

(b)   Yes. At full saturation 150 g of Hb would carry 200 ml O_2.

(c)   Yes.

(d)   No. An arterio-venous (a-v) difference of 20 ml per litre, at a resting oxygen usage of 250 ml per min, means that the cardiac output would have to be 12.5 litres per min. Although cardiac output is likely to be higher than normal with this degree of hypoxia, it would not be as high as this. The a-v difference is more likely to be, say, 40 ml per litre (mixed venous oxygen 110 ml per litre) allowing 250 ml per min uptake from a cardiac output of 6.25 litres per min.

(e)   Yes. From the haemoglobin dissociation curve, this is the oxygen tension equivalent to 75% saturation of Hb.

6.22

(a)   No. A typical normal value is 5×10^{12} per litre.

(b)   No. This is too high (normally 140–150 g per litre).

(c)   No. This is also too high (normally close to 0.45 litre per litre).

(d)   No. MCV is given by haematocrit divided by RBC count, which is $0.6/10^{13}$ or 60 femtolitres.

(e)   Yes. MCH is given by Hb concentration divided by RBC count which is $220/10^{13}$.

6.23

(a)   No. Microcytosis means that the average volume of the erythrocytes is low. Consequently the MCV is the measurement needed to make the diagnosis; this requires packed cell volume (PCV) as well as the red cell count.

(b)   No. Anaemia means a reduction in the concentration of haemoglobin in the blood. This is measured directly by the haemoglobin (g per litre of blood) and is also indicated, less directly, by the red cell count (cells per litre of blood). In anaemia, cells may be small, normal or larger than normal.

(c)   Yes. Hypochromia means a reduction in the concentration of haemoglobin in the erythrocytes and is measured directly by the MCHC (given as haemoglobin in g per decilitre of cells).

(d)   Yes. Leucocytosis means a raised white cell count.

(e)   No. Erythrocyte fragility is measured by suspending samples of blood in solutions containing graded concentrations of sodium chloride and noting the osmolarity below which haemolysis occurs. The packed cell volume means the volume of red cells contained in a given volume of blood.

6.24

(a)   Yes.
(b)   Yes.
(c)   Yes.
(d)   Yes.
(e)   Yes.

6.25

(a)   Yes. The erythrocytes are negatively charged and this results in mutual repulsion, tending to prevent clotting. The negatively-charged heparin molecules enhance this effect.
(b)   Yes. By the inverse mechanism of (a).
(c)   No. Platelets are necessary for the intrinsic clotting process, but clotting can occur as a result of the release of chemicals into the blood from damaged tissue ('extrinsic clotting').
(d)   No. Vitamin K acts on the liver to promote the formation of pro-thrombin. It does not itself have any direct effect on blood clotting.
(e)   No. The amount required would kill the patient before its anti-coagulant action was effective.

6.26

(a)   Yes.
(b)   Yes. The fibrinogen in plasma forms fibrin in the whip and is thereby removed.
(c)   Yes. In a clean glass vessel the platelets adhere to the glass and disintegrate, promoting clotting. In a vaseline coated vessel the platelets adhere less readily, so that clotting is delayed.
(d)   Yes. By precipitating the calcium ions in blood as calcium citrate.
(e)   No. Dicoumarol acts as an anticoagulant *in vivo* by preventing synthesis in the liver of prothrombin; it has no anticoagulant effect *in vitro*.

6.27

(a)   No. Group O is the universal **donor** group because the red cells possess no A or B antigen.
(b)   Yes.
(c)   Yes.
(d)   Yes. A severe transfusion reaction involves extensive intravascular haemolysis and this leads to jaundice.
(e)   Yes. For A and B agglutinogens, agglutination occurs in the cold and in the absence of complement; such antibodies are called 'complete' antibodies.

6.28

(a)   No. If the mother is Rh negative, she is genotype rh/rh. If the father is phenotype Rh positive but genotype Rh/rh (heterozygous), then the child has a 50% chance of being rhesus negative, and therefore not at risk.

(b)   Yes. Previous sensitization of the mother by a Rh-positive baby results in the second Rh-positive child being more at risk than the first.

(c)   No. It requires repeated exposure of Rh-negative subjects to the Rh antigen for antibodies to be generated.

(d)   Yes. It is only the incomplete antibodies that cross the placental barrier although maternal antibodies are both complete and incomplete.

(e)   No. This would exacerbate the haemolysis of the baby's cells by maternal antibodies.

7 Heart

Electrical activity, ECG	7.1–7.10
Mechanical events of cardiac cycle	7.11–7.27
Pressure–volume relationships	7.28–7.37
Miscellaneous and applied	7.38–7.49

QUESTIONS

Electrical activity

7.1 **With reference to the electrical events in the cardiac cycle:**
(a) the ventricular action potential lasts about 0.3 seconds at rest.
(b) high extracellular potassium may result in ventricular fibrillation.
(c) the QRST complex of the ECG has the same wave form as that which would be recorded from a microelectrode inside a ventricular muscle fibre.
(d) vagal stimulation reduces the rate of depolarization in pacemaker cells during diastole.
(e) the upstroke of the ventricular action potential is due to an increase in potassium permeability of the muscle membrane.

7.2 **With respect to the spread of excitation through the normal human heart:**
(a) the frequency of generation of action potentials is greater in the cells of the sino-atrial node than in those of the atrioventricular node.
(b) there is a delay of 60–100 msec between action potentials in the atrial muscle and those in the ventricular muscle.
(c) conduction through the Purkinje system is about five times as fast as conduction through the atrial muscle.
(d) the duration of the action potential in a ventricular muscle fibre is about the same as in a skeletal muscle fibre.
(e) the action potential lasts longest in the ventricular muscle fibres which are excited first.

7.3 **Concerning the activation of the heart:**
(a) Purkinje fibres are modified cardiac muscle fibres.
(b) the Purkinje fibre system originates in the sino-atrial node.
(c) the influence of Purkinje fibres on cardiac muscle is via chemical synapses.
(d) propagation of the electrical signal through the thickness of the ventricle walls is via Purkinje fibres.
(e) in bundle branch block, the region of myocardium previously excited by that branch fails to contract.

7.4   **With reference to the normal human heart:**

(a)   the only connection for the spread of excitation from atria to ventricles is via the atrio-ventricular node.

✗ (b)   if the spread of excitation from atria to ventricles is blocked, the ventricles cease to beat indefinitely.

✗ (c)   R and T waves of opposite polarity occur as a result of a slowing of spread of the wave of excitation through the myocardium.

✗ (d)   depression of the ST segment of the ECG can occur transiently during angina pectoris.

✗ (e)   left axis deviation leads to an abnormally large R-wave in lead I (left arm–right arm).

7.5   **Concerning the healthy human heart:**

(a)   the R wave of the ECG is generated by depolarization in the atrioventricular A-V node.

(b)   the S wave of the ECG is generated by depolarization of the bundle of His.

(c)   there is a delay of about 200 msec between the impulse in the A-V node and depolarization of the apex of the heart.

(d)   the last part of the ventricle to be activated is the epicardium of the apex.

(e)   the T wave of the ECG occurs at the beginning of the absolute refractory period of the ventricle.

✗**7.6**   **The three traces in Figure 7.6 show records from the standard leads of an electrocardiogram (ECG). In these traces:**

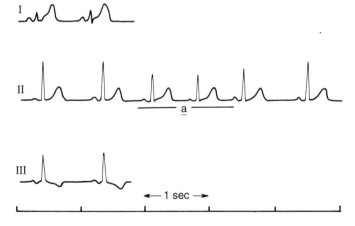

(a)   period **a** corresponds to inspiration.

(b)   when the heart rate changes during the record (lead II), the P–T interval changes less than the T–P interval.

(c)   the record could have been taken from a patient with a denervated heart.

(d)   the conduction time between the sino-atrial and the atrioventricular nodes is greater than normal.

(e)   the direction of the electrical vector at the time of ventricular depolarization is approximately the same as that at the time of ventricular repolarization.

7.7   Concerning the electrocardiogramn (ECG) of an adult human:

(a)   the P wave coincides with depolarization of the atria.

(b)   the Q wave coincides with repolarization of the atria.

(c)   a P–R interval of 0.3 seconds indicates impaired conduction.

(d)   the R wave coincides with depolarization of the apex of the heart.

(e)   during the isopotential (isoelectric) phase between the S and T waves, the intracellular potential in ventricular muscle cells is positive with respect to the interstitial fluid.

✗ **7.8   Concerning the event that gave rise to the ECG waveform X in Figure 7.8:**

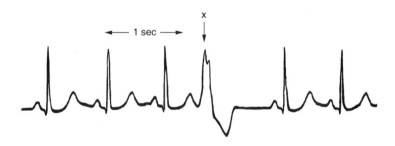

(a)   it originated from a ventricular ectopic focus.

(b)   it reset the cardiac rhythm.

(c)   both heart sounds would have been present.

(d)   the path of spread of excitation through the ventricle was like that in a normal cardiac cycle.

(e)   the duration of the action potential in a given ventricular muscle fibre was longer than normal.

7.9   With reference to the ECG:

(a)   the QRS complex is produced by depolarization of the ventricles.

(b)   the Q–T interval gives an approximate indication of the duration of ventricular systole.

(c)   the aortic valve is closed at the time of the P wave.

(d)   the first heart sound occurs at about the same time as the P wave.

(e)   the second heart sound occurs at about the same time as the QRS complex.

7.10 **In the adult human ECG represented in Figure 7.10, are the following statements true?**

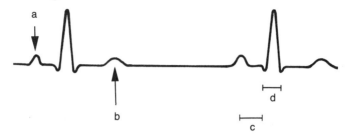

(a) judging by the interval between T and P relative to the duration of the whole cycle, the pulse rate is likely to be nearer 60 than 120 beats per minute.

(b) at the time corresponding to arrow a, the rate of filling of the ventricles would be at its peak.

(c) the arrow b indicates a time at which there is a rise in potassium permeability in ventricular muscle cells.

(d) the line c represents the period during which the atria are contracting.

(e) the line d represents the duration of ventricular systole.

Mechanical events of the cardiac cycle

7.11 **Concerning the cardiac cycle of a normal young healthy adult human who is reclining and breathing quietly:**

(a) the peak pressure in the right ventricle is about 25 mmHg.

(b) the lowest pressure in the right ventricle is about 10 mmHg.

(c) the mean jugular venous pressure is about 10 mmHg.

(d) the peak of the V wave of the ACV complex occurs immediately before the atrioventricular valve opens.

(e) the first heart sound occurs early in atrial systole.

7.12 **With reference to the mechanical events in the cardiac cycle in a normal adult human:**

(a) the left ventricle ejects more blood per beat than the right ventricle.

(b) the mitral valve opens when the left atrial pressure exceeds the left ventricular pressure.

(c) during strenuous work in a healthy subject, the left ventricle may contain, at the end of diastole, twice as much blood as it does at rest.

(d) the pulmonary valve opens when the right ventricular pressure reaches 20–25 mmHg.

(e) during a single cardiac cycle, there are two phases when both the atrio-ventricular valve and the aortic valve are closed.

7.13   Figure 7.13 represents a record of pressure changes in the right ventricle in a normal resting adult human:

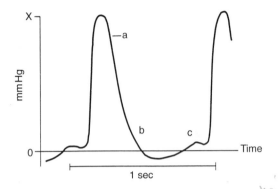

1 sec

(a)   the pressure X could be 50 mmHg.
(b)   during the phase from a to b, the ventricle is relaxing isometrically.
(c)   near b, the pulmonary valve would open.
(d)   during the phase from b to c, the atrioventricular valve would be open.
(e)   the peak of the pressure curve is simultaneous with the R deflection of the ECG.

7.14   **Suppose that Figure 7.13 now represents a record of pressure changes in the left ventricle in a normal resting adult human.**
(a)   the pressure X could be 125 mmHg.
(b)   during the phase from a to b, the ventricle is ejecting blood.
(c)   at b, the aortic valve would close.
(d)   at c, the aortic valve would be open.
(e)   the peak of the pressure curve is simultaneous with the P deflection of the ECG.

7.15   **In a young healthy adult, reclining at rest:**
(a)   the first heart sound occurs at the end of the phase of isometric (isovolumetric) contraction of the ventricles.
(b)   the second heart sound occurs at the end of the phase of isometric relaxation.
(c)   at the end of the diastole, the 2 ventricles together hold about 20% of the total blood volume.
(d)   the mean pulmonary arterial pressure is about 12 mmHg.
(e)   the jugular venous pulse gives an indication of right atrial filling pressure.

7.16 **Concerning the cardiac cycle in a normal person at rest:**
(a) the lowest pressure in the right ventricle is typically 10 mmHg.
(b) the highest pressure in the left atrium is typically 70 mmHg.
(c) the atrioventricular valves close when the ventricular pressures exceed the atrial pressures.
(d) atrial contraction is essential for ventricular filling.
(e) the wall of the aorta is stretched during the ejection of blood from the left ventricle.

LOVE YA LOADS + LOADS

7.17 **Concerning the cardiac cycle:**
(a) there is a phase in the cardiac cycle in which all the blood to be expelled into the aorta during systole is contained in the left ventricle.
(b) there is a phase in the cardiac cycle in which all the blood to be expelled into the aorta during systole is contained in the left atrium.
(c) the left ventricle shows a phase of isovolumetric contraction.
(d) the left atrium shows a phase of isovolumetric contraction.
(e) if the ventricular contractility and heart rate are unchanged, the volume of blood flowing through the left atrium during one cardiac cycle is equal to the left ventricular stroke volume.

7.18 **Concerning the cardiac cycle:**
(a) blood flows into the atria throughout the cardiac cycle.
(b) blood flows from atria to ventricles throughout the cardiac cycle.
(c) blood flows from the left ventricle to the aorta throughout the cardiac cycle.
(d) blood flows from the aorta to the large arteries throughout the cardiac cycle.
(e) the flow of blood in all arteries is pulsatile.

7.19 **During the cardiac cycle in a normal human adult at rest, with a blood pressure of 120/70 mmHg:**
(a) the lowest pressure in the left ventricle is 70 mmHg.
(b) the maximum pressure difference across the aortic valve is 120 mmHg.
(c) the maximum pressure difference across the mitral (left atrioventricular) valve is close to 120 mmHg.
(d) the maximum pressure difference across the tricuspid (right atrioventricular) valve is about 25 mmHg.
(e) the volume of blood in the left atrium decreases during ventricular systole.

7.20   Concerning the arterial blood pressure:
(a)   the pressure falls to its lowest value during ventricular diastole.
(b)   the peak pressure occurs during ventricular systole.
(c)   the magnitude of the peak pressure is close to the highest pressure in the left ventricle.
(d)   the magnitude of the lowest pressure is close to the lowest pressure in the left ventricle.
(e)   in a small artery such as the radial artery, the blood pressure is about one half the value in the aorta.

7.21   In a normal human adult at rest:
(a)   the rate of flow of blood from the left ventricle to the aorta is approximately constant throughout the ejection phase.
(b)   during the cardiac cycle, the volume of blood contained in the ventricles is highest during the phase of isovolumetric relaxation.
(c)   during the phase of isovolumetric relaxation of the ventricles, the volume of blood in the atria is constant.
(d)   during a single cardiac cycle, there is a phase when both the atrioventricular valve and the aortic valve are open.
(e)   during diastole, the pressure in each ventricle is equal to or lower than that in the corresponding atrium.

7.22   In a healthy average-sized man:
(a)   at rest, during each cardiac cycle about 70 ml of blood is ejected from each ventricle.
(b)   at rest the end-systolic volume of each ventricle is around 70 ml.
(c)   in exercise, the whole of the increase in stroke volume is achieved by an increase in the end-diastolic volume.
(d)   athletic training results in an increase in resting end-systolic volume.
(e)   athletic training results in an increase in resting stroke volume.

7.23   In Figure 7.23, the curves show the relation between the stroke work of the left ventricle (i.e. the stroke volume multiplied by the average ventricular pressure during ejection) and the pressure in the ventricle at the end of diastole. They represent two states of contractility. Are the following statements true?

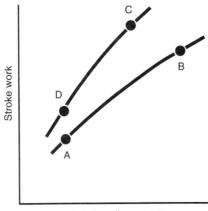

End-diastolic pressure

(a) the volume of blood in the ventricle at the end of diastole would be greater at B than at A.

(b) the change from A to B exemplifies Starling's law of the heart.

(c) at D, contractility is less than at A.

(d) a change from curve AB to curve DC could be produced by stimulating the sympathetic nerve supply to the heart.

(e) a change from A to C could be produced by a change in posture from lying to standing.

7.24 **Figure 7.24 represents the waveform of the aortic pressure in a normal subject at rest. Are the following statements true?**

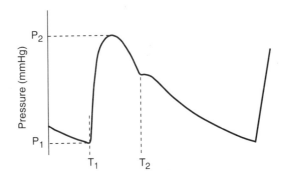

Time

(a) P_1 is typically 5 mmHg.
(b) P_2 is typically 120 mmHg.
(c) T_1 corresponds to the closure of the mitral valve.
(d) T_2 corresponds to the opening of the aortic valve.
(e) T_2 corresponds to the QRS complex of the ECG.

7.25   Figure 7.25 shows the pressure waveform in the right atrium in a normal subject at rest.

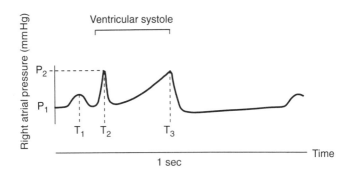

(a) P_1 is typically 0 mmHg.
(b) P_2 is typically 40 mmHg.
(c)   wave T_1 corresponds to atrial systole.
(d)   wave T_2 is produced by bulging of the pulmonary valve into the right ventricle.
(e)   wave T_3 is due to venous filling of the atrium.

7.26   With further reference to Figure 7.25:
(a)   the value of P_1 increases during inspiration.
(b)   at T_1, the tricuspid valve opens.
(c)   at T_3, the tricuspid valve closes.
(d)   between T_2 and T_3, the right ventricle expels blood.
(e)   between wave T_3 and wave T_1 of the following cardiac cycle, the pressure in the atrium is close to that in the ventricle.

7.27   Figure 7.27 shows the pressure waveform in the left atrium and the atrial volume in a normal subject at rest. With reference to the atrial volume changes:

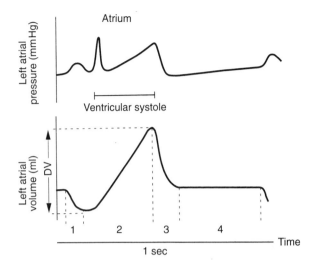

(a)   the fall in volume in phase 1 is due to the left ventricle sucking blood out of the atrium.

(b)   the rise in volume in phase 2 is due to the fact that blood entering the atrium cannot move on into the ventricle.

(c)   the fall in volume in phase 3 is due to blood leaking back into the pulmonary veins.

(d)   the constant volume in phase 4 indicates that no blood is entering or leaving the atrium.

(e)   the change in volume DV during the cardiac cycle is the same as the stroke volume of the left ventricle.

Pressure–volume relationships

7.28   Figure 7.28 shows how the pressure and volume of a ventricle change with respect to one another during the cardiac cycle. Are the following statements true?

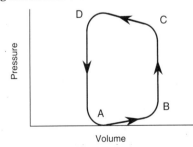

(a)   the curve between A and B is part of the passive pressure–volume relation of the ventricle.

(b)   between B and C the ventricle fills with blood.

(c)   ejection of blood from the ventricle occurs between C and D.

(d)   the area of the loop gives an indication of the work done by the ventricle during one cardiac cycle.

(e)   at D the atrioventricular valve opens.

7.29   **Figure 7.29 shows pressure–volume relations in the left ventricle of a normal human at rest. The loop 1–2–3–4 represents the sequence of changes in pressure and volume during one cardiac cycle:**

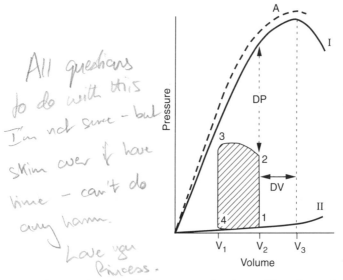

All questions to do with this I'm not sure – but skim over & have time – can't do any harm.

Love you Princess.

(a)   the curve 2–3 represents the phase of isovolumetric contraction of the ventricles.

(b)   the duration of phase 4–1 would be greater than the total duration of the rest of the loop.

(c)   the volume change from 4 to 1 is about 10 ml.

(d)   the pressure at point 2 could be 70 mmHg.

(e)   the shaded area represents the cardiac output.

7.30   **In Figure 7.29, the solid curve I represents the peak systolic pressures that would be developed if the isolated left ventricle were to contract isovolumetrically at successively greater initial volumes; curve II shows the corresponding pressures and volumes during diastole. The loop 1–2–3–4 represents, on the same scale, one normal cardiac cycle *in vivo* in a healthy adult human.**

(a)   the point V_2 represents the end-systolic volume.
(b)   at point 3 the aortic valve opens.
(c)   at point 4 the mitral valve opens.
(d)   the rate of ejection of blood from the ventricle would be lower if DP were smaller.
(e)   increase in the pulmonary venous pressure will result in the pressure-volume loop moving to the right.

7.31   With further reference to Figure 7.29:
(a)   the pressure at point 2 is the aortic diastolic pressure.
(b)   a change in the position of the pressure–volume relation for active cardiac muscle from curve I to curve A signals that the contractility of the heart is increased.
(c)   if, in a subject at rest, the end-diastolic volume is V_2, sustained increase in the pulmonary venous pressure will increase the value of V_2.
(d)   when the end-diastolic volume is at V_3, the ventricle pumps with greater force than at any other end-diastolic volume.
(e)   a person with an end-diastolic volume at V_3 is on the verge of cardiac failure.

7.32   With further reference to Figure 7.29:
(a)   the volume $(V_2 - V_1)$ represents the stroke volume.
(b)   the pressure at point 2 is typically 70 mmHg.
(c)   the duration of phase 1 to 2 is about 0.4 sec.
(d)   the first heart sound occurs at a time corresponding to point 1 on the pressure loop.
(e)   if the heart were failing as a pump, the loop 1–2–3–4 would shift to the left.

7.33   With further reference to Figure 7.29, in a healthy subject:
(a)   with exercise, curve I moves to curve A.
(b)   exercise would shift the line 1–2 to the left.
(c)   exercise would depress the level of segment 2–3.
(d)   exercise would shift the line 3–4 to the left.
(e)   at rest, the trained athlete will have a smaller value of DV than an untrained person of similar stature.

7.34   With further reference to Figure 7.29:
(a)   if V_3 represents the end-diastolic volume of a patient, increase in the pulmonary venous pressure will increase the force of ventricular contraction.

(b)   if an increase in pulmonary venous pressure were to cause a decrease in cardiac contractility, this would provide an effective compensatory mechanism for pumping excess blood from the venous to the arterial side of the circulation.

(c)   if V_3 represents the end-diastolic volume of a patient, increase in the pulmonary venous pressure will result in an increase in stroke volume.

(d)   if V_3 represents the end-diastolic volume of a patient, sustained increase in the pulmonary venous pressure will result in the pressure–volume loop moving progressively to the right until the patient dies.

(e)   for a heart that is operating with an end-diastolic volume at V_3, blood-letting helps the failing heart.

7.35   With further reference to Figure 7.29:
(a)   adrenaline administration moves curve I to curve A.
(b)   in congestive cardiac failure, administration of an agent that moves curve I to the dashed line tends to improve the cardiac condition.
(c)   in a patient with myocardial damage, curve I moves down.
(d)   in a patient with a transplanted heart in physiological adaptations, the curve I may move curve A.
(e)   in a patient whose heart rate is held constant by a cardiac pacemaker, if a pharmacological agent is administered that moves curve I to curve A, the pressure–volume loop of the cardiac cycle moves to the left.

7.36   With further reference to Figure 7.29:
(a)   sympathetic activity would move curve I to curve A.
(b)   administration of atropine would move curve I to curve A.
(c)   agents that inhibit the sodium pump move curve I to curve A.
(d)   a decrease in the myocardial intracellular calcium concentration would move curve I to curve A.
(e)   an agent that blocks calcium channels would move curve I to curve A.

7.37   Concerning the left ventricle during various phases of the cardiac cycle:
(a)   during the ejection phase of a healthy heart, the myocardium is moving along the Starling relationship in the direction of increasing the potential strength of contraction.
(b)   the faster the rate of ejection of blood from the ventricle, the greater the rate of rise of intraventricular blood pressure.
(c)   for a given tension developed by the wall of the ventricle, the intraventricular blood pressure is greater if the volume of the ventricle is greater.
(d)   a premature heart beat develops a greater peak systolic pressure than a normal heart beat.
(e)   for a given end-diastolic volume, the amount of blood expelled by the ventricle by an extrasystole originating from an ectopic focus in the ventricular myocardium is greater than for an atrial extrasystole.

Miscellaneous and applied

7.38   With reference to cardiac muscle fibres:
(a)   when the sodium pump is starved of adenosine triphosphate (ATP), the addition of ATP to the extracellular solution restores the efflux of sodium ions.
(b)   the beneficial effect of cardiac glycosides on myocardial contractility is attributable to stimulation of the sodium pump.
(c)   the presence of potassium ions in the extracellular solution is essential for the operation of the sodium pump.
(d)   the action of cardiac glycosides is reinforced when the extracellular potassium concentration is high.
(e)   cardiac glycosides decrease the intracellular calcium ion concentration.

7.39   With reference to cardiac muscle fibres:
(a)   the beneficial effects of the cardiac glycosides are primarily to increase the heart rate.
(b)   the cardiac glycosides administered to a subject with a failing heart increase the end-diastolic volume of the left ventricle.
(c)   there is a specific calcium pump, independent of the sodium pump, to extrude calcium from the ventricular muscle fibres.
(d)   excitation-contraction coupling in the heart is primarily due to entry of sodium ions during the cardiac action potential.
(e)   the increase in calcium concentration in the myocardial fibres is due mainly to influx across the cell membrane.

7.40   With respect to the human heart:
(a)   the spread of excitation through the wall of the ventricles is from the endocardial surface outwards.
(b)   the first heart sound is shorter than the second.
(c)   the ejection of blood from the ventricles occurs between the first and the second heart sounds.
(d)   in exercise, systole shortens more than diastole.
(e)   in the resting subject, denervation of the heart would result in a rise in heart rate.

7.41   Concerning the heart:
(a)   the heart stops beating immediately if nerve impulses via its autonomic innervation are blocked.
(b)   the force of ventricular contraction is increased by sympathetic stimulation.
(c)   the heart rate is increased by vagal stimulation.
(d)   the diameter of the arterioles in the coronary circulation is mainly controlled by neural influences.
(e)   the blood supply to the cardiac musculature is completely interrupted during systole.

7.42   **Increased activity of the vagus nerve supplying the mammalian heart:**
(a)   can produce cardiac arrest.
(b)   has little effect on contractility of the ventricles.
(c)   accelerates depolarization of cells of the sino-atrial node.
(d)   increases the conduction time between the atria and ventricles.
(e)   is ineffective after previous treatment of the heart with atropine.

7.43   **During a Valsalva's manoeuvre (forced expiration against a closed glottis) there is an increase in:**
(a)   venous return to the heart.
(b)   the intrathoracic pressure.
(c)   the heart rate.
(d)   the cerebrospinal fluid (CSF) pressure.
(e)   the cardiac output.

7.44   **With reference to the human heart:**
(a)   the P–Q interval of the ECG is a measure of the conduction time along the Purkinje fibres.
(b)   ventricular systole has the same duration as the QRS complex.
(c)   in normal resting conditions, the influence of the sympathetic nerve supply on the sino-atrial node predominates over that of the parasympathetic.
(d)   the left ventricular pressure rises by 8–10 mmHg during the phase of isometric contraction.
(e)   the rate of emptying of the left ventricle is fairly uniform throughout the ejection phase of ventricular systole.

7.45   **Noradrenaline acts on the heart to cause:**
(a)   tachycardia.
(b)   increased potassium conductance of the membranes of pacemaker cells.
(c)   increased concentration of free calcium in the myoplasm.
(d)   increased strength of cardiac contraction.
(e)   increased duration of the cardiac action potential.

7.46   **Concerning the heart in a normal subject:**
(a)   at rest, the duration of diastole equals that of systole.
(b)   at rest, the left ventricular end-diastolic volume is typically 140 ml.
(c)   at rest, about 90% of the end-diastolic blood volume is ejected during systole.
(d)   in exercise, the stroke volume may increase 10-fold.
(e)   myocardial tissue has about the same number of capillaries per unit mass as skeletal muscle.

✗ **7.47** **Concerning the control of the heart beat:**
  (a) if the brain-stem ceases to function, the heart stops beating immediately.
  (b) the initiation of heart beats normally depends on bursts of action potentials in the motor nerves innervating the heart.
  (c) neuromuscular blockade interrupts the beating of the heart.
  (d) the innervation of the heart is via end-plates on the myocardial fibres.
  (e) a denervated heart can beat spontaneously.

7.48 **As a result of deformity of the aortic valve, it may not be able to close completely. In this situation:**
  (a) during ventricular diastole, blood flows from the aorta into the left ventricle.
  (b) there is likely to be a higher pulse pressure than normal.
  (c) for a given cardiac output, the left ventricle must do more work than usual.
  (d) the left ventricle exhibits a phase of isovolumetric relaxation.
  (e) in each complete cardiac cycle, more blood enters the left ventricle than leaves it.

SKIM IT THROUGH but DO not WORRY ABOUT IT

✗ **7.49** **Features of right ventricular failure include:**
  (a) ascites (accumulation of fluid in the peritoneal cavity).
  (b) enlargement of the liver.
  (c) peripheral cyanosis.
  (d) pulmonary oedema.
  (e) increase in the diffusion barrier between the alveolar gas and blood in pulmonary capillaries.

ANSWERS

7.1
  (a) Yes.
  (b) Yes. For this reason hyperkalaemia can be fatal.
  (c) No. Consult diagrams of action potential in ventricular muscle: the ECG deflections are maximal when there is a change in potential recorded from muscle fibre: ECG is isoelectric during the plateau of action potential.
  (d) Yes. This is the effect of acetylcholine – the rate of change of the pacemaker potential is slowed, so that it takes longer to reach threshold.
  (e) No. It is due to an increase in sodium permeability followed by a slower increase in calcium permeability.

7.2

(a) Yes. This is why the sino-atrial node is normally the pacemaker.

(b) Yes. The interval includes the delay in the region of the atrio-ventricular node.

(c) Yes.

(d) No. The action potential lasts more than 10 times longer in ventricular muscle than in skeletal muscle.

(e) Yes.

7.3

(a) Yes.

(b) No. It originates in the bundle of His.

(c) No. The communication from cell to cell is via nexuses which allow direct electrical propagation from cell to cell.

(d) No. Propagation through the ventricular walls is direct from cell to cell of the ventricular muscle itself.

(e) No. The region of myocardium previously excited by Purkinje fibres will be activated more slowly via neighbouring muscle cells.

7.4

(a) Yes.

(b) No. If the spread of excitation from atria to ventricles is blocked, usually a focus somewhere in the ventricle starts its own autonomous rhythm, at a lower frequency than the atrial rhythm.

(c) Yes. A normal speed of propagation of excitation through the myocardium is a prerequisite for the normal situation, in which the R and T waves have the same polarity.

(d) Yes. The inadequate coronary blood flow during angina pectoris causes temporary depolarisation of the deep layers of the myocardium and a transient depression of the ST segment.

(e) Yes.

7.5

(a) No. The R wave is generated by depolarization of the ventricles.

(b) No. Depolarization of the bundle of His occurs at the time of the beginning of the R wave.

(c) No. The delay is much shorter than this – normally typically 10–15 msec.

(d) No. The base of the ventricle is activated last.

(e) No. The T wave represents repolarization, which is towards the end of the absolute refractory period.

7.6

(a) Yes. Heart rate increases during inspiration (respiratory sinus arrhythmia).

(b)   Yes. This reflects a greater change in the duration of diastole than of systole.

(c)   No. Because the heart rate obviously varies with respiration; the denervated heart does not exhibit sinus arrhythmia. Also, the heart rate would be about 100 beats per minute in a denervated heart.

(d)   No. The P–R interval is less than 0.2 sec, which is the upper limit of normal.

(e)   No. The two vectors are approximately at right angles to each other.

7.7

(a)   Yes.

(b)   Yes. Repolarization of the atria does coincide with the Q wave, but it cannot be identified in the ECG because it is obscured by the ventricular complex.

(c)   Yes. 0.2 sec is the upper limit of normal.

(d)   Yes.

(e)   Yes. This represents the 'plateau' of the ventricular action potential, during which the muscle remains depolarized.

7.8

(a)   Yes. The abnormal wave reflects ventricular excitation, which lasts longer than a normal R wave because propagation is not via the normal fast Purkinje fibre route.

(b)   No.

(c)   Yes. The mechanical events of the abnormally arising beat would have the components that give rise to the two main heart sounds.

(d)   No. The spread of excitation started at some point in the ventricular muscle, and therefore spread differently; the deflection X is much wider than the normal QRS complex.

(e)   No. A rough indication of the duration of excitation in the ventricle is given by the Q–T interval, and this is about 0.25 sec for both the normal and the abnormal complexes. Wherever its excitation comes from, there is no reason for variation in the duration of the action potential in a muscle fibre.

7.9

(a)   Yes.

(b)   Yes.

(c)   Yes. It is closed between T and R approximately.

(d)   No. The first sound, coincident with closure of the atrioventricular valves, occurs just after the QRS complex, i.e. at the start of ventricular contraction.

(e)   No. The second sound, coincident with closure of the aortic and pulmonary valves, occurs immediately after the T wave, i.e. at the start of ventricular relaxation.

7.10

(a)   Yes. T–P represents most of diastole, which is longer than the remainder of the cycle at rest. It would be relatively shorter if heart rate were as high as 120.

(b)   No. The ventricles fill most rapidly in early diastole.

(c)   Yes. During repolarization (T wave), potassium permeability is high and potassium entry into cells brings about repolarization of the cardiac muscle membrane.

(d)   Yes. Atrial contraction is initiated by the electrical activity reflected in the P wave.

(e)   No. Ventricular systole starts with the QRS complex, but continues longer, until the repolarization, reflected by the T wave.

7.11

(a)   Yes. This is a normal peak systolic pressure in the right ventricle and pulmonary artery.

(b)   No. The right ventricular pressure varies from about zero during ventricular diastole to 20–25 mmHg at the peak of ventricular systole.

(c)   No. The mean jugular venous pressure is between +2 cm and −2 cm of blood or saline (equivalent to a range of <0.5 mmHg).

(d)   Yes. The V wave of the ACV complex is due to the filling of the right atrium from the great veins, which precedes the opening of the atrioventricular valves at the end of ventricular relaxation.

(e)   No. The first heart sound occurs early in ventricular systole: at this time, the atria have finished active contraction.

7.12

(a)   No. There may be small discrepancies beat by beat, but over several beats, or over several seconds, the output of each ventricle must be the same (except for a small physiological shunt; this amounts to around 2% of the cardiac output).

(b)   Yes. This pressure difference is what causes it to open.

(c)   No. The stroke volume can increase up to twice the resting value, but this is partly or mostly because of extra emptying, rather than extra filling.

(d)   No. The pulmonary valve opens when the right ventricular pressure reaches the falling (diastolic) pressure in the pulmonary artery, which is 8–10 mmHg.

(e)   Yes. During isovolumetric contraction and during isovolumetric relaxation, both the atrio-ventricular valve and the aortic valve are closed.

7.13

(a)   No. The right ventricular and pulmonary artery pressures rise to only 20–25 mmHg during systole.

(b)   Yes. The pulmonary valve will have closed near a, so the ventricle is relaxing without filling (i.e. isovolumetrically) until the pressure falls below that in the right atrium.

(c)   No. The pulmonary valve is closed in this phase of the cardiac cycle (see (b)).

(d)   Yes. This is the filling phase; ventricular pressure is below atrial pressure between b and c and the atrioventricular valve is open; the valve will not close until the ventricle starts to contract and raises the ventricular pressure above atrial, after c.

(e)   No. The peak of the pressure curve is during ventricular contraction, but later than the QRS complex.

7.14

(a)   Yes. This is the same as the systolic blood pressure.

(b)   No. a to b represents isovolumetric relaxation.

(c)   No. The aortic valve closes at a.

(d)   No.

(e)   No. The peak of the pressure curve occurs during the isoelectric phase of the ECG between the QRS complex and the T wave. The P wave signals atrial excitation.

7.15

(a)   No. The first heart sound occurs as the atrioventricular valves close at the start of isovolumetric contraction.

(b)   No. The second heart sound occurs as the aortic and pulmonary valves close, at the start of isovolumetric relaxation.

(c)   No. At the end of the diastole, the 2 ventricles together hold typically 280 ml blood and the total blood volume is typically 5.5 litres.

(d)   Yes. Taking pulmonary artery pressure as 20/8 mmHg; like mean systemic blood pressure, mean pulmonary artery pressure is closer to diastolic than to systolic.

(e)   Yes. There are no valves between the jugular vein and the right atrium, so atrial pressure changes are reflected in the jugular pulse.

7.16

(a)   No. The lowest pressure in the right ventricle is around zero; 8–10 mmHg is the pressure in the right ventricle at which the pulmonary valve will open.

(b)   No. The pressure in the left atrium reaches less than 10 mmHg at its highest.

(c)   Yes.

(d)   No. For example, ventricular filling continues when the atria cease to contract rhythmically in the condition of atrial fibrillation.

(e)   Yes.

7.17

(a)   Yes. This is true during the phase of isovolumetric contraction, when both the atrioventricular and the aortic valves are closed.

(b)   No. Blood is flowing continuously during diastole through the atria into the ventricles until ventricular contraction starts, raising the ventricular pressure and closing the atrioventricular valves.

(c)   Yes. Between the closure of the atrioventricular and the opening of the aortic valves.

(d)   No. See (b). Atrial contraction simply gives a 'boost' to continuous diastolic ventricular filling.

(e)   Yes.

7.18

(a)   Yes.

(b)   No. Only during ventricular diastole.

(c)   No. Only during the ejection phase of ventricular systole.

(d)   Yes. Flow is much faster during systole, but the elastic recoil of the aortic wall maintains onward flow during diastole.

(e)   Yes. Because of (d), the flow is pulsatile.

7.19

(a)   No. The lowest ventricular pressure is around zero.

(b)   No. 120 mmHg can be taken to be the systolic aortic pressure. When the aortic valve closes, the pressure in the aorta has already fallen to a value between systolic and diastolic. At this time the ventricular pressure is dropping rapidly to zero, so the greatest pressure difference across the aortic valve is more like 90–100 mmHg. Immediately before the valve is opened again, as ventricular pressure rises from zero, the pressure difference rapidly decreases from aortic diastolic pressure (60–70 mmHg).

(c)   Yes. The highest pressure in the left ventricle is the same as the aortic systolic pressure; at this time the left atrial pressure is slightly above zero.

(d)   Yes. The highest pressure in the right ventricle is the same as the pulmonary systolic pressure; at this time the right atrial pressure is slightly above zero.

(e)   No. Blood continues to enter the atria during systole.

7.20

(a)   No. The pressure in the aorta is still falling during the isovolumetric phase of ventricular contraction.

(b)   Yes.

(c)   Yes.

(d)   No. The left ventricular pressure falls to zero after the aortic valve closes, while the arterial blood pressure falls only to the diastolic value of 70–80 mmHg.

(e)   No. The mean arterial pressure falls off only by a few mmHg along the branching system, and the pulse pressure tends to increase.

7.21

(a)   No. The rate of ejection is greatest initially.

(b)   No. The volume contained during isovolumetric relaxation is the end-systolic, or residual volume: the smallest during the cycle.

(c)   No. Blood flows into the atria during the whole cycle.

(d)   No. There is no phase in the cardiac cycle when both the atrioventricular valve and the aortic valve are open.

(e)   Yes. During diastole, the atrioventricular valves are open, allowing ventricular filling; pressure cannot therefore be higher in the ventricle than in the corresponding atrium.

7.22

(a)   Yes. A heart rate of 70+ and a stroke volume of 70 ml accounts for a cardiac output of 5 litres per minute.

(b)   Yes. The residual volume is about the same as the ejected volume.

(c)   No. Most of the increase is due to greater emptying, rather than greater filling of the ventricles, i.e. decrease in end-systolic volume.

(d)   No. Training results in the resting cardiac output being maintained at a lower heart rate and greater stroke volume by means of greater emptying: a smaller end-systolic volume.

(e)   Yes. See (d).

7.23

(a)   Yes. The greater end-diastolic pressure would be due to greater filling.

(b)   Yes. The curve A–B shows that stroke work increases with end-diastolic pressure, which is equivalent to stroke volume increasing with length or stretch of the ventricular muscle fibres.

(c)   No. At D, stroke work is greater than at A for the same end-diastolic pressure. This implies an increase in contractility: stroke volume would be greater without an increase in filling.

(d)   Yes. Sympathetic stimulation increases contractility.
(e)   No. A change from lying to standing will decrease the filling pressure for the heart.

7.24
(a)   No. P_1 is the diastolic arterial pressure and is typically 70 mmHg.
(b)   Yes.
(c)   No. T_1 corresponds to the opening of the aortic valve. The mitral valve has been closed since the start of isovolumetric contraction of the ventricle.
(d)   No. T_2 corresponds to the closure of the aortic valve.
(e)   No. The QRS complex of the ECG is the electrical complex preceding ventricular contraction and occurs before T_1 in the figure.

7.25
(a)   Yes.
(b)   No. P_2 is typically 5 mmHg.
(c)   Yes. This is called the A wave.
(d)   No. Wave T_2 is produced by bulging of the tricuspid valve into the right atrium; it is called the C wave, c for closure of the tricuspid valve.
(e)   Yes. Wave T_3 is due to venous filling of the atrium during the phase when the tricuspid valve is closed. The fall in pressure thereafter is due to opening of the tricuspid valve and drainage of blood from right atrium to right ventricle.

7.26
(a)   No. During inspiration the intrathoracic pressure is below atmospheric and so the value of the whole sequence, including P_1, falls during inspiration.
(b)   No. At T_1, the tricuspid valve is already open.
(c)   No. At T_3, the tricuspid valve opens.
(d)   Yes.
(e)   Yes.

7.27
(a)   No. The fall in volume in phase 1 is at the time of atrial systole and is due to the atrium pumping out blood, mainly into the left ventricle.
(b)   Yes. Phase 2 corresponds to venous filling of the atrium.
(c)   No. The fall in volume in phase 3 is due to opening of the mitral valve and blood moving from left atrium to left ventricle.

(d)   No. The constant volume in phase 4 reflects the fact that the rate of blood entering the atrium from the pulmonary veins is equal to the rate of blood leaving the atrium to enter the ventricle.

(e)   No. The total amount of blood entering or leaving the atrium in one cardiac cycle equals the ventricular stroke volume. The atrium never holds all this blood at any instant of time.

7.28

(a)   Yes.

(b)   No. The volume is constant from B to C. This represents the phase of isovolumetric contraction.

(c)   Yes. The volume decreases from C to D. This is the ejection phase.

(d)   Yes. The dimensions of pressure $\times$ volume are $N.m^{-2} \times m^3 = Nm$, which are the units of work.

(e)   No. At D the ventricle is starting to relax isovolumetrically. The pressure is still much higher than in the atrium; the atrioventricular valve does not open until the ventricular pressure has fallen below that in the atrium, as it approaches A.

7.29

(a)   No. The phase 1 to 2 represents isovolumetric contraction.

(b)   Yes. This represents ventricular filling.

(c)   No. It is around 70 ml (= stroke volume).

(d)   Yes. This represents aortic diastolic pressure.

(e)   No. The shaded area represents the work done by the left ventricle during one cardiac cycle.

7.30

(a)   No. Point V_2 represents the end-diastolic volume.

(b)   No. At point 3 the aortic valve closes.

(c)   Yes.

(d)   Yes. The length of the line DP represents the extra force the left ventricle could develop if it continued to contract isometrically instead of ejecting blood.

(e)   Yes. Increase in the pulmonary venous pressure leads to an increase in ventricular filling, an increase in end-diastolic volume and hence will result in the pressure–volume loop moving to the right.

7.31

(a)   Yes. This is the point at which the aortic valve opens and so corresponds to the lowest pressure in the aorta during the cardiac cycle.

(b)   Yes. If the pressure–volume relation changes from curve I to curve A, then at a given volume, the ventricle exerts a greater pressure, i.e. the contractility of the heart is increased.

(c)   Yes. Sustained increase in the pulmonary venous pressure results in an increase in end-diastolic volume; because the heart is operating on the rising part of the pressure-volume relationship, this increases the force of contraction and hence increases the stroke volume.

(d)   Yes. When the end-diastolic volume is at V_3, the difference between the curves representing diastole and systole is greatest and so the ventricle pumps with greater force than at any other end-diastolic volume.

(e)   Yes. When the end-diastolic volume is at V_3, the slightest increase in end-diastolic volume will push the ventricle on to the downhill part of the Starling curve, i.e. into cardiac failure.

7.32

(a)   Yes. This is the amount by which the ventricular volume decreases during expulsion of blood during one cardiac cycle and is thus the stroke volume.

(b)   Yes. This is the diastolic arterial blood pressure.

(c)   No. The phase 1 to 2 is the phase of isovolumetric contraction and lasts about one-twentieth of a second.

(d)   Yes.

(e)   No. If the heart were failing as a pump, the loop 1–2–3–4 would shift to the right.

7.33

(a)   Yes. With exercise, the release of catecholamines into the blood moves curve I to curve A.

(b)   No. Exercise would shift the line 1–2 to the right due to increased pulmonary venous pressure consequent on increased venous return.

(c)   No. In exercise, there is an increase in arterial blood pressure, so the level of segment 2–3 is elevated, not depressed.

(d)   Yes. Due to increased contractility of the myocardium, exercise shifts the line 3–4 to the left.

(e)   No. Training results in an increase in DV, with a consequent increase in the cardiac reserve.

7.34

(a)   No. The force of ventricular contraction is indicated by the difference in pressure between that reached at the start of the ejection phase and curve I. If the end-diastolic volume is V_3, increase in the pulmonary venous pressure will increase the end-diastolic volume to a value above V_3, and the force of ventricular contraction will decrease.

(b)   No. If an increase in pulmonary venous pressure caused a decrease in cardiac contractility, the ability of the heart to pump out the excess venous blood would be reduced, not increased.

(c)   No. By the same argument as (b), if the end-diastolic volume is V_3, an increase in the pulmonary venous pressure will result in a decrease in stroke volume.

(d)   Yes. For each cardiac cycle, the blood is less able to pump out blood, so less is removed from the venous side. This means that the venous pressure rises further, pushing the end-diastolic volume ever further to the right. This is the phase of cardiac decompensation.

(e)   Yes. Blood-letting reduces the volume of circulating blood, reduces the pulmonary venous pressure and can pull the failing heart back on to the physiological part of the pressure–volume curve, i.e. end-diastolic volume less than V_3.

7.35

(a)   Yes.

(b)   Yes. A move from curve I to curve A indicates that the heart is contracting more strongly. In congestive cardiac failure, this effect can bring the pressure–volume loop of the cardiac cycle to the left and hence back to the compensated (physiological) part of the working curve.

(c)   Yes. A decrease in contractility of the heart is signalled by curve I moving down.

(d)   Yes. In a patient with a transplanted heart in physiological adaptations, for instance those resulting in the increase in concentration of circulating catecholamines, the curve I moves to curve A.

(e)   Yes. In a patient whose heart rate is held constant by a cardiac pacemaker, if a pharmacological agent is administered that moves curve I to curve A, this signals an increase in cardiac contractility; the ventricle expels blood more forcibly and so the pressure–volume loop of the cardiac cycle moves to the left.

7.36

(a)   Yes.

(b)   No. Atropine blocks muscarinic receptors for acetylcholine and there are very few of these on ventricular muscle cells. Any effect would be in the opposite direction, of decreasing cardiac contractility.

(c)   Yes. Calcium extrusion depends on exchange with sodium ions. If the sodium pump is inhibited, the sodium concentration gradient across the membrane is reduced so calcium extrusion is depressed. The intracellular calcium concentration rises and this enhances myocardial contractility.

(d)   No. The opposite is true; an increase in the myocardial intracellular calcium concentration would cause the shift in the curve from I to A. This is the mechanism of the shift produced by sympathetic stimulation.

(e)   No. An agent that blocks calcium channels would reduce calcium entry with the cardiac action potential and so reduce cardiac contractility; the curve would move down, not up.

7.37

(a)   No. The trajectory representing the ejection phase is from right to left in Figure 7.29, i.e. in the direction of decreasing strength of contraction.

(b)   No. The opposite is true. A low rate of ejection indicates a slow rate of shortening of ventricular muscle and a corresponding high rate of rise of intraventricular blood pressure.

(c)   No. By the law of Laplace, at constant wall tension, in a sphere, the pressure is inversely proportional to the radius. So for the ventricle, for a given tension developed by the wall of the ventricle, the intraventricular blood pressure is smaller if the volume of the ventricle is greater.

(d)   No. For a premature heart beat, there has been less time than usual for the ventricle to fill. So the cardiac contraction is less forceful and expels less blood than usual and the peak pressure achieved is correspondingly reduced.

(e)   No. An extrasystole originating from an ectopic focus in the ventricular myocardium results in excitation spreading through the ventricle in a sequence that is not as well suited as normal for expelling blood; an extrasystole from an atrial focus spreads through the ventricle in the same sequence as for a normal beat. Therefore, for a given end-diastolic volume, the stroke volume of a ventricular extrasystole is less than for an atrial extrasystole.

7.38

(a)   Yes. ATP is needed as the immediate energy source for sodium extrusion against the electrochemical gradient; when the sodium pump is starved of ATP, the addition of ATP to the extracellular solution restores the efflux of sodium ions.

(b)   No. The beneficial effect of cardiac glycosides on myocardial contractility is attributable to inhibition of the sodium pump.

(c)   Yes. The sodium pump exchanges intracellular sodium for extra-cellular potassium, so the presence of potassium ions in the extracellular solution is essential for the operation of the sodium pump.

(d)   No. A low extracellular potassium concentration depresses the sodium pump, which in turn reinforces the action of cardiac glycosides.

(e)   No. Cardiac glycosides increase the intracellular calcium ion concentration.

7.39

(a)   No. The beneficial effects of the cardiac glycosides are primarily to increase the strength of contraction of the heart, not to have an effect on heart rate.

(b)   No. The cardiac glycosides administered to a subject with a failing heart, by increasing the strength of contraction, decrease the end-diastolic volume of the left ventricle.

(c)   No. In the myocardial cells, calcium extrusion is by means of an exchange mechanism with sodium; calcium leaves in return for sodium entry. So the energy for calcium extrusion is derived from the sodium pump. There is no specific calcium pump, independent of the sodium pump, to extrude calcium from the ventricular muscle fibres.

(d)   No. Excitation-contraction coupling in the heart is primarily due to entry of calcium ions during the cardiac action potential.

(e)   No. There is some influx of calcium during the action potential; this triggers a much greater release from intracellular stores. So the increase in calcium concentration in the myocardial fibres is due mainly to this release from intacellular stores.

7.40

(a)   Yes. The Purkinje fibres run subendocardially, so this muscle is activated first.

(b)   No. The first heart sound (lub) is longer than the second (dupp).

(c)   Yes. The second heart sound is due to the closure of the aortic and pulmonary valves and signals the end of the phase of ejection of blood from the ventricles.

(d)   No. Diastole shortens when heart rate increases. Systole shortens less, although the shortening is significant.

(e)   Yes. The vagal slowing effect is predominant over the sympathetic, so removal of both influences would lead to a higher heart rate.

7.41

(a)   No. The heart generates its own autonomous rhythm (in the sino-atrial node) and continues to beat if nerve impulses via its autonomic innervation are blocked.

(b)   Yes.

(c)   No. The heart rate is decreased by vagal stimulation. Indeed there may be cardiac arrest.

(d)   No. The diameter of the arterioles in the coronary circulation is mainly controlled by humoral influences (local and circulating chemical factors). Neural influences are much less significant.

(e)   No. The force of the myocardial contraction is sufficient during systole to reduce the overall flow, because of the squeezing of vessels in the inner part of the wall of the left ventricle: this muscle receives most of its blood flow during diastole; the outermost muscle, however, has a greater flow during systole.

7.42

(a)   Yes.

(b)   Yes.

(c)   No. Vagal (parasympathetic) stimulation has the opposite effect.

(d)   Yes.

(e)   Yes.

7.43

(a)   No. The venous return is impeded by the increase in intrathoracic pressure.

(b)   Yes.

(c)   Yes. The increase in intrathoracic pressure reduces the transmural pressure across the wall of aortic arch, and hence the stretch of the baroreceptors; there are therefore reflex increases in heart rate and peripheral resistance, as long as the manoeuvre is maintained.

(d)   Yes. The raised intrathoracic pressure causes back pressure in the jugular veins, which are in direct communication with the cerebral venous sinuses; the intracranial pressure, measured as CSF pressure, therefore rises.

(e)   No. Cardiac output decreases because of the reduction in venous return.

7.44

(a)   No. The activity is being conducted through the atria at this time.

(b)   No. The QRS complex signals depolarization of various regions of the ventricular system, systole continues until repolarization, at the T wave. So ventricular systole lasts much longer than the QRS complex.

(c)   No. The other way round: if both are blocked, the heart rate rises.

(d)   No. It must rise from around zero to the aortic diastolic pressure, which means a rise of at least 60 mmHg.

(e)   No. The rate of emptying reaches a high peak immediately after opening of the aortic valve and declines very rapidly from that peak.

7.45

(a)   Yes.

(b)   No. Noradrenaline causes a decrease in the potassium conductance of the membranes of pacemaker cells; this contributes to the increase in rate of depolarization and is part of the mechanism of the tachycardia.

(c)   Yes.

(d)   Yes.

(e)   No. The duration of the cardiac action potential is decreased.

7.46

(a)   No. At rest, the duration of diastole is about twice that of systole.

(b)   Yes.

(c)   No. At rest, about 50% of the end-diastolic blood volume is ejected during systole.

(d)   No. The maximum increase in stroke volume in exercise is about two and a half-fold.

(e)   No. Both cardiac and skeletal muscle have one capillary per muscle fibre, but since skeletal muscle fibres are thicker than cardiac muscle fibres, there are about six times as many capillaries per unit mass in myocardial tissue.

7.47

(a)   No. The heart can continue to beat – but not indefinitely – without a functional brain-stem if breathing is artificially maintained.

(b)   No. The initiation of heart beats depends on the heart's own rhythmically discharging pacemaker in the sino-atrial node.

(c)   No. Neuromuscular blockade affects the action of skeletal muscle only.

(d)   No. End-plates are a feature of the innervation of skeletal muscle only.

(e)   Yes. Although pacemaker discharge frequency is normally regulated by autonomic innervation, it will continue at its own inherent frequency if denervated.

7.48

(a)   Yes. During ventricular diastole, the pressure in the aorta exceeds that in the left ventricle, so with an incompetent aortic valve, blood flows from the aorta into the left ventricle.

(b)   Yes. The diastolic pressure in the aorta tends to be lower than usual due to leakage of blood from aorta to left ventricle during diastole. As a result, there is likely to be a higher pulse pressure than normal.

(c)   Yes. In addition to its normal work, the left ventricle must pump out blood that leaks back during diastole.

(d)   No. Isovolumetric relaxation depends on both inlet and outlet valves being closed.

(e)   No. This implies accumulation of blood in the ventricle, which would occur only in left ventricular failure.

7.49

(a)   Yes. Right ventricular failure leads to a build-up in pressure in the systemic veins, one result of which is ascites.

(b)   Yes. Due to venous engorgement.

(c)   Yes. Due to low cardiac output, and hence greater deoxygenation of blood in the tissues.

(d)   No. See (e).

(e)   No. This would be the case in left ventricular failure.

Be comfortable with this one but do not worry — you're great

8 Circulation

QUESTIONS

Flow in tubes and blood vessels

8.1   The flow (volume per unit time) through blood vessels:
(a)   varies directly with the pressure difference from one end to the other.
(b)   varies directly with the square of the radius.
(c)   varies directly with the length of the vessel.
(d)   varies inversely with the viscosity of the fluid.
(e)   is directly proportional to velocity (distance/time).

8.2   Blood is pumped at constant pressure P_1 through an isolated artery as shown in Figure 8.2.

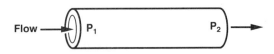

(a)   the flow would be decreased by increasing P_2.
(b)   the flow would be decreased by adding more packed cells to the blood.
(c)   the flow would be decreased by stretching the vessel lengthways.
(d)   the flow would be decreased by pharmacologically paralysing the vascular smooth muscle.
(e)   with the vascular smooth muscle pharmacologically paralysed, the flow would be decreased by increasing pressures P_1 and P_2 by the same amount.

8.3   In Figure 8.3, liquid is being pumped at a constant volume per minute along a tube in the direction shown by the arrow.

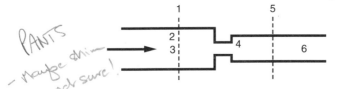

(a)   the flow (in ml per min) across plane 1 equals that across plane 5.
(b)   the mean velocity of flow across plane 1 equals that across plane 5.
(c)   the kinetic energy per gram of fluid is greater at plane 1 than at plane 5.
(d)   turbulence is more likely to occur at point 4 than point 6.
(e)   if the liquid is blood and the flow at plane 1 is laminar, the packed cell volume (PCV) at 3 is greater than at 2.

8.4   In a system of rigid cylindrical tubes represented by lines in Figure 8.4, fluid is flowing into tube A. A divides into B and C, of equal length. These latter then join to form tube D; against each tube is indicated its resistance.

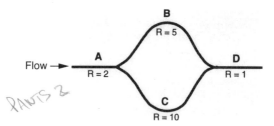

(a)   the volume flow (ml per min) is the same in tube A as in tube D.
(b)   the volume flow (ml per min) in B and C together equals that in tube A.
(c)   the volume flow (ml per min) in tube B is half that in tube C.
(d)   the velocity of flow (cm per min) is the same in tube A as in tube D.
(e)   the pressure at the end of tube A is less than the pressure at the start of tube D.

8.5   **With further reference to Figure 8.4:**
(a)   the resistance across tubes B and C (from the end of A to the start of D) is 15 units.
(b)   the total resistance from the start of tube A to the end of tube D is less than 3 units.
(c)   the pressure drop from the beginning to the end of B is the same as that from the beginning to the end of C.
(d)   deduced from the relative resistances of the tubes, the diameter of tube B is twice that of tube C.
(e)   the average transit time of the liquid is shorter via tube B than via tube C.

8.6 This question is about flow in cylindrical tubes. For each part of the question, you are to decide whether the relationship shown in the sketch diagram below left is appropriate for the feature described below right.

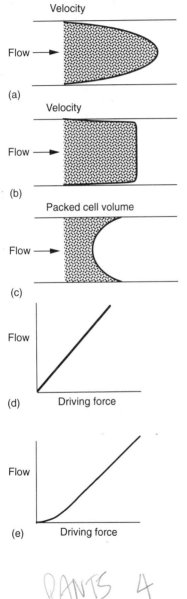

(a) flow velocity profile for a stream of an aqueous solution.

(b) flow velocity profile for a stream of blood.

(c) packed cell volume (PCV) profile for a moving stream of blood.

(d) relationship between driving force and flow for an aqueous solution.

(e) relationship between driving force and flow for blood.

PANTS 4

Check your pants
but not too
thoroughly

8.7   Figure 8.7 represents an arteriole, a venule and a capillary bed.
The resistances of all five capillaries are equal. The pressures in
the arteriole and in the venule remain constant.

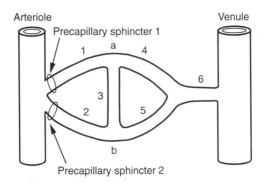

(a)   with both precapillary sphincters open, blood flows in capillary 3 from
a to b.
(b)   constriction of precapillary sphincter 2 reduces the blood flow through
capillary 2.
(c)   if precapillary sphincter 2 constricts but sphincter 1 is relaxed, the
blood flow in capillary 3 is from a to b.
(d)   the direction of flow in capillary 3 can be reversed by changes
in the relative state of constriction of precapillary sphincters 1
and 2.
(e)   the direction of flow in capillary 5 can be reversed by changes
in the relative state of constriction of precapillary sphincters 1
and 2.

8.8   With further reference to Figure 8.7:
(a)   the summed flow through capillaries 1 and 2 equals that through
capillaries 4 and 5.
(b)   the summed flow through capillaries 1 and 2 equals that through
capillary 6.
(c)   if sphincter 1 closes, the flow through capillary 2 increases.
(d)   if either sphincter 1 or 2 closes, the flow through capillary 6 will
drop.
(e)   if sphincter 1 closes, the pressure in capillary network at site b will
drop.

8.9 A length of elastic artery is connected as shown in Figure 8.9A to a pump and a rigid tube. As the piston rises, fluid is pumped into the artery at a constant rate. Valves a and b arrange that, as the piston rises, the fluid is pumped into the artery and as the piston falls, there is no backflow of fluid from the artery. The time-course of flow into the artery is shown in Figure 8.9B.

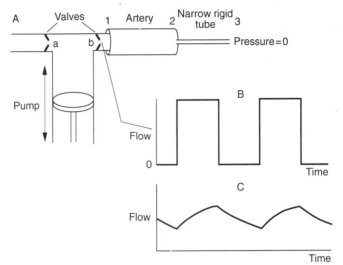

(a) as the pump piston rises and fluid is forced into the artery, the artery bulges.

(b) at every instant of time, the flow at position 1 is the same as at position 2.

(c) the average flow (volume per unit time) over several strokes of the pump is the same at position 1 as at position 2.

(d) Figure 8.9C could represent the flow at position 3.

(e) the maximum rate of flow at the outlet occurs at the start of ejection of fluid from the pump to the artery.

8.10 With further reference to Figure 8.9:

(a) the capacity of the rigid tube varies during the pump cycle.

(b) the pressure in the artery at position 1 is at zero during the part of the cycle when valve b is closed.

(c) the pressure in the artery at position 1 is at a constant level when valve b is open.

(d) the pressure in the artery at position 2 follows the same time course as the flow shown in Figure 8.9C.

(e) the effect of the arrangement set up in Figure 8.9A is to smooth the flow at the outflow of the rigid tube.

8.11 With further reference to Figure 8.9, if the rigid tube is replaced by another rigid tube of the same length but smaller diameter, by comparison with the situation with the wider tube:

(a) the average pressure at position 1 in the artery is greater.

(b) the average volume of the artery throughout a pump cycle is greater.

(c) the average speed of flow of fluid (in m per sec) through the rigid tube 3 is greater.

(d) at position 3, the fluctuation in flow expressed as a fraction of the mean flow is raised.

If this situation is used as an analogy to the circulation, with the rigid tube replaced by an arteriole:

(e) when an arteriole dilates, the fluctuation in blood flow in the capillaries it supplies becomes more pronounced.

8.12 With further reference to Figure 8.9, if the elastic artery from a young individual is replaced by a sclerotic artery from an aged individual, then by comparison with the elastic artery:

(a) the sclerotic artery will bulge more during the pump cycle.

(b) during each pump cycle, the pressure at 1 will rise to a higher level.

(c) during each pump cycle, the pressure at 1 will fall to a lower level.

(d) the oscillation in pressure at position 2 will be greater.

(e) the smoothing of flow will be more effective.

Blood vessel types, peripheral circulation

8.13 Capillaries:

(a) contain at any one time about 50% of the blood volume.

(b) are of a diameter approximately the same as that of a red blood cell.

(c) show an increased permeability in the presence of histamine.

(d) in the lungs are mostly separated from alveolar epithelium only by thin basement membranes.

(e) in the brain allow free exchange of hydrogen ions between plasma and interstitial fluid.

8.14 Concerning precapillary sphincters:

(a) they consist of smooth muscle cells.

When a precapillary sphincter closes:

(b) the mean capillary hydrostatic pressure rises.

(c) there is a net movement of fluid from the capillary lumen to the interstitial fluid.

(d) the colloid osmotic pressure of the luminal fluid rises.

(e) the flow of lymph from the tissue supplied by the capillary network rises.

8.15 **Concerning the capillaries in a particular vascular bed, if the venous pressure rises while the mean arterial blood pressure remains constant:**

(a) there is an increase in the rate of blood flow through the capillaries.

(b) there is an increase in the mean luminal pressure in the capillaries.

(c) there is an increase in the formation of tissue fluid.

(d) there is an increase in the colloid osmotic pressure of blood in the capillaries.

(e) there is passive distension of the capillaries.

8.16 **Concerning the peripheral circulation:**

(a) the velocity of blood flow (in cm per sec) is greater in the great veins than in the large arteries.

(b) the velocity of blood flow (in cm per sec) is greater in the capillaries than in the arterioles.

(c) capillaries are about 1 mm in length.

(d) capillaries are about 6 μm in diameter.

(e) the velocity of blood flow in capillaries is about 1 mm per sec.

8.17 **Concerning the peripheral circulation:**

(a) the walls of systemic arterioles contain proportionally more smooth muscle than any other type of blood vessel.

(b) most of the peripheral resistance is provided by the capillaries.

(c) arterioles are about 1 mm long.

(d) arterioles are about 1 mm in diameter.

(e) at any instant, more than half the blood in the circulation is in the veins.

8.18 **Concerning the peripheral circulation:**

(a) the total cross-sectional area of the systemic capillaries is greater than that of the systemic arteries.

(b) there are more arterioles than capillaries.

(c) in the supine posture, the mean systemic blood pressure decreases progressively around the peripheral circulation from aorta to venae cavae.

(d) the velocity of blood flow decreases progressively around the peripheral circulation from aorta to venae cavae.

(e) exchange of materials across the walls of vessels occurs mainly in the arterioles.

8.19   With respect to different types of blood vessels:

(a)   veins are more compliant than arteries of similar size (i.e. distend more for a given increase in intravascular pressure in the physiological range).

(b)   the wall of a capillary consists of endothelium and basement membrane only.

(c)   capillaries in all regions of the body show fenestrations in their walls.

(d)   all arterial vessels have smooth muscle in their walls.

(e)   arteries and arterioles are the only blood vessels innervated by sympathetic nerve fibres.

8.20   With reference to capillaries:

(a)   fenestrations are present in the renal glomerular capillaries.

(b)   cerebral capillaries have microscopically visible 'leaks'.

(c)   when skeletal muscle is active, there are more capillaries open than when it is at rest.

(d)   the diameter of a capillary in skeletal muscle is usually about twice the diameter of a red blood cell.

(e)   capillaries in the dermis actively constrict in response to sympathetic stimulation.

8.21   In capillaries in resting skeletal muscle (given that the extra-vascular hydrostatic pressure is equal to atmospheric pressure):

(a)   the mean hydrostatic pressure difference across the capillary wall would be 25 mmHg typically.

(b)   at the arteriolar end, there is a net movement of fluid from lumen to interstitial fluid.

(c)   at the venous end, the hydrostatic pressure of the blood exceeds its colloid osmotic pressure.

(d)   all the water that leaves the blood as it passes along the capillary is returned to the circulation via the lymphatic system.

(e)   the net loss of fluid from the blood as it passes along capillaries is about 10% of its volume.

8.22   Concerning the flow of blood in vessels:

(a)   at very low flow rates, the viscosity of blood is lower than at high flow rates.

(b)   in a vessel subserving autoregulation, increase in intraluminal pressure causes the vessel to dilate.

(c)   in an elastic artery, increase in intraluminal pressure leads to a fall in the resistance of the artery.

(d)   if there is a widespread replacement of elastic tissue in the walls of arteries by collagen, the pulse pressure rises.

(e)   in muscle, the change from rest to rhythmic contraction is accompanied by a rise in the rate of lymph formation.

8.23 **Concerning structure of blood vessels:**
(a)   there is a higher proportion of elastic tissue in the wall of an arteriole than in the wall of the aorta.
(b)   for blood vessels of similar diameter, the muscle layer is thicker in an artery than in a vein.
(c)   in their passage through capillaries, erythrocytes may become distorted.
(d)   veins actively constrict in response to sympathetic stimulation.
(e)   fenestrated capillaries are characteristic of brain tissue.

Cardiac output, blood pressure and peripheral resistance

8.24 **Does the change on the left imply that the change on the right must also have occurred?**
(a)   a fall in total peripheral resistance with constant mean blood pressure.   rise in cardiac output.
(b)   a fall in diastolic pressure with constant mean blood pressure.   fall in systolic pressure.
(c)   a rise in heart rate with constant cardiac output.   rise in stroke volume
(d)   vasodilatation in a localized vascular bed with constant mean blood pressure.   vasodilatation in other vascular beds.
(e)   vasoconstriction in a localized vascular bed and fall in flow to that bed.   fall in mean blood pressure.

8.25 **Concerning cardiac output, arterial blood pressure and peripheral resistance:**
(a)   if the heart rate increases and there is no increase in the venous return, the cardiac output is unchanged.
(b)   if at a given heart rate the arterial pressure rises and the diastolic pressure falls by the same amount, the mean arterial blood pressure stays the same.
(c)   if the cardiac output rises and there is no change in mean arterial blood pressure, the peripheral resistance must have risen.
(d)   if haemoconcentration occurs and there is no change in cardiac output or in peripheral vasodilatation/constriction, the mean arterial blood pressure must have risen.
(e)   if the contractility of the heart increases with no change in venous return, the end-diastolic volume increases.

Equations might be handy here.

8.26   Concerning the dynamics of the circulation:
(a)   the resistance of a rigid cylindrical tube is inversely proportional to the square of its diameter.
(b)   the arterioles contribute most of the resistance of the vascular bed.
(c)   the pulse pressure measured in a medium-sized artery is less than that in the aorta.
(d)   if the elastic tissue in the large arteries is replaced by inelastic tissues, the pulse pressure rises.
(e)   if the mean arterial blood pressure remains constant and the arterioles supplying a small vascular bed constrict, then the pressure in the capillaries supplied by those arterioles rises.

8.27   Concerning flow, resistance and pressure:
(a)   if the mean blood pressure remains constant when the peripheral resistance falls, the cardiac output must have remained constant.
(b)   if the mean blood pressure remains constant when the diastolic pressure falls, the systolic pressure must have risen.
(c)   if the cardiac output remains constant and the heart rate falls, the stroke volume must have fallen.
(d)   if the diastolic pressure remains constant and the pulse pressure rises, the systolic pressure must have risen.
(e)   if, in a local vascular bed, the flow decreases with no change in its vascular resistance, the cardiac output must have fallen.

8.28   With reference to the regulation of arterial blood pressure and cardiac output:
(a)   if cardiac output decreases, the arterial blood pressure will necessarily also be decreased.
(b)   during muscular exercise, the total peripheral resistance is unchanged.
(c)   increase in the force of ventricular contraction is one effect of an increase in sympathetic activity.
(d)   the main factor causing the increase in blood flow to exercising muscles is an increase in arterial blood pressure.
(e)   blood flow to the heart muscle (coronary flow) varies with the cardiac output.

8.29   With reference to the regulation of arterial blood pressure and cardiac output:
(a)   mean arterial pressure rises significantly during moderately severe sustained isometric exercise.
(b)   tilting a normal person from the horizontal to the vertical position results in an increase in heart rate.
(c)   constriction of veins is one of the responses to decreased arterial baroreceptor stimulation.
(d)   when the arterial blood pressure falls, ventilation decreases.
(e)   a decrease in ventricular end-systolic volume is one effect of an increase in sympathetic activity.

8.30 **Concerning the circulation:**
(a) the total peripheral resistance of the systemic circulation is more than five times greater than that of the pulmonary circulation.
(b) a rise in intracranial pressure leads to a reflex fall in mean arterial blood pressure.
(c) myogenic autoregulation of blood flow in a tissue is produced principally by venular smooth muscle.
(d) during inspiration, the right ventricular stroke volume increases.
(e) during inspiration, the left ventricular stroke volume increases.

8.31 **For each pair of statements, the change described on the left has occurred. Does this imply that the change on the right must also have occurred?**
(a) a fall in diastolic pressure with constant mean blood pressure — rise in systolic pressure.
(b) a fall in total peripheral resistance with constant mean blood pressure — fall in cardiac output.
(c) a fall in heart rate with constant cardiac output — rise in stroke volume.
(d) vasodilatation in a small vascular bed with constant mean blood pressure — vasoconstriction in other vascular beds.
(e) vasoconstriction in a small vascular bed and fall in flow to that bed — fall in cardiac output.

8.32 **In a normal human subject, if the change on the left has occurred, does this mean that the change on the right has also occurred?**
(a) increase in heart rate with constant venous return — fall in stroke volume.
(b) increase in mean blood pressure — reduction in mean firing rate of baroreceptors in the carotid sinuses.
(c) increase in mean firing rate of baroreceptors in the carotid sinuses — reduction in activity of the medullary vasomotor centre.
(d) increase in activity in the sympathetic innervation of the heart — increased contractility of ventricular musculature.
(e) tilting from the horizontal to the upright position — decrease in cardiac output.

8.33 **Suppose that the vascular resistance in a small structure S remained the same but the flow of blood through S decreased. Given that the venous pressure remains constant, is it true that the following necessarily occurred also?**

(a) the mean blood pressure has fallen.
(b) the cardiac output has fallen.
(c) the total peripheral resistance has fallen.
(d) the lymph flow from S has increased.
(e) if the oxygen consumption of S is unchanged, the oxygen extracted from each ml of blood passing through S decreases.

Blood pressure regulation

8.34 **Concerning the human heart and circulation:**

(a) if the venous return to the heart decreases, the cardiac output can be maintained constant by a rise in heart rate alone.
(b) increased stimulation of atrial baroreceptors results in reflex tachycardia.
(c) increased activity in arterial baroreceptors results in reflex tachycardia.
(d) in a normal standing adult, the mean arterial blood pressure at ankle level is at least 50 mmHg greater than that in the aortic arch.
(e) the reflex responses produced by tilting a normal human from the horizontal to the upright position include a fall in total peripheral resistance.

8.35 **If both carotid sinus nerves are cut, there is an increase in:**

(a) heart rate.
(b) mean arterial blood pressure.
(c) total peripheral resistance.
(d) activity of parasympathetic nerve fibres supplying the heart.
(e) ventilation.

8.36 **The graph represents a record of intra-arterial pressure from a healthy individual:**

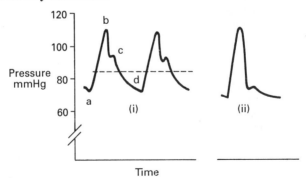

Time

(a) the dotted line is a good approximation to the mean arterial pressure.
(b) the rate of change of pressure from a to b is related to the force of contraction of the left ventricle.
(c) during the period b to c, the left ventricle would be relaxing isovolumetrically.
(d) the rate of change of pressure from c to d depends only on the peripheral resistance.
(e) record (ii) is from a more peripheral artery than record (i).

8.37   When a normal person lies down:
(a) heart rate settles to a higher level than when standing.
(b) venous return is immediately increased.
(c) cerebral blood flow settles to a higher level than when standing.
(d) blood flow in the apices of the lungs increases.
(e) lower limb veins constrict actively.

8.38   If arterial blood pressure falls, reflex effects mediated by arterial baroreceptors include:
(a) constriction of cerebral arterioles.
(b) constriction of muscle arterioles.
(c) constriction of veins.
(d) decrease in ventilation.
(e) increase in force of ventricular contraction.

8.39   Cardiovascular changes that usually occur within two minutes if a normal human subject is tilted from the horizontal to the 60° head-up position, with minimal activity of the leg muscles, are:
(a) net transfer of blood from intrathoracic reservoirs (lungs and great veins) to abdominal and leg veins.
(b) reduction of the end-diastolic volumes of right and left ventricles.
(c) increase in total peripheral resistance.
(d) increased rate of discharge of carotid sinus baroreceptors.
(e) increase in cardiac output.

8.40 Figure 8.40 represents a record of arterial blood pressure in an anaesthetized animal. Could the following produce the effects shown?

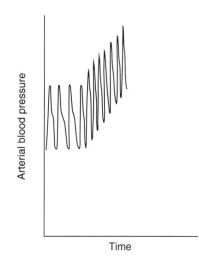

Time

(a) occlusion of the carotid arteries proximal to the carotid sinus.
(b) direct electrical stimulation of the carotid sinus nerves.
(c) direct stimulation of the peripheral ends of the divided vagus nerves.
(d) noradrenaline injection into the femoral vein.
(e) tilting the animal to head-up.

Regional blood flow

8.41 Myogenic autoregulation of blood flow in a tissue:
(a) tends to keep the blood flow constant despite changes in mean arterial blood pressure.
(b) is due to induction of contraction in smooth muscle in response to stretch.
(c) tends to keep the blood flow constant despite changes in metabolic activity of the tissue.
(d) depends on neural innervation of the blood vessels.
(e) is enhanced by anoxia.

8.42 **With respect to blood flow in different regions:**
(a) blood flow to the brain varies with the arterial blood pressure.
(b) blood flow to the myocardium is greater during diastole than during systole.
(c) blood flow to the kidneys is high relative to their oxygen requirement.
(d) voluntary hyperventilation increases the blood flow to the brain.
(e) the increase of skeletal muscle blood flow during exercise is mainly due to decreased sympathetic noradrenergic vasoconstriction.

8.43 **Concerning the hepatic portal venous system:**
(a) it joins two sets of capillaries lying in series with each other.
(b) it provides a means of transferring products of digestion from the alimentary tract direct to the liver.
(c) the control of secretion of insulin by the pancreas is aided by the direct passage of glucose absorbed from the intestine to the pancreas via the portal vein.
(d) the portal vein is the main route for the transfer of the products of fat absorption to the liver.
(e) during digestion of a meal, the hydrogen ion concentration of portal venous blood is greater than that of mixed venous blood.

8.44 **Cerebral blood flow:**
(a) varies little, overall, in normal physiological circumstances.
(b) is regulated mainly by the autonomic nervous system.
(c) increases if there is an increase in arterial PCO_2.
(d) decreases if the mean arterial blood pressure falls below about 85 mmHg.
(e) decreases if there is any increase above normal intracranial pressure.

8.45 **Concerning regional blood flow:**
(a) blood flow to the skin increases during heavy muscular work.
(b) blood flow to the myocardium increases when heart rate increases.
(c) in a hot environment, the arterio-venous difference for oxygen across the vascular bed of the skin is smaller than in a cold environment.
(d) at rest, blood in the coronary sinus (myocardial venous blood) has a lower oxygen content than the whole body average (mixed venous blood).
(e) at rest, blood in the renal vein has a lower oxygen content than the whole body average (mixed venous blood).

8.46   Concerning blood flow in the lungs:
(a)   blood flow in the pulmonary arteries is regulated by changes in the pulmonary vascular resistance.
(b)   the pulmonary vessels contain at any one time about a third of the blood volume.
(c)   the tissues of the lungs receive their blood supply from the pulmonary arteries.
(d)   bronchial veins drain into the pulmonary veins.
(e)   lymph flow from the lungs increases when pulmonary capillary pressure increases.

Miscellaneous

8.47   Oedema in the legs can be caused by:
(a)   cardiac failure with raised venous pressure.
(b)   decreased plasma albumin level.
(c)   raised systemic arterial blood pressure due to arteriolar constriction.
(d)   lymphatic obstruction in the legs.
(e)   lack of movement of the legs in the sitting posture.

8.48   Concerning the lymphatic system:
(a)   most of the lymph in the body is produced in lymph nodes.
(b)   the lymphatic system drains most of the plasma protein that escapes from blood in the capillary beds.
(c)   the rate of lymph flow from a tissue is equal to the gross rate of movement of fluid out of its capillaries.
(d)   brain tissue is drained by lymphatics.
(e)   the lymphatics which take up absorbed fat from the alimentary tract transport it directly to the liver.

ANSWERS

8.1
(a)   Yes.
(b)   No. Flow varies with the fourth power of the radius.
(c)   No. Flow varies inversely with the length of the vessel.
(d)   Yes.
(e)   Yes. But for the same flow, fluid travels more slowly in a wider vessel: velocity varies with flow and inversely with cross-sectional area.

8.2

(a) Yes. Increasing P_2 (simulating an increase in venous pressure) decreases the pressure drop across the artery and so decreases the flow.

(b) Yes. Adding more packed cells to the blood increases its viscosity.

(c) Yes. Stretching the vessel lengthways increases its length and decreases its diameter; both these factors will lead to an increase in resistance and hence a decrease in flow.

(d) No. Paralysing the vascular smooth muscle will result in dilatation and hence an increase in flow.

(e) No. If pressures P_1 and P_2 are increased by the same amount, this will increase the diameter of the vessel, decrease its resistance, and hence increase, not decrease, flow.

8.3

(a) Yes.

(b) No. For the same volume flow, the velocity of flow varies inversely with the cross-sectional area of the tube; since the tube is narrower at plane 5, the velocity is greater.

(c) No. Kinetic energy is proportional to the square of the velocity; it is therefore greater across plane 5.

(d) Yes.

(e) Yes.

8.4

(a) Yes. Since the system of tubes is rigid, the volume flow is the same in tube A as in tube D.

(b) Yes. The total flow from A divides between B and C, so the volume flow in B and C together equals that in tube A.

(c) No. Since B has half the resistance of tube C, the flow rate in B is twice that in C.

(d) No. The flow (in ml per min) is the same in both A and D, but since tube D is wider than tube A, the velocity of flow is less in tube D than in tube A.

(e) No. The pressure falls progressively along the path of flow and so will be greater at the end of tube A than at the start of tube D.

8.5

(a) No. Tubes B and C are in parallel, so the resistance across them is less than either. It can be calculated from the formula:
$1/R = 1/R1 + 1/R2$.

(b) No. The total resistance from the start of tube A to the end of tube D equals the sum of the resistances of A, of B and C combined (as in part (a)) and of D. Since A and D contribute 3 units, the total resistance must be greater than this.

(c)   Yes. The beginning and end of tubes B and C are connected so that the pressure drop across each must be the same.

(d)   No. The resistance of a cylindrical tube is inversely proportional to the fourth power of the diameter. So the ratio of diameters is the fourth root of 1/2.

(e)   Yes. In a cylindrical tube of diameter d:

Flow is directly proportional to d^4
Cross-sectional area is directly proportional to d^2
Average speed is proportional to flow divided by cross-sectional area, or d^2

So the transit time is inversely proportional to d^2. Clearly the diameter of tube B exceeds that of tube C, so the transit time is shorter in B than in C.

8.6

(a)   Yes. The parabolic profile is that given for laminar flow of an aqueous solution.

(b)   Yes. Blood gives this profile, as does any suspension of particles. The erythrocytes aggregate in the middle of the stream.

(c)   No. The aggregate of erythrocytes described in (b) is surrounded by a thin layer of fluid almost free of erythrocytes. So the PCV is close to zero at the walls and rises rapidly to a constant value across the path of the flow. The shape of the PCV profile is very like that shown in diagram B.

(d)   Yes. For an aqueous solution, there is a linear relation between driving force and flow.

(e)   Yes. For blood, for low driving forces and low flow rates, the ratio of flow to driving force is less than for high driving forces. This is because as the velocity increases, the erythrocytes form an aggregate surrounded by a plasma collar that provides an efficient low-viscosity lubricant to flow. The effective viscosity of blood is thus higher at lower flow rates, a phenomenon known as 'the anomalous viscosity of blood'.

8.7

(a)   No. Due to the symmetrical arrangement of five capillaries each with the same resistance, with both precapillary sphincters open there will be no pressure drop across capillary 3 and therefore no flow.

(b)   Yes.

(c)   Yes. If precapillary sphincter 2 constricts, the pressure in capillary 1 is greater than in capillary 2. Blood flow in capillary 3 is therefore from a to b.

(d)   Yes.
(e)   No. If sphincter 1 is closed, flow is through capillary 2 and thence divides between capillaries 3 and 5; in capillary 5, flow is from left to right. If sphincter 2 is closed, flow is through capillary 1 and thence divides between capillaries 3 and 4; the flow in capillary 3 continues through capillary 5 and is still from left to right in capillary 5. The direction of flow in capillary 5 cannot be reversed by changes in the relative state of constriction of precapillary sphincters 1 and 2.

8.8

(a)   Yes. This is true whether or not there is flow in capillary 3.
(b)   Yes. All blood entering capillaries 1 and 2 must leave through capillary 6.
(c)   Yes. With both sphincters open, all blood entering capillary 2 proceeds along capillary 5 and 6; none passes along capillary 3, so capillary 3 could be blocked off without altering the flow. The downstream resistance from point 2 is thus the sum of resistances of capillaries 5 and 6. With sphincter 1 closed, capillary 3 becomes available to carry some of the blood passing along capillary 2, which will divide into streams along capillaries 5 and 3. The overall downstream resistance for blood leaving capillary 2 will be less, so the flow will be increased.
(d)   Yes. Because closing of either sphincter increases the resistance of the capillary bed and therefore reduces flow, all of which must traverse capillary 6.
(e)   Yes. The resistance of capillary 2 is in series with a downstream resistance between point b and the venule. The pressure drop from arteriole to venule is constant. If sphincter 1 closes, the resistance of capillary 2 itself is unchanged but the total resistance downstream of capillary 2 is reduced. Therefore, the pressure at b is reduced by closure of sphincter 1.

8.9

(a)   Yes. As the pump piston rises and fluid is forced into the artery, the elasticity of the artery wall behaves like a sausage-shaped balloon and the artery bulges.
(b)   No. During the ejection phase of the cycle, the bulging of the artery acts as a store of blood. So during ejection, the flow at 2 is less than the flow at 1 and during the phase when valve b is closed, the artery recoils and maintains some flow through the rigid tube.
(c)   Yes.

(d)   Yes. Figure 8.9C shows the smoothing of outflow resulting from the elasticity of the arterial wall coupled with the resistance of the rigid tube.

(e)   No. The maximum rate of flow at the outlet occurs when the bulging of the artery is at its maximum, i.e. at the end of the phase of fluid ejection from the pump.

8.10

(a)   No. Since the tube is rigid, its capacity does not vary during the pump cycle.

(b)   No. During the ejection phase, the wall of the artery has bulged and this stores energy which maintains the pressure in the artery at position 1 during the part of the cycle when valve b is closed.

(c)   No. When valve b is open, the pump pumps fluid at a constant rate into the artery. The artery therefore bulges more and more during the ejection phase and the pressure rises.

(d)   Yes. Since the rigid tube acts as a constant resistance, we can apply Ohm's law to it. This tells us that the pressure drop across the rigid tube is proportional to the flow through it. So the pressure at position 2 follows the same time course as the flow shown in Figure 8.9C.

(e)   Yes. This point arises from the previous sequence.

8.11

(a)   Yes. Since the rate of flow, imposed by the pump, is constant and the total resistance of the system has risen, the average pressure at position 1 in the artery rises.

(b)   Yes. Fluid is being pumped into the artery at the same rate but output is being impeded by a higher resistance. Therefore the average volume of the artery throughout a pump cycle is greater.

(c)   Yes. The total volume flow through the system imposed by the pump is unchanged, and the speed of flow is inversely proportional to the cross-sectional area of the tube. So reduction in the diameter of the tube results in an increase in speed.

(d)   No. The time constant of the rise and fall of outflow equals the capacitance of the artery multiplied by the resistance of the rigid tube. A rise in resistance therefore results in an increase in the time constant. The flow rises and falls more slowly with the thinner tube and so the fluctuation in flow expressed as a fraction of the mean flow is reduced.

(e)   Yes. Arteriolar dilatation results in a reduction in its resistance and, by the converse of (d), there is an increase in fluctuation of outflow. This change may be so pronounced that the outflow changes from being continuous to being pulsatile.

8.12

(a)   No. The sclerotic vessel is more rigid than the elastic vessel and so will bulge less during the pump cycle.

(b)   Yes. Since the sclerotic artery wall does not expand so much, a given inflow during the ejection phase will result in the pressure at 1 rising to a higher level than for the elastic artery.

(c)   Yes. During the phase of no inflow to the artery, the stiffer walls of the sclerotic artery will not maintain the pressure so effectively as for the elastic artery and so the pressure at 1 will fall to a lower level.

(d)   Yes. The result of (b) and (c) is that the oscillation in pressure at position 2 will be greater for the sclerotic than for the elastic artery.

(e)   No. The smoothing of flow will be less effective.

8.13

(a)   No. This is about 10 times too much.

(b)   Yes.

(c)   Yes. This accounts for local swelling in response to injury.

(d)   Yes.

(e)   No. The blood–brain barrier prevents free exchange of charged particles.

8.14

(a)   Yes. A precapillary sphincter is a circular thickening of the arteriolar smooth muscle around the origin of a network of capillaries.

(b)   No. When the precapillary sphincter closes, this provides an upstream resistance to flow through the capillary so the mean capillary hydrostatic pressure falls.

(c)   No. Due to the decrease in luminal hydrostatic pressure, the gradient is from interstitial fluid to lumen and this is the direction in which fluid moves.

(d)   No. As a result of (c), the luminal fluid is diluted and its colloid osmotic pressure falls.

(e)   No. The cessation of formation of interstitial fluid means that the flow of lymph from the tissue decreases.

8.15

(a)   No. If the pressure across the capillaries decreases, the flow decreases.

(b)   Yes. An increase in venous pressure with no change in arterial pressure implies an increase in the mean luminal pressure in the capillaries.

(c)   Yes. Because of the increased luminal pressure, there is an increase in the formation of tissue fluid.

(d)   Yes. Because of ultrafiltration of luminal plasma, there is an increase in the colloid osmotic pressure of blood in the capillaries.

(e)   Yes. Because of the increased luminal pressure, there is passive distension of the capillaries.

8.16

(a)   No. The flow in veins is slower than in arteries. Although the flow in litres per minute entering and leaving the heart must be the same, the capacity of veins is greater, and so the flow is slower.

(b)   No. Flow is faster in arterioles, again because their capacity is smaller.

(c)   Yes, but very variable.

(d)   Yes. Just large enough for the transit of erythrocytes.

(e)   Yes.

8.17

(a)   Yes.

(b)   No. Most of the peripheral resistance is provided by the arterioles, which are therefore called the resistance vessels.

(c)   No. Arterioles are about 10 mm long.

(d)   No. Arterioles range from about 10–200 μm in diameter.

(e)   Yes. Since at any instant of time, about 60% of the blood in the circulation is in the veins, the veins are called the capacitance vessels.

8.18

(a)   Yes.

(b)   No.

(c)   Yes.

(d)   No. It becomes slower in capillaries, but speeds up again in veins.

(e)   No. Exchanges are mainly across the capillary walls.

8.19

(a)   Yes. Veins distend more, with very little pressure increase, up to the point of fullness, when pressure increases rapidly.

(b)   Yes.

(c)   No. This is true only in certain regions, e.g. in endocrine glands.

(d)   Yes.

(e)   No. Veins are also sympathetically innervated.

8.20

(a)   Yes.

(b)   No. They have tight junctions between the endothelial cells which contribute to blood–brain barrier function.

(c)   Yes.

(d)   No. Capillaries are about the same diameter or smaller: red blood cells are sometimes distorted in their passage through.

(e)   No. They cease to fill when precapillary sphincters constrict.

8.21

(a)   Yes.

(b)   Yes.

(c)   No. The reverse is true.

(d)   No. Most of the water filtered at the arteriolar end of the capillary returns to the blood at the venular end of the capillary, as the balance of forces changes direction.

(e)   No. The net loss is less than 1%.

8.22

(a)   No. At high flow rates, the formed elements in blood form a plug, with a thin layer of plasma between the plug and the vessel wall. This causes a reduction in viscosity. So at very low flow rates, the viscosity of blood is higher than at high flow rates.

(b)   No. In a vessel subserving autoregulation, increase in intraluminal pressure causes the vessel to constrict, thus maintaining a constant flow rate.

(c)   Yes. Increase in intraluminal pressure in an elastic artery distends the artery and so leads to a fall in its resistance.

(d)   Yes. If there is a widespread replacement of elastic tissue in the walls of arteries by collagen, the resilience of the artery wall is reduced, there is less stretching of the wall during the ejection of blood from the ventricle and the pulse pressure rises.

(e)   Yes. The change from rest to rhythmic contraction in muscle results in dilatation in muscle arterioles, a rise in capillary pressure and so a rise in the rate of lymph formation.

8.23

(a)   No. The wall of the aorta contains much elastic tissue, connected with its function of passive stretching during ventricular systole, partially storing the stroke volume, and its passive recoil during diastole which provides a continuous flow of blood to the tissues throughout the cardiac cycle. The walls of arterioles are rich in smooth muscle connected with the function of being a resistance vessel whose diameter can be controlled for appropriate regional distribution of blood. So there is a lower, not a higher, proportion of elastic tissue in the wall of an arteriole than in the wall of the aorta.

(b)   Yes. It is typical of blood vessels that the muscle layer is thicker in an artery than in a vein.

(c)   Yes.

(d)   Yes.

(e)   No. Capillaries in brain tissue impede the transfer of fluid and solutes; fenestrations are found in capillaries where there is a large flow of fluid, e.g. glomerular capillaries.

8.24

(a)   Yes. Mean blood pressure (MBP) = cardiac output (CO)/total peripheral resistance (TPR), so given that MBP is constant, CO must have risen if TPR has fallen.

(b)   No. Given that MBP is maintained, and diastolic BP has fallen, systolic BP must have risen.

(c)   No. CO = HR × SV, so if the one has gone up the other must have gone down.

(d)   No. Constant MBP with localized vasodilatation implies that there is some vasoconstriction elsewhere, an increase in cardiac output, or both. (There could also be vasodilatation in other vascular beds, if the cardiac output had increased sufficiently to maintain the MBP).

(e)   No. Local vasoconstriction reduces flow in the vascular bed at constant MBP.

8.25

(a)   Yes. The cardiac output equals the venous return. If the venous return does not increase along with heart rate, the stroke volume becomes smaller – there is less time for filling in each diastolic period.

(b)   No. The mean arterial blood pressure over the cycle is closer to diastolic than to systolic (at resting heart rate, mean blood pressure = diastolic pressure + 1/3 pulse pressure). So if the arterial pressure rises and the diastolic pressure falls by the same amount, the mean arterial blood pressure falls.

(c)   No. Mean arterial blood pressure = cardiac output × peripheral resistance. So if the cardiac output rises with no change in mean arterial blood pressure, the peripheral resistance must have fallen.

(d)   Yes. Haemoconcentration results in an increase in the viscosity of the blood. This increases the resistance term in the equation that relates flow, pressure and resistance. So if the flow is unchanged through the same vascular resistance, the pressure must have increased.

(e)   No. If the contractility of the heart were to increase with no change in venous return, the heart would contract more forcefully and expel more blood for a few cycles, so both the end-systolic and the end-diastolic volumes would decrease.

8.26

(a)   No. Resistance is inversely proportional to the fourth power of the diameter.

(b)   Yes.

(c)   No. Due to reflection of the pressure wave from branch points of the arterial tree, the pulse pressure is greater in a medium-sized artery than in the aorta.

(d)   Yes. Reduced elasticity causes both less distension (higher systolic pressure) and less recoil (lower diastolic pressure).

(e)   No. The pressure in the capillaries will fall in this situation.

8.27

(a)   No. Since mean blood pressure is proportional to cardiac output × peripheral resistance, the cardiac output must have risen.

(b)   Yes. Because mean blood pressure equals diastolic pressure plus one-third pulse pressure.

(c)   No. Since cardiac output equals heart rate × stroke volume, the stroke volume must have risen.

(d)   Yes.

(e)   No. The perfusion pressure must have fallen. Since this depends on cardiac output × total peripheral resistance, the fall could be due to any combination of changes in these variables.

8.28

(a)   No. A decrease in cardiac output can be compensated by an increase in peripheral resistance, so that arterial blood pressure is unchanged.

(b)   No. In exercise, although the systolic blood pressure (BP) increases, the mean BP is relatively unaltered. This implies that the increase in cardiac output is balanced by a comparable decrease in peripheral resistance.

(c)   Yes.

(d)   No. The main factor is a decrease in the vascular resistance in the muscle itself, together with mean arterial blood pressure maintained at or above the resting level by the increase in cardiac output.

(e)   Yes.

8.29

(a)   Yes. During isometric exercise, the contracted muscles squeeze the blood vessels within the muscles and there is a reflex increase in mean arterial blood pressure.

(b)   Yes. Tilting from the horizontal to the vertical position results in pooling of blood in the lower extremities, simulating a mild haemorrhage. The slight fall in systemic arterial blood pressure leads to a reflex rise in heart rate.

(c)   Yes. Decreased arterial baroreceptor stimulation leads to a reflex increase in sympathetic tone, with venoconstriction as one important component.

(d)   No. When the arterial blood pressure falls, ventilation is reflexly stimulated.

(e)   Yes. Increase in sympathetic activity increases the heart rate and strength of contraction. Both cause a decrease in ventricular end-systolic volume.

8.30

(a)   Yes. The equation cardiac output = mean arterial pressures/total resistance applies to both pulmonary and systemic circulations. If mean systemic BP is 90–100 mmHg, and mean pulmonary arterial pressure is 12–15 mmHg, then the ratio of resistances is typically about 6:1.

(b)   No. A severe rise in intracranial pressure leads to a rise in arterial blood pressure.

(c)   No. Myogenic autoregulation – constriction in response to a rise in pressure, and dilatation to a fall in pressure – is a function of arterioles.

(d)   Yes. During inspiration, an increase in right ventricular filling causes an increase in right ventricular stroke volume.

(e)   No. During inspiration the expansion of the lungs increases the capacity of the pulmonary vessels; this accommodates the greater right ventricular sroke volume so the filling of the left ventricle and its stroke volume do not increase.

8.31

(a)   Yes. This should be self-evident.

(b)   No. The cardiac output must have risen, by the same factor as the fall in total peripheral resistance, if blood pressure has not changed.

(c)   Yes.

(d)   No. Vasodilatation in a small vascular bed would have a very small lowering effect on blood pressure if nothing else were to change; but a similarly small increase in cardiac output could maintain the blood pressure.

(e)   No. A fall in flow to a vascular bed where there is vasoconstriction will occur without any change in blood pressure or cardiac output. (If the vascular bed concerned were of significant size, the constriction might cause a rise in blood pressure with reflex reduction in cardiac output.

8.32

(a)   Yes. The ventricles fill to a lesser extent during each diastole, so the stroke volume is reduced.

(b)   No. The baroreceptors respond to stretch, so firing increases when the blood pressure increases.

(c)   Yes. This is the part of the reflex response to a rise in blood pressure that leads to peripheral vasodilatation.

(d)   Yes.

(e)   Yes. This manoeuvre reduces the venous return, the filling pressure for the ventricle, and therefore the cardiac output.

8.33

(a)   Yes. This must be the cause of the reduction in flow.

(b)   No. A fall in blood pressure is not necessarily due to a fall in cardiac output – there could have been a fall in vascular resistance elsewhere.

(c)   No. A fall in blood pressure is not necessarily due to a fall in total peripheral resistance – there could have been a fall in cardiac output.

(d)   No. Lymph flow from S depends on the hydrostatic pressure in its capillary. If the arterial pressure has decreased and the pressure drop across arterioles is unchanged (vascular resistance unchanged) then the pressure in the capillaries must have fallen.

(e)   No. The blood flow is lowered, therefore a greater fraction of its oxygen must be extracted to maintain the uptake per minute.

8.34

(a)   No. Except for transient differences due to changes in the volume of blood held in the heart itself and in the lungs, left ventricular output equals venous return to the right atrium.

(b)   Yes. This is a protective reflex against an excessive rise in central venous pressure.

(c)   No. Such activity signals an increase in arterial blood pressure; the reflex effects include a fall in heart rate.

(d)   Yes. The mean blood pressure at the ankle is approximately the mean aortic blood pressure plus the pressure exerted by the column of blood from the aortic arch to the ankle. A column of blood 1 m high exerts a pressure of approximately 1000 mm H_2O, equivalent to $1000/13.6$ $= 80$ mmHg. (13.6 is the density of Hg.)

(e)   No. The pooling of blood in the veins of the legs and consequent reduction in venous return, cardiac output and arterial blood pressure results in reflex increase in sympathetic tone. One effect of this is arteriolar vasoconstriction, with a consequent increase in total peripheral resistance.

8.35

(a)   Yes. See (c).

(b)   Yes. See (c).

(c)   Yes. These are all sympathetically-mediated components of the increase in activity of the vasomotor and cardio-accleratory centres, released from inhibition by carotid sinus input (it 'looks as though' there has been a drop in blood pressure).

(d)   No. As sympathetic activity is enhanced, activity in parasympathetic nerve fibres to the heart is reduced.

(e)   No. The carotid bodies as well as the carotid sinuses have had their afferent nerve pathway interrupted. A small component of the drive to breathe is lost, so ventilation is a little depressed.

8.36

(a)   Yes. The mean pressure during the cardiac cycle is nearer to diastolic than systolic, and is approximately diastolic plus one-third pulse pressure.

(b)   Yes. The rise of pressure during ventricular systole is related to the force of contraction, but it will also be modified by the compliance of the arterial tree and the total peripheral resistance.

(c)   No. The ventricle is still ejecting blood into the aorta between b and c, that is until the dicrotic notch which signifies the point of closure of the aortic valve.

(d)   No. The fall-off of pressure in diastole will be related to both the peripheral resistance and the elastic recoil of the arteries.

(e)   Yes. In a more peripheral artery, the pulse pressure is greater but the mean pressure is a little lower than in a more central artery.

8.37

(a)   No. Heart rate becomes slower; venous return increases, cardiac output increases, rising blood pressure stimulates baroreceptors.

(b)   Yes.

(c)   No. Cerebral blood flow remains unchanged: a higher blood pressure would be accompanied by 'autoregulatory' vasoconstriction in the brain.

(d)   Yes. Gravity determines blood flow distribution to a great extent in the lungs. The perfusion pressure to the apices increases.

(e)   No. Constriction of lower limb veins occurs on standing.

8.38

(a)   No. Cerebral vessels dilate by autoregulation when blood pressure falls.

(b)   Yes. The skeletal muscle arterioles are an important part of the total peripheral resistance.

(c)   Yes. This is an important response to reduced arterial blood pressure, reducing the volume of the circulation, increasing ventricular filling and therefore cardiac output.

(d)   No. There may be an increase in ventilation, and it will be mediated by the chemoreceptors, not the baroreceptors.

(e)   Yes. This is a component of the responses mediated by an increase in sympathetic activity.

8.39

(a)   Yes.

(b)   Yes.

(c)   Yes. This is part of the baroreceptor reflex which restores arterial blood pressure after an initial fall.

(d)   No. The fall in blood pressure reduces the rate of discharge.

(e)   No. The cardiac output decreases and remains at a lower level than when horizontal. The heart rate increases reflexly, but stroke volume remains lower.

8.40

(a)   Yes. Occlusion of the carotid arteries proximal to the carotid sinus simulates a fall in arterial blood pressure and initiates pressor reflex effects.

(b)   No. Direct electrical stimulation of the carotid sinus nerves simulates a rise in arterial blood pressure and initiates reflexes to reduce the blood pressure.

(c)   No. Direct stimulation of the peripheral ends of the divided vagus nerves inhibits the heart, causing a fall in heart rate and hence in cardiac output and blood pressure.

(d)   No. The record shows a rise in both blood pressure and heart rate. Noradrenaline injection into the femoral vein causes a rise in blood pressure and, via the carotid sinus and aortic baroreceptor mechanism, the raised blood pressure causes a reflex fall in heart rate.

(e)   No. Tilting the animal to head-up results in pooling of blood in the dependent regions of the body. This simulates a mild haemorrhage and there would be an initial fall in blood pressure. Thereafter, there would be reflex responses to restore the blood pressure and heart rate.

8.41

(a)   Yes. This is the function of this physiological mechanism.

(b)   Yes. This is the mechanism of myogenic autoregulation.

(c)   No. Myogenic autoregulation buffers the effect of changing blood pressure, keeping flow constant when metabolic activity is constant; other mechanisms cause blood flow to vary to match changing tissue requirements for oxygen.

(d)   No. It is by definition inherent and independent of nerve supply.

(e)   No. The mechanism is paralysed by anoxia.

8.42

(a)   No. There is pressure autoregulation in the brain, maintaining near-constant flow when blood pressure changes.

(b)   Yes. Ventricular contraction diminishes flow, particularly to the innermost muscle.

(c)   Yes. Although the tubular cells have a high oxygen consumption, the renal blood flow is still relatively much higher and the arterio-venous oxygen difference is small; the high flow accords with the functions of filtration and reabsorption.

(d)   No. Hyperventilation reduces arterial PCO_2.

(e)   No. Sympathetic cholinergic and beta-adrenergic effects assist vasodilatation but the main factors are local metabolites.

8.43

(a)   Yes. The portal vein drains blood from the capillaries of the small intestine with those of the liver, i.e. it joins two sets of capillaries lying in series with each other.

(b)   Yes. The transfer of the products of digestion from the alimentary tract direct to the liver is the primary function of the portal venous system.

(c)   No. The portal vein does not drain into the pancreas.

(d)   No. The main route for the transfer of the products of fat absorption is from intestinal lymphatics via the thoracic duct into the left internal jugular vein. Thence these products must find their way to the liver via the general circulation.

(e)   No. During digestion of a meal, hydrogen ions are secreted into the lumen of the stomach and this is accompanied by alkalinization of the blood draining the stomach and entering the portal vein. Consequently, the hydrogen ion concentration of portal venous blood is less than that of mixed venous blood.

8.44

(a)   Yes. Although flow to different regions of the brain varies with their activity (e.g. localized parts of the motor cortex during voluntary movements) this makes no significant difference to the overall flow, which is normally near constant.

(b)   No. Blood flow in the brain is regulated mainly by local factors, myogenic and metabolic, and to some extent by intrinsic nerves.

(c)   Yes. Cerebral blood vessels dilate strongly to any increase in arterial PCO_2. Because CO_2 moves freely across the blood–brain barrier, an increase raises the interstitial acidity, and relaxes the vascular smooth muscle. The blood flow therefore increases.

(d)   No. This is within the autoregulatory range: vessels dilate and maintain near-constant blood flow until mean arterial pressure falls to about 60 mmHg; below this, the flow decreases.

(e)   No. At constant mean arterial blood pressure (BP), any increase in intracranial pressure (ICP) decreases the effective perfusion pressure; but there is autoregulatory vasodilatation, similar to that when the arterial BP itself falls. A progressive rise in ICP eventually reduces blood flow, although a reflex increase in arterial BP (the so-called cerebral ischaemic reflex) helps to maintain it.

8.45

(a) Yes. Skin blood flow increases because of the increase in core temperature, allowing additional heat loss.

(b) Yes. Although the shortening of diastole relative to systole tends to impede blood flow over the cardiac cycle, vasodilatation more than compensates for this.

(c) Yes. Because skin blood flow increases, serving heat loss rather than metabolic requirement, less oxygen is extracted per ml of blood, so the arterio-venous difference decreases.

(d) Yes. Even with the body at rest, the myocardium has a higher oxygen extraction ratio than the average; when its oxygen requirement increases, this is met by an increase in blood flow rather than an increase in extraction.

(e) No. At rest, the renal blood flow is high relative to its oxygen needs. This is because of the need to remove a large amount of fluid in the glomerular filtrate without causing an undue increase in viscosity of the blood of the efferent arterioles. As a result, the oxygen content of blood in the renal vein is more than the whole body average.

8.46

(a) No. The pulmonary blood flow is imposed by the cardiac output, varying with whatever factors are causing cardiac output to vary. The pulmonary vascular resistance changes in the opposite direction to alterations in pulmonary blood flow, so that the pulmonary arterial pressure alters very little. This is quite different from the systemic vascular beds.

(b) No. The fraction of the blood in the pulmonary vessels is little more than one-fifth – close to 1 litre out of the typical 5 litres. Of this about one-tenth (100 ml) is traversing the alveolar capillaries. The capacity can vary considerably, particularly of the pulmonary veins.

(c) No. The tissues of the lungs receive a systemic blood supply from the bronchial arteries, from the aorta.

(d) Yes. This adds a small amount of systemic venous blood to the oxygenated blood in the pulmonary veins, accounting for a component of the alveolar-arterial difference for oxygen.

(e) Yes. Any increase in pulmonary capillary pressure causes a greater loss of fluid into the interstices among alveoli; these drain to the lymphatic vessels and the lymph flow increases (note that there is no accumulation of fluid – pulmonary oedema – until or unless the increase in fluid extravasation is severe).

8.47

(a) Yes. Raised venous pressure engenders increased capillary pressure, which promotes the formation of oedema.

(b) Yes. Decreased plasma albumin reduces the plasma colloid osmotic pressure and thus promotes oedema formation.

(c) No. In this situation the pressure and osmotic relations in the leg tissues are balanced as in normal subjects. There is greater arterial pressure, but a greater drop from arteries to capillaries.

(d) Yes. Blockade of lymphatic drainage promotes oedema formation.

(e) Yes. The relatively high venous pressure in the legs in the sitting subject raises the capillary pressure and so favours the formation of oedema.

8.48

(a) No. Lymph is formed by drainage of tissue fluid, in turn derived from net loss from capillaries.

(b) Yes.

(c) No. The major fraction of fluid moving out of capillaries is reabsorbed into them.

(d) No. There are no lymphatics in the central nervous system.

(e) No. They drain, with the rest of the lymphatic system, into the great veins in the thorax.

9 Haemorrhage

QUESTIONS

9.1 Features of severe non-fatal haemorrhage include:
(a) reduced cardiac output.
(b) bradycardia.
(c) increased urinary output.
(d) cutaneous vasoconstriction.
(e) sweating.

9.2 Features of severe non-fatal haemorrhage include:
(a) reduced arterial blood pressure.
(b) reduced pulse pressure.
(c) net movement of fluid from interstitial fluid to plasma.
(d) hypoventilation.
(e) pupillary constriction.

9.3 12 hours after a severe non-fatal haemorrhage there is:
(a) haemodilution.
(b) an increase in blood concentration of adrenaline.
(c) an increase in blood concentration of aldosterone.
(d) an increase in blood concentration of vasopressin.
(e) an increase in blood concentration of haemopoietin.

9.4 Features of severe non-fatal haemorrhage include:
(a) pink skin.
(b) warm skin.
(c) thirst.
(d) increased blood concentration of atrial natriuretic factor (ANF).
(e) cyanosis.

9.5 One hour after a severe non-fatal haemorrhage there is:
(a) an increase in respiratory minute volume.
(b) an increase in urine osmolarity.
(c) an increase in plasma colloid osmotic pressure.
(d) an increase in packed cell volume.
(e) an increase in oxygen carrying capacity of the blood.

9.6   In haemorrhagic shock there is:
(a)   an increase in renal inulin clearance.
(b)   an increase in renal para-amino hippuric acid (PAH) clearance.
(c)   an increase in core temperature.
(d)   an increase in plasma renin concentration.
(e)   an increase in the total peripheral resistance.

9.7   Following moderate blood loss (e.g. 500 ml):
(a)   the arterial blood pressure may be normal.
(b)   skin vessels are constricted.
(c)   lymph flow from peripheral tissues is diminished.
(d)   the maintenance of brain blood flow is mediated by cerebral vasoconstriction.
(e)   the hypothalamic osmoreceptors are stimulated.

9.8   A normal 50 kg woman loses 1 litre of blood:
(a)   her blood volume is depleted by about 35%.
(b)   the loss of erythrocytes would amount to approximately 5×10^{12}.
(c)   heart rate would be likely to be over 100 beats per minute.
(d)   immediately after the haemorrhage, the haematocrit value would be increased.
(e)   the absorption of iron from the intestinal tract would subsequently increase.

9.9   The immediate effects of the sudden loss of 1500 ml of blood in a 70 kg person are likely to include a DECREASE of:
(a)   the packed cell volume.
(b)   the haemoglobin concentration in the blood.
(c)   venous return.
(d)   the rate of discharge from the carotid sinus (baroreceptors).
(e)   the rate of discharge of the right atrial pressure receptors.

ANSWERS

9.1
(a)   Yes. Due to reduced blood volume, the venous pressure, and therefore the filling pressure, for the heart is low, and ventricular stroke volume is reduced.
(b)   No. There is tachycardia as a component of the reflex response to haemorrhage.
(c)   No. Vasoconstriction of the renal afferent arterioles occurs, with a resultant oliguria.
(d)   Yes. Cutaneous vasoconstriction is one of the effects of the reflexly increased sympathetic output.

(e)   Yes. Sweating is another effect of massive increase in sympathetic output due to discharge of the sympathetic innervation of sweat glands.

9.2

(a)   Yes. The blood pressure is reduced as a consequence of the reduced volume of circulating blood.

(b)   Yes. This reflects the reduced stroke volume of the heart.

(c)   Yes. The arteriolar vasoconstriction leads to a reduction in hydrostatic pressure in capillaries and hence a net movement of fluid into the plasma. This is part of the homeostatic response, and contributes by returning the blood volume towards normal.

(d)   No. There is more likely to be hyperventilation.

(e)   No. There is pupillary dilatation due to sympathetic activity.

9.3

(a)   Yes. This is due to movement of fluid from the interstitial compartment to the plasma compartment.

(b)   to (e). Yes. These are all components of the endocrine response to haemorrhage.

9.4

(a)   No. After a haemorrhage the skin is white due to cutaneous vasoconstriction.

(b)   No. The skin is cold due to vasoconstriction and evaporation of sweat.

(c)   Yes. This is a response to hypovolaemia.

(d)   No. The pressure in the atria falls and consequently there is a reduction in the release of atrial natriuretic factor.

(e)   Yes. Hypovolaemia results in depression of cardiac output, and hypoperfusion of tissues leads to cyanosis.

9.5

(a)   Yes. Respiration is stimulated.

(b)   Yes. The anti-diuretic response to diminished circulatory volume is accompanied by an increase in urine osmolarity.

(c)   No. There is haemodilution and hence a decrease in plasma colloid osmotic pressure.

(d)   No. There is haemodilution and hence a decrease in packed cell volume.

(e)   No. There is haemodilution and hence a decrease in oxygen carrying capacity of the blood.

9.6

(a)   No. The glomerular filtration rate is reduced, so the renal inulin clearance is reduced.

(b)   No. The renal blood flow is reduced, so the renal PAH clearance
        is reduced.
(c)   No. Because of sweating, the core temperature tends to fall.
(d)   to (e). Yes. These are all hormonal responses to hypovolaemia.

9.7

(a)   Yes. Compensation for a slow, moderate blood loss can be con-
        tinuous and complete – as blood is lost there is vasoconstriction in
        the skin and splanchnic areas, and venoconstriction which reduces
        the capacity of the circulation; heart rate is also increased, so that
        cardiac output and blood pressure can be maintained.
(b)   Yes. See (a).
(c)   Yes. Capillary blood pressure will be reduced, so transudation
        diminishes, so lymph flow diminishes.
(d)   No. This would not make sense. If the arterial blood pressure is
        normal or low, constriction would diminish the brain blood flow
        further; cerebral vasodilatation accompanies any fall in arterial blood
        pressure.
(e)   No. There is nothing happening that could increase extracellular
        osmolarity.

9.8

(a)   Yes. At 50 kg she will have a blood volume of 3–4 litres.
(b)   Yes. 5×10^{12} erythrocytes per litre of blood is a typical normal
        value.
(c)   Yes. Compensatory reflex mechanisms, via an increased sympathetic
        outflow, increase the heart rate.
(d)   No. The first compensation for the reduced blood volume is a transfer
        of fluid from the interstitial compartment, which results from lowered
        capillary blood pressure; this dilutes the red cell mass, so haematocrit
        decreases.
(e)   Yes. Iron absorption is varied according to requirement. If the total
        body iron is diminished by blood loss, more is absorbed for
        haemopoiesis.

9.9

(a)   and (b) No. These effects depend on the transfer of interstitial fluid
        to the plasma and they take some time.
(c)   Yes.
(d)   Yes. The fall in blood pressure reduces the stimulus.
(e)   Yes. Because of the fall in atrial pressure.

10 Muscular work and exercise

Cardiorespiratory adjustments	10.1–10.8
Changes in other systems	10.9–10.11

QUESTIONS

Cardiorespiratory adjustments

10.1 During any rhythmic exercise (e.g. running):

(a) the maximal heart rate that can be reached decreases with fitness.

(b) training increases the amount of work that can be done at a given heart rate.

(c) the cardiac output can increase by a factor of 15.

(d) pulmonary vascular resistance increases.

(e) the diastolic blood pressure increases considerably.

10.2 With reference to adjustments in exercise:

(a) an increase in muscle blood flow begins after the first half minute of exercise.

(b) cerebral blood flow increases if the exercise causes systolic arterial blood pressure to rise.

(c) body temperature may rise measurably.

(d) lymph flow from the exercising muscles increases.

(e) visceral blood flow decreases.

10.3 Strenuous exercise in a healthy subject might typically:

(a) increase the transit time of blood through the pulmonary capillaries.

(b) increase the heart rate to three times the resting value.

(c) increase the stroke volume to three times the resting value.

(d) increase the systolic blood pressure.

(e) increase the splanchnic vascular resistance.

10.4 Comparing the uptake of oxygen during muscular activity with that at rest:

(a) if oxygen uptake by the whole body is trebled, the diffusing capacity of the lungs must be trebled.

(b) more oxygen is usually taken in from each litre of inspired air.

(c) more oxygen is extracted from each litre of circulating blood.

(d) more oxygen is transported to the tissues in each litre of blood.

(e) the increase in the rate of oxygen uptake in the lungs is assisted by an increase in the PO_2 difference between mixed venous blood and alveolar gas.

10.5 **When oxygen consumption is increased from its resting value by a factor of 10 in exercise:**

(a) the rate of oxygen delivery to the tissues (cardiac output × oxygen content in arterial blood) is multiplied by 10.

(b) the oxygen saturation of arterial blood is increased.

(c) the oxygen content in mixed venous blood is decreased by a factor of 10.

(d) the PO_2 of mixed venous blood would be around 40 mmHg.

(e) the PO_2 of the blood leaving the working muscles is lower than that of mixed venous blood.

10.6 **At progressively higher work rates on a cycle ergometer:**

(a) the pulmonary ventilation increases linearly in proportion to work rate up to the point of exhaustion.

(b) the oxygen consumption increases linearly in proportion to work rate until about 50% of maximal work rate is reached.

(c) plasma lactate concentration starts to rise steeply at about 50% of the maximal work rate.

(d) the respiratory exchange ratio (CO_2 output/O_2 uptake) decreases.

(e) plasma potassium concentration rises progressively.

10.7 **An endurance exercise training regime is likely to lead to an increase in:**

(a) capillary density in exercised muscles.

(b) number of muscle fibres in exercised muscles.

(c) cross-sectional area of exercised muscles.

(d) arterial blood pressure at a given work load.

(e) vital capacity.

10.8 **With reference to different types of muscular work or exercise:**

(a) during strenuous effort that is isometric (static) there is usually a significant rise in mean arterial blood pressure.

(b) isometric contraction at 40% of the instantaneous maximal voluntary force of contraction (MVC) can be sustained for at least 10 minutes.

(c) 'concentric' contractions (with muscle shortening) are more liable to cause muscle damage than 'eccentric' contractions (with muscle lengthening).

(d) an all-out effort lasting 30 seconds involves predominantly anaerobic muscle metabolism.

(e) the rise in plasma lactate concentration which accompanies strenuous exercise is reversed immediately the exercise stops.

Changes in other systems

10.9 **During heavy prolonged muscular work or exercise:**
(a)   muscle uses up its glycogen store.
(b)   blood glucose concentration falls progressively from the start.
(c)   circulating catecholamines promote gluconeogenesis.
(d)   arterial carbon dioxide tension increases.
(e)   plasma lactate concentration increases.

10.10 **Concerning thermoregulation in exercise:**
(a)   body temperature may rise by up to 5°C during strenuous exercise.
(b)   the most effective means of heat loss in exercise is by radiation from warm skin.
(c)   for maximal cooling, sweat should be wiped off as promptly as possible.
(d)   a healthy person exercising in unaccustomed heat may produce about 1 litre of sweat per hour.
(e)   exercise training at high ambient temperature leads to a reduction in the sweating rate.

10.11 **With reference to fluid exchange in exercise:**
(a)   net loss of 1–2 litres of body water can significantly diminish athletic performance.
(b)   exercise stimulates the secretion of anti-diuretic hormone.
(c)   taking a sugary drink immediately beforehand is a good way of providing energy for exercise.
(d)   thirst is a good guide to the water deficit during exercise.
(e)   water is absorbed more rapidly during exercise than at rest.

ANSWERS

10.1
(a)   No. Young healthy individuals have approximately the same maximal heart rate (around 190) however fit or unfit they are; the difference is in the severity of exercise at which they reach that rate.
(b)   Yes. This is partly because training improves the possible increase in stroke volume so that cardiac output is greater at a given heart rate; partly also because the work done at a given cardiac output is increased by more effective oxygen extraction in the working muscles.

(c)   No. Cardiac output may increase by about × 5. Since oxygen supply can increase by a factor of 15, greater extraction from the blood must account for × 3.

(d)   No. It decreases as the cardiac output increases.

(e)   No. The diastolic blood pressure tends to decrease in rhythmic exercise because of the lowering of peripheral resistance by vasodilatation in the muscles.

10.2

(a)   No. Vasodilatation is virtually immediate when muscle activity starts.

(b)   No. Total cerebral blood flow does not change appreciably: if the mean arterial blood pressure rises, brain blood flow is prevented from rising by autoregulatory cerebral vasoconstriction. (Modern methods of mapping regional cerebral blood flow show a localized increase in those areas of the brain 'switched on' during motor activity in exercise: this is a small localized adjustment of blood flow, meeting the needs of increased neuronal metabolism.)

(c)   Yes.

(d)   Yes. Both capillary blood pressure (because of arteriolar dilatation) and surface area (because of opening of more channels), are greater than at rest; more fluid leaves the bloodstream, and the muscle pump assists an increase in lymph flow.

(e)   Yes. Cardiovascular adjustments to exercise include splanchnic vasoconstriction, part of a series of changes that tend to divert blood flow from temporarily inessential areas to skeletal muscle. (This 'diversion', however, is a very small contribution to the muscle blood flow, compared with the increase in cardiac output.)

10.3

(a)   No. The transit time of blood through the pulmonary capillaries would be decreased.

(b)   Yes. Say from 60 to 180 beats per min.

(c)   No. The stroke volume may double, but not treble. Resting stroke volume is about the same as the resting residual volume. In exercise it increases by both greater filling and greater emptying.

(d)   Yes.

(e)   Yes. There is depression of gastro-intestinal and hepatic metabolic function in the presence of increased sympathetic activity of exercise;

concomitantly the splanchnic blood flow is reduced by an increase in vascular resistance.

10.4

(a)   No. The diffusion rate of oxygen from lungs to blood in ml per min must clearly be trebled. The diffusing capacity is defined as the rate of transfer per mmHg PO_2 difference across the alveolar–capillary membrane. The increase in diffusion rate is achieved both by an increase in the pressure gradient (because mixed venous oxygen goes down) and an increase in diffusing capacity (because the area of the alveolar–capillary interface increases).

(b)   Yes. The mixed expired oxygen percentage decreases. With increased tidal volume, a greater fraction of the expired volume comes from the alveolar regions, where the oxygen percentage remains close to its resting value; the mixture with gas exhaled unchanged from the dead space therefore has a lower oxygen percentage than at rest.

(c)   Yes. The extra oxygen supply to exercising muscles is obtained partly by extra blood flow, and partly by extraction of a greater fraction of the oxygen from the blood.

(d)   No. Haemoglobin cannot carry more oxygen per litre since it is normally virtually saturated at rest.

(e)   Yes.

10.5

(a)   No. The rate of oxygen delivery to the tissues is increased, but not by a factor of 10. Cardiac output can typically increase only about five times (except in the highly trained) and the oxygen content of the blood is already at its maximum at rest.

(b)   No. Because haemoglobin is virtually fully saturated at rest, arterial oxygen content remains the same in exercise.

(c)   No. The typical mixed venous oxygen content at rest is 150 ml per litre of blood. One-tenth would be 15 ml per litre or 7.5% saturation. Even blood from the working muscles will not be as desaturated as this, and it mixes with blood from other parts of the body that are extracting much less oxygen than the muscles. The mixed venous oxygen content is unlikely to fall below about 25% saturation, or 50 ml per litre. Thus the oxygen extraction (shown by the arterio-venous difference) for the whole body can increase up to about three times from 50 ml per litre at rest to 150 ml per litre in exercise. Combined with a five-fold increase in cardiac output, this could allow a 15-fold increase in oxygen consumption. For a 10-fold increase, cardiac output and oxygen extraction must both increase; the proportion that each contributes may vary, e.g. with training.

(d)   No. This is the typical mixed venous PO_2 at rest. It decreases during exercise.

(e)   Yes.

10.6

(a)   No. From a level of exercise about 50% of maximal oxygen consumption, the ventilation starts to rise more steeply, leading to hypocapnia.

(b)   No. Oxygen consumption continues to increase linearly with work rate until it flattens out at its maximum, close to exhaustion, even though anaerobic glycolysis is significantly contributing to the effort from about 50% of the maximum.

(c)   Yes. This is known as the lactate (or anaerobic) threshold, when a significant increase in lactate is measurable in the blood, reflecting anaerobic glycolysis in the working muscles.

(d)   No. At increasing work rate, the respiratory exchange ratio increases; more CO_2 is lost from the body partly because of its release from bicarbonate by the lactacidaemia.

(e)   Yes.

10.7

(a)   Yes.

(b)   No. The muscles get bigger, but by increase in size of fibres.

(c)   Yes.

(d)   No. The arterial blood pressure at a given work load is more likely to decrease.

(e)   No. Vital capacity is unlikely to increase: the lungs and breathing capacity are not normally limiting factors in exercise.

10.8

(a)   Yes. Both systolic and diastolic blood pressure rise in most individuals during contractions above 20–30% of maximal voluntary contraction force.

(b)   No. A contraction of 40% MVC can only be sustained for about two minutes.

(c)   No. Eccentric contractions are more liable to cause damage to the stretched muscle fibres.

(d)   Yes.

(e)   No. The rise in plasma lactate continues for several minutes after the end of a strenuous effort as more is released from recovering muscles.

10.9

(a)   Yes. This is the first fuel to be used.

(b)   No. Blood glucose is maintained or increased implying a greater mobilization that more than matches the increase in muscle utilization in the early stages. Later, as fatty acids are mobilized and liver glycogen stores diminish, blood glucose may decrease.

(c)   Yes. Both direct sympathetic stimulation and circulating catecholamines stimulate gluconeogenesis.

(d)   No. Arterial PCO_2 is kept normal initially, by an appropriate increase in alveolar ventilation. It decreases at higher levels of exercise when the 'ventilatory threshold' is reached because of an additional stimulus to ventilation, generally attributed to lactic acidaemia.

(e)   Yes. The anaerobic component of metabolism releases lactic acid, causing decreased plasma pH and increased plasma lactate.

10.10

(a)   No. This would be lethal. Body temperature may rise by up to 3°C.

(b)   No. The most effective means of heat loss is by evaporation of sweat.

(c)   No. Wiping off the sweat defeats the purpose of evaporative cooling of the skin.

(d)   Yes.

(e)   No. Acclimatization by exercising in hot surroundings leads to an increase in sweating rate, allowing a greater evaporative heat loss.

10.11

(a)   Yes.

(b)   Yes. For this reason, water drunk just prior to exercise does not produce the diuresis it would produce at rest.

(c)   No. Taking a sugary drink stimulates insulin secretion, which diminishes both the availability of plasma glucose to exercising muscle and the mobilization of fatty acids.

(d)   No. Taking the amount of water dictated by thirst alone does not meet the deficit due to sweating during strenuous exercise; this is partly because salt is lost as well as water.

(e)   No. The reduction in visceral blood flow and gastric motility in exercise delays stomach emptying and intestinal absorption. Any solute causes still further delay.

11 Special senses, somaesthetic receptors

Vision and visual pathways	11.1–11.18
Hearing	11.19–11.22
Somaesthetic receptors, receptors in general and sensory function	11.23–11.29

QUESTIONS

Vision and visual pathways

11.1 Concerning human vision:

(a) with near-threshold light stimuli to the dark adapted eye, stimuli exactly on the visual axis are less easily seen than those slightly off the visual axis.

(b) the normal dark-adapted subject can recognize the colour of near-threshold light stimuli.

(c) in a well-illuminated room, an emmetrope with one dioptre of accommodation looks with one eye at a page of writing held at 30 cm. His facility of reading will improve if he looks through a disc with a pinhole in the middle.

(d) the direct pupillary light reflex depends on the integrity of the visual area of the cerebral cortex.

(e) if a normal subject changes his focus point from 25 cm to infinity, there is an accompanying constriction of the pupils.

11.2 Concerning vision and eye movements:

(a) a lesion of the 6th cranial nerve results in inward deviation of the ipselateral eyeball.

(b) when a subject reads, his eyes move smoothly to scan the page.

(c) if a subject watches an object moving at a constant velocity, his eyes move smoothly to follow the object.

(d) the lateral semicircular canals are more closely connected with the eye muscles causing lateral eye movements than with those causing vertical eye movements.

(e) nystagmus can be induced in a normal subject without stimulation of the semicircular canals.

11.3 **Concerning normal human vision:**
(a)   for most normal humans, visual input is necessary for accurate alignment of the visual axis.
(b)   during dark-adaptation, the sensitivity of the eye increases by about 10-fold.
(c)   dark adaptation depends principally on pupillary dilatation.
(d)   the lens contributes more than the anterior surface of the cornea to the refractory power of the eyeball.
(e)   if the eyes are open under water, they can form focused images of an illuminated underwater object on the retinae.

11.4   **Figure 11.4 shows pathways concerned with vision and pupillary reflexes:**

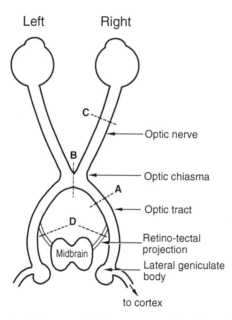

(a)   a lesion at A will cause a left homonymous hemianopia.
(b)   a lesion at B will cause a bitemporal heteronymous hemianopia.
(c)   with a lesion at C, light shone into the left eye will cause pupillary constriction in the right eye (consensual light reflex).
(d)   lesions at D will abolish the direct light reflexes on both sides.
(e)   lesions at D will abolish the reflex pupillary constriction with accommodation (the accommodation-convergence reflex) on both sides.

11.5 **Concerning the ciliary muscles and accommodation of the eye:**

(a) the increase in power of the eye needed for near vision is achieved mainly by an increase in curvature of the posterior surface of the lens.

(b) contraction of the ciliary muscle causes the lens to get thinner.

(c) ciliary muscle is multiple-unit smooth muscle.

(d) circulating adrenaline causes the ciliary muscle to contract.

(e) the nerve supply to the ciliary muscle runs with the optic nerve.

11.6 **An individual has 1 dioptre (1 D) of hypermetropia (hyperopia) and his range of accommodation is 2 dioptres: (1 D = 1/focal length in metres):**

(a) his near point is 1 m in front of his cornea.

(b) his far point is 1 m behind his cornea.

(c) he can clearly see distant objects.

(d) if his accommodation is paralysed by atropine applied to the eye, he can clearly see objects 1 m in front of him.

(e) if his accommodation is paralysed, a +3 D spectacle lens will allow him to see clearly an object 50 cm in front of him.

11.7 **Consider an emmetropic individual whose range of accommodation is 2 dioptres:**

(a) his near point is 1 m in front of his cornea.

(b) his far point is 1 m behind his cornea.

(c) he can clearly see distant objects.

(d) if his accommodation is paralysed by atropine applied to the eye, he can clearly see objects 1 m in front of him.

(e) if his accommodation is paralysed, a +2 D spectacle lens will allow him to see clearly an object 50 cm in front of him.

11.8 **Under dim illumination, the pupil diameters of a patient are both 8 mm. On illumination of the right eye with a pen torch, both pupils constrict to 3 mm. On illumination of the left eye, both pupils constrict to 6 mm. The following conditions would account for these observations:**

(a) a lesion of the left optic nerve.

(b) a lesion of the left oculomotor nerve.

(c) a lesion of the occipital lobe of the left cerebral hemisphere.

(d) an opacity of the lens of the left eye.

(e) loss of brain-stem function.

11.9   Concerning the nerve supply to the intrinsic eye muscles:
(a)   the dilator pupillae is supplied by the sympathetic nervous system.
(b)   the sympathetic nerve supply to the eye leaves the central nervous system at the level of the thoracic spinal cord.
(c)   the sympathetic fibres run from the spinal cord to the eye muscles without synaptic relay.
(d)   the parasympathetic nerve supply to the eye leaves the central nervous system at the level of the medulla oblongata.
(e)   the cholinergic receptors at the neuro-effector junction between the parasympathetic nerve fibres and smooth muscle are of the nicotinic type.

11.10   Concerning the eye and vision:
(a)   in a myopic ('short-sighted') subject, the image of an object on the horizon falls behind the retina.
(b)   in a myopic subject, the near point is further away than normal.
(c)   visual acuity depends on rods.
(d)   the rods and cones are visible through an ophthalmoscope.
(e)   a subject without cones is colour blind.

11.11   The eye contains two distinct sets of photoreceptors – the rods and the cones:
(a)   the rod system is specialized to respond in low levels of illumination.
(b)   the highest density of rods is found in the peripheral retina.
(c)   the convergence of many visual receptors on to a single bipolar neurone provides a structural basis for visual sensitivity.
(d)   the convergence of many visual receptors on to a single bipolar neurone provides a structural basis for visual acuity.
(e)   the terminals of the optic nerve fibres directly innervate the photoreceptors.

11.12   Concerning the eye and vision:
(a)   when parallel light rays pass from the air to the cornea, the light rays diverge.
(b)   atropine applied to the eye causes everything to appear dimmer.
(c)   atropine applied to the eye improves visual acuity.
(d)   the intermittent movement of the visual image on the retina caused by saccadic eye movements is essential for a person to be able to see.
(e)   a focal lesion in the primary visual area of the cortical convexity results in loss of vision in part of the ipselateral peripheral visual field.

11.13 Concerning the eye and vision:
(a)   the optic nerve contains axons of retinal ganglion cells.
(b)   the primary visual cortex lies in the parietal lobe of the cerebral cortex.
(c)   the part of the cerebral cortex to which an object lying on the visual axis projects is on the cortical convexity.
(d)   the fovea of one eye is represented in the visual areas of both cerebral hemispheres.
(e)   pupillary constriction is caused by increased activity in sympathetic nerves.

11.14 Concerning nystagmus:
(a)   the visual image is suppressed during the fast phase of nystagmus.
(b)   the fast phase is a ramp movement.
(c)   the fast phase of nystagmus depends on the integrity of the cerebral cortex.
(d)   the fast phase of nystagmus is in a direction such as to stabilize the visual image on the retina.
(e)   nystagmus occurs only if the eyes are open.

11.15 Concerning the eyes:
(a)   with damage to the optic nerve on one side, the pupils are symmetrical in size.
(b)   with damage to the oculomotor nerve on one side, the pupils are symmetrical in size.
(c)   if a point of light is presented in the peripheral visual field, the direction of gaze moves to bring the light on to the visual axis.
(d)   if the sympathetic innervation of one eye is interrupted, the pupillary response of that eye to light is abolished.
(e)   meningeal irritation may lead to pupillary constriction.

11.16 Concerning the eye:
(a)   the oculomotor nerve contains the motor nerve fibres responsible for blinking.
(b)   blinking is produced by smooth muscle.
(c)   the levator palpebrae superioris muscle contains smooth muscle fibres.
(d)   overactivity of the sympathetic nerve supply to the head results in drooping of the eyelid.
(e)   the parasympathetic nerve supply to the eye runs in the optic nerve.

11.17 In a subject who has suffered severe damage to the occipital cortex of one cerebral hemisphere:
(a) with both eyes open, the subject's peripheral visual field is as extensive as that of a normal person.
(b) there is a loss of foveal vision.
(c) a light shone on to part of the retina that evokes no vision can nevertheless evoke a direct light reflex.
(d) a light shone on to part of the retina that evokes no vision can nevertheless evoke a consensual light reflex.
(e) convergence with accommodation is present.

11.18 With reference to vision:
(a) the pupillary light reflex is dependent on the integrity of the midbrain.
(b) in a normal person, when light is shone into only one eye, both pupils constrict.
(c) dark adaptation is complete when the sensitivity of the cones has settled at a new level.
(d) vision in dim light is defective in vitamin D deficiency.
(e) the image of the visual field formed by the eye on the retina is inverted.

Hearing

11.19 Concerning the ear
(a) the receptor cells of the cochlea have efferent innervation.
(b) in the normal healthy subject, the cavity of the middle ear is filled with fluid.
(c) the differential sensitivity to a change in pitch at a given intensity above threshold is linearly related to frequency.
(d) the otolith organs are sensitive to the orientation of the head in space.
(e) the receptors in the semicircular canals are sensitive to gravitational forces.

11.20 With reference to hearing in a normal subject:

(a)   contraction of the tensor tympani muscle decreases sound transmission through the middle ear.

(b)   if two tones of equal amplitude, each with a frequency of 200 Hz but differing in phase by 1 msec, are heard by the two ears, the subject can detect this difference.

(c)   the intensity threshold for hearing is relatively independent of the frequency of a sound, in the range 50 Hz to 12 kHz.

(d)   the just perceptible difference in intensity of a 1 kHz tone is relatively independent of the intensity level at which it is tested.

(e)   the percentage change in frequency of a sine wave sound that is just detectable is less than the percentage change in amplitude of the sound.

11.21 With respect to the ear and hearing:

(a)   the lever system of the ossicles of the middle ear serves to amplify the movement of the ear drum.

(b)   high-pitched sounds are detected by receptors at the apical end of the cochlea.

(c)   the foot-plate of the stapes fits into the oval window.

(d)   contraction of the stapedius muscle causes an increase in the apparent intensity of a sound.

(e)   a subject in whom the middle ear ossicles become fixed will still be able to hear in the same ear the sound from a vibrating tuning fork held against his mastoid promontory.

11.22 Which of the following statements about the threshold of hearing curve are true?

(a)   the maximum sensitivity occurs in the range 1–3 kHz.

(b)   the threshold increases as the frequency of the tone is decreased below 1 kHz.

(c)   the lowest tone that a normal person can hear is 100 Hz.

(d)   the frequency of the highest note that a normal person can hear decreases as he ages.

(e)   if a vibrating tuning fork is placed firmly on the skin over the mastoid bone of a normal subject and its vibration is allowed to decrease until it just ceases to be audible, the subject will still be able to hear the note when the fork is held to his pinna.

Somaesthetic receptors, receptors in general and sensory function

11.23 Concerning cutaneous sensation in the human:
(a) a human can sense cold in skin in which the only sensory nerve endings are naked nerve endings.
(b) the distribution of touch sensitivity is punctate.
(c) skin receptors transmit to the spinal cord via axons that conduct at about 100 m/sec.
(d) two-point discrimination is better developed in the skin of the forefinger than in that of the arm.
(e) Pacinian corpuscles lie in the epidermis.

11.24 Figure 11.24 shows the membrane potential for a stretch receptor before, during and after a stretch.

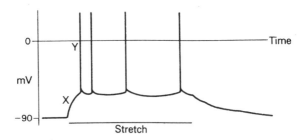

Are the following statements correct?
(a) the initial response to stretch (at X) is a generator potential.
(b) the initial response is a depolarization.
(c) stretch produces at Y a high amplitude generator potential.
(d) stretch produces a train of action potentials, which demonstrates adaptation.
(e) the peak voltage of the action potentials depends on the duration of the stimulus.

11.25 Concerning cutaneous sensation:
(a) the presence in skin of Meissner's corpuscles is necessary for the sense of touch.
(b) nociceptive nerve endings lie in the epidermis.
(c) Pacinian corpuscles are temperature receptors.
(d) in the skin, there are separate receptors for hot and cold.
(e) a receptor sensitive principally to cold and one principally sensitive to touch may connect with a common sensory nerve fibre.

11.26 Concerning sensation:
(a) in non-glabrous skin, the sensation of touch is mediated by free nerve endings.
(b) a single point on the skin can be sensitive to both pain and touch.
(c) the conjunctiva of the eye-ball is devoid of sensory receptors.
(d) a rapidly adapting receptor signals the rate of change of strength of a stimulus rather than its absolute intensity.
(e) skin sensitivity to change in temperature is important in reflex regulation of skin blood flow.

11.27 Concerning receptors:
(a) nociceptors have unencapsulated endings.
(b) the lamellae of a Pacinian corpuscle protect the nerve endings from mechanical distortion.
(c) the Pacinian corpuscle exhibits adaptation in its response to a maintained deformation.
(d) in all general (somaesthetic) senses, the receptor is the ending of the sensory nerve fibre itself.
(e) for special senses, the receptor is in most cases a modified epithelial cell.

11.28 There are sensory receptors in:
(a) the meninges.
(b) the cerebral cortex.
(c) the hypothalamus.
(d) the basal ganglia.
(e) the medulla oblongata.

11.29 Are these associations appropriate?
(a) activation of muscle spindle receptors — tapping the patellar tendon.
(b) cone photoreceptor — acuity of vision.
(c) rod photoreceptor — visual sensitivity.
(d) Pacinian corpuscle — heat receptor.
(e) free cutaneous nerve ending — Group 1A sensory nerve fibre.

ANSWERS

11.1
(a) Yes. Because the fovea, on the visual axis, is devoid of rods, which are the elements responsible for vision in dim light.
(b) No. Because in this situation cones are not excited.

(c)   Yes. The writing is closer than the subject's near point. The pinhole results in only the central part of the lens being used for focusing and this improves the resolving power of the eye.

(d)   No. The pathways for the pupillary reflexes pass from the optic tract to the midbrain without traversing the cortex.

(e)   No. The opposite occurs. The pupil dilates for distant, and constricts for close, objects.

11.2

(a)   Yes. The rectus externus muscle is supplied by the 6th cranial nerve and paralysis of this muscle results in inward rotation of the eye ball.

(b)   No. These movements are jerky; they are known as saccades.

(c)   Yes. Such tracking movements are smooth if the movement being followed is smooth.

(d)   Yes. The placement of the lateral canal allows detection of rotation of the head in the horizontal plane and hence the compensatory eye movements are lateral movements.

(e)   Yes. For instance, optokinetic nystagmus.

11.3

(a)   Yes. The Maddox rod test shows that if the fine detail of visual input to one eye is disturbed, the result is a non-alignment of the visual axes.

(b)   No. The factor is around 10 000.

(c)   No. Dark adaptation is principally due to retinal factors and it takes up to an hour.

(d)   No. The anterior surface of the cornea provides two-thirds of the refractory power of the eye.

(e)   No. This so reduces the refractory power of the eye that even an object at a great distance cannot be focused on the retina.

11.4

(a)   Yes. The right half of each retina is denervated causing blindness in the left half of the visual field of both eyes, i.e. a left homonymous hemianopia. 'Homonymous' means corresponding parts of the visual field in both eyes. 'Hemianopia' means that half of the visual field is lost.

(b)   Yes. The inner half of each retina is denervated causing blindness in both temporal and visual fields. 'Heteronymous' means different parts of the visual fields in the two eyes.

(c)   Yes. The efferent limb of the arc is via the 3rd nerve.

(d)   Yes. The pathway for the direct light reflex is via the retinotectal projection.

(e) No. This reflex depends on pathways from the oculomotor nuclei to the Edinger-Westphal nucleus and thence via III to the pupil; it does not depend on the retinotectal projection.

Note: A lesion at D causes loss of light reflexes but spares the accommodation-convergence reflex, a condition known as the Argyll-Robertson pupil.

11.5

(a) No. The increase in power of the eye is achieved mainly by an increase in curvature of the anterior, not the posterior, surface of the lens.

(b) No. Contraction of the ciliary muscle reduces the tension on the suspensory ligaments of the lens, allowing it to become thicker.

(c) Yes. Multiple-unit smooth muscle is smooth muscle in which the muscle units can be separately controlled by the motor nerves.

(d) No. The ciliary muscle is innervated by the parasympathetic nervous system.

(e) No. It runs with the oculomotor nerve.

11.6

(a) Yes. Since he has 1 dioptre of hypermetropia and 2 dioptre of accommodation, when fully accommodated his eye has strength of 1 dioptre: it is therefore focused 1 m ahead, which, by definition, is his near point.

(b) Yes. The 'far point' is, by definition, the point from which rays are brought to a focus on the retina by the relaxed (unaccommodated) eye.

(c) Yes. He exerts 1 dioptre of accommodation to focus on distant objects.

(d) No. If accommodation is paralysed, the refractive power is too weak to bring any real object to a focus on the retina.

(e) Yes. With a +3 D spectacle lens, the power of his eye is 2 dioptres, so the eye will be focused on objects 50 cm away.

11.7

(a) No. Near point = 0.5 m in front of his cornea.

(b) No. The definition of an emmetrope is that his far point is at infinity.

(c) Yes.

(d) No. If his accommodation is paralysed, his eyes are focused on infinity and so objects 1 metre ahead are not seen clearly.

(e) Yes. The power of the eye plus spectacle lens is then 2 dipotres, so it is focused 0.5 m = 50 cm ahead of him.

11.8

(a)   Yes. A lesion of the left optic nerve would reduce the afferent discharge when the left eye was illuminated and so reduce reflex effects.

(b)   No. A lesion of the left oculomotor nerve, carrying the para-sympathetic innervation of the dilator pupillae muscle, would influence the pupillary constriction of the left eye only.

(c)   No. A lesion of the occipital lobe of the left cerebral hemisphere would not interfere with light reflexes.

(d)   Yes. An opacity of the lens of the left eye would reduce the illumination falling on the left retina and so reduce reflex effects of illuminating the left eye.

(e)   No. With no brain-stem function there would be no light reflexes at all because the oculomotor nuclei lie in the brain-stem. The pupils would be fixed and dilated.

11.9

(a)   Yes.

(b)   Yes.

(c)   No. There is a synapse on the pathway; this synapse lies in the superior cervical ganglion.

(d)   No. It leaves at the level of the midbrain.

(e)   No. The receptors are muscarinic, i.e. blocked by atropine. Atropine therefore leads to unopposed sympathetic dilatation.

11.10

(a)   No. In a myopic subject, the image of an object on the horizon falls in front of the retina.

(b)   No. In a myopic subject, the near point is closer than normal.

(c)   No. Visual acuity, the ability to discriminate two points of light that are close together, depends on cones.

(d)   No. The rods and cones are far too small to be seen through an ophthalmoscope.

(e)   Yes. Colour vision depends on cones.

11.11

(a)   Yes.

(b)   Yes. The highest density of rods is found in the annulus surrounding the macula lutea, i.e. in the peripheral retina.

(c)   Yes. As a result of the convergence of many visual receptors on to a single bipolar neurone, the effects of activation of neighbouring sensory elements can summate, thus providing a structural basis for visual sensitivity.

(d)   No. The convergence of many visual receptors on to a single bipolar neurone operates against spatial discrimination, i.e. against acuity.

(e)   No. The photoreceptors connect directly with bipolar cells which in turn form synaptic connection with retinal ganglion cells; these are the cell bodies of the optic nerve fibres.

11.12

(a)   No. When parallel light rays pass from the air to the cornea, the light rays are converged.

(b)   No. Atropine applied to the eye causes pupillary dilatation and everything appears brighter to the subject.

(c)   No. The image produced by a lens is clearest if light rays pass only through the central portion of the lens; the pupillary dilatation caused by atropine thus reduces visual acuity.

(d)   Yes. If an image is thrown on to the retina via a mirror mounted on a contact lens and a projector is used to project a visual stimulus in such a way that the retinal image is stationary, the subject perceives the image when the projector is first switched on, but then the perception of the image rapidly fades (with a time constant of less than 1 sec). Vision depends on the intermittent movement of the visual image on the retina caused by saccadic eye movements.

(e)   No. A focal lesion in the primary visual area of the cortical convexity results in loss of vision in part of the contralateral peripheral visual field.

11.13

(a)   Yes.

(b)   No. The primary visual cortex lies in the occipital lobe of the cerebral cortex.

(c)   No. The part of the cerebral cortex to which an object lying on the visual axis projects is on the medial aspect of the cerebral hemisphere.

(d)   Yes. The fovea of one eye is represented in the visual areas of both cerebral hemispheres, but a point in the peripheral visual field projects only to one hemisphere.

(e)   No. Pupillary dilatation is caused by increased activity in sympathetic nerves. This is easy to remember, since dilatation of the pupils is a feature of 'fight or flight', a sympathetic response.

11.14

(a)   Yes. The perception of visual images requires the suppression of the image during the fast phase of nystagmus just as during other saccadic eye movement.

(b)   No. It is a saccadic movement.

(c)   Yes.

(d)   No. The slow phase of nystagmus is in a direction such as to stabilize the visual image; the fast phase occurs to bring the visual axis rapidly back towards the midline when the axis has deviated maximally during the slow phase.

(e)   No. Nystagmus occurs, for instance, if the eyes are closed and the subject is rotated on a Barany chair. This can be detected by electrodes placed to pick up the retinocorneal potential.

11.15

(a)   Yes. The pupils are symmetrical in size so long as the efferent innervation is normal.

(b)   No. With damage to the oculomotor nerve on one side, the pupils are asymmetrical in size because the oculomotor nerve contains the parasympathetic innervation of the eye.

(c)   Yes.

(d)   No. If the sympathetic innervation of one eye is interrupted, that eye will still show some degree of pupillary response to light mediated via the parasympathetic innervation.

(e)   Yes. Meningeal irritation may cause 'pin-point' pupils and this presents a difficulty to the doctor in trying to assess cranial nerve function with tests of pupil reactions.

11.16

(a)   No. The facial nerve is the motor nerve involved.

(b)   No. The orbicularis oculi muscle, responsible for blinking, is skeletal muscle.

(c)   Yes. This component is also known as Muller's muscle. Loss of sympathetic function ('Horner's syndrome') therefore includes a drooping eyelid, as well as pupillary constriction, on the affected side.

(d)   No. The smooth muscle of the levator palpebrae superioris is sympathetically innervated; contraction of this muscle retracts the upper lid, which is the opposite of drooping.

(e)   No. It runs with the oculomotor nerve.

11.17

(a)   No. With severe damage to the occipital cortex of one cerebral hemisphere, even with both eyes open the subject will not be able to see anything in the visual field to the side of the visual axis opposite to the side of the lesion. Foveal vision will be spared.

(b)   No. Foveal vision is represented in both hemispheres and will be spared.

(c)   Yes. The direct light reflex depends on pathways through the brain-stem, pathways which do not traverse the cerebral cortex. So a light shone on to part of the retina that evokes no vision will evoke a direct light reflex.

(d)   Yes. Just as in (c), a light shone on to part of the retina that evokes no vision evokes a consensual light reflex via brain-stem pathways.

(e)   Yes. The real image formed by the refractory power of the eye is inverted.

11.18

(a)   Yes. The motor nuclei for the pupillary muscles lie in the midbrain, so the pupillary light reflex is dependent on the integrity of the midbrain.

(b)   Yes.

(c)   No. Vision in dim illumination depends on rods, not cones. So dark adaptation is complete when the sensitivity of the rods, not the cones, has settled at a new level.

(d)   Yes. The visual pigments are derived from vitamin D, so vision in dim light is defective in vitamin D deficiency.

(e)   Yes. The pupillary accommodation reflex is dependent on the cerebral cortex.

11.19

(a)   Yes. The receptor cells of the cochlea are unusual in that they have an efferent innervation; it is via the olivo-cochlear bundle.

(b)   No. In the normal healthy subject, the cavity of the middle ear is filled with air.

(c)   No. The differential sensitivity to pitch (frequency) is the percentage change in frequency that can just be detected. It is fairly constant over a wide range of frequencies.

(d)   Yes. The otolith organs contain otoliths (ear stones) that act like tiny plumb lines and provide information about the direction of linear acceleration. If the head is stationary, this direction is the direction of the gravitational field; the otoliths provide information about the direction of 'down-ness'.

(e)   No. The receptors in the semicircular canals are sensitive to angular movements of the head and not to linear acceleration.

11.20

(a)   Yes.

(b)   Yes. The auditory system is sensitive to a phase difference of this magnitude.

(c)   No. The intensity threshold is least at about 1 kHz, and rises steeply for frequencies below or above this.

(d)   No. The just perceptible difference in intensity rises with the intensity level at which it is tested.

(e)   Yes. The difference between the two is at least three-fold in most people.

11.21

(a)   No. It is the force that is amplified; the amplitude of movement is reduced.

(b)   No. High frequencies are detected by receptors close to the oval window.

(c)   Yes.

(d)   No. Contraction of the stapedius muscle reduces the effectiveness of mechanical transmission through the ossicles.

(e)   Yes. The energy of the sound waves is conducted directly to the receptors through the bone.

11.22

(a)   Yes.

(b)   Yes.

(c)   No. The lowest tone that a normal person can hear is around 30 Hz.

(d)   Yes.

(e)   Yes. Bone conduction is very efficient in carrying sound energy and the fact that the subject will still be able to hear the note when the fork is held to his pinna after it ceases to be audible with bone conduction is a witness to the high efficiency of the pinna in collecting sound energy and of the auditory ossicles in matching the auditory signal to the impedance of the cochlear mechanism.

11.23

(a)   Yes. For instance, the skin of the ear lobe contains only free nerve endings and yet cooling is readily appreciated.

(b)   Yes. For all types of cutaneous sensation including touch, each nerve ending innervates a small region of skin and in between nerve endings there are regions of skin that are insensitive to touch, i.e. the distribution of touch sensitivity is punctate.

(c)   No. The only nerve fibres in the human that conduct at this speed are group 1A afferents from muscle spindle receptors.

(d)   Yes.

(e)   No. They lie in the dermis.

11.24

(a)   Yes.

(b)   Yes.

(c)   No. The high amplitude voltage excursion is an action potential.

(d)   Yes. The first two action potentials occur in rapid succession; the interval between successive impulses increases. This is adaptation.

(e)   No. The action potential peak voltage is constant, consistent with its 'all or none' nature.

11.25

(a)   No. Non-glabrous (hairy) skin is devoid of Meissner's corpuscles but is sensitive to touch.

(b)   Yes. Nociceptive nerve endings are the only sensory nerve endings that lie in the epidermis.

(c)   No. Pacinian corpuscles are deformation receptors.

(d)   Yes. Different modalities are served by different receptors.

(e)   No. If this were the case, the central nervous system would not be able to discriminate between cold and touch; this discrimination depends on different modalities transmitting along different lines.

11.26

(a)   Yes. In non-glabrous skin, all nerve endings are free nerve endings.

(b)   Yes. The receptive fields of receptors of different modality frequently overlap.

(c)   No. The conjunctiva is extremely sensitive; it is richly endowed with free nerve endings.

(d)   Yes.

(e)   Yes.

11.27

(a)   Yes.

(b)   No. The lamellae of a Pacinian corpuscle transmit mechanical distortion to the nerve endings.

(c)   Yes. The Pacinian corpuscle typically generates one or two impulses in its afferent nerve fibre at the onset of distortion, and thereafter, when the distortion is maintained, there is no afferent discharge.

(d)   Yes.

(e)   Yes. This is true of visual, auditory, balance and taste receptors. The exception is olfaction, where the receptors are the cell bodies of the primary afferent neurones.

11.28

(a)   Yes. The meninges are very sensitive to stretch.

(b)   No. The cerebral cortex is devoid of sensory receptors.

(c) Yes. The hypothalamus contains elements sensitive to osmolality, temperature, etc.

(d) No. The basal ganglia are devoid of sensory receptors.

(e) Yes. The medulla oblongata contains receptors sensitive to the pH of the cerebral interstitial fluid.

11.29

(a) Yes. Tapping the patellar tendon stretches the muscle spindles and activates their receptors.

(b) Yes. Acuity of vision (the ability to distinguish two points of light that are close to each other) is mediated by cones.

(c) Yes. For most parts of the visual spectrum, the rods are sensitive at intensities of illumination below those at which cones are excited. So rods mediate sensitivity of vision.

(d) No. Pacinian corpuscles are deformation receptors, not heat receptors.

(e) No. Primary muscle spindle receptors connect with Group 1A sensory nerve fibres.

12   Excitable tissues: nerve and muscle

Resting potential and action potential	12.1–12.10
Nerve fibre types	12.11–12.14
Division of nerve	12.15–12.18
Nerve: general	12.19–12.20
Neuromuscular transmission	12.21–12.25
Skeletal muscle	12.26–12.38
Cardiac muscle	12.39–12.41
Smooth muscle	12.42–12.47
Muscle in general	12.48–12.49

QUESTIONS

Resting potential and action potential

12.1 The equilibrium potential across a cell membrane for an ionic species:
(a) is the membrane potential at which there is no net movement of these ions across the membrane, assuming the ion to be permeant.
(b) is the voltage that the membrane potential would assume if the membrane were permeable to that ion and to no others.
(c) would be zero if the concentration of the ion on one side of the membrane were 10 times its concentration on the other side.
(d) is necessarily zero if the ion is impermeant.
(e) has approximately the same value for sodium and potassium ions in resting nerve fibres.

12.2 The equilibrium potential of a given ion across a membrane is:
(a) the membrane potential that would be required to balance the concentration gradient for that ion.
(b) directly proportional to the difference in concentration of the ion on the two sides of the membrane.
(c) the resting potential across the membrane.
(d) the membrane potential that would be reached if the membrane were equally permeable to all ions.
(e) the same as the equilibrium potential for all other ions with the same charge.

12.3   Concerning membrane phenomena:

(a)   the equilibrium potential for an ion is the potential that would exist across the membrane if the membrane were permeable only to that ion.

(b)   if the membrane potential is the same as the equilibrium potential for a particular ion, then when membrane channels that allow that ion to pass are opened, there is a large net influx of the ion into the intracellular fluid.

(c)   when membrane channels that allow an ion to pass are opened, there is an increase in the rate of to and fro movement of the ion across the membrane.

(d)   the movement of an uncharged molecule across the cell membrane is unaffected by the membrane potential.

(e)   membrane current is carried by free electrons.

12.4   Concerning the movement of ions across the membrane of a nerve fibre:

(a)   when the fibre has been at rest for a long period of time, for any ion the rate of efflux equals the rate of influx.

(b)   during the upstroke of the action potential, there is a net flow of current across the cell membrane.

(c)   at the peak of the action potential when the membrane potential is momentarily unchanging, there is a net flow of current across the cell membrane.

(d)   at the peak of the action potential, the rate of efflux of potassium equals the rate of influx.

(e)   during the downstroke of the action potential, the membrane conductance for potassium is higher than in the axon at rest.

12.5   Concerning a nerve fibre:

(a)   at rest, the inside of the nerve fibre is positive to the outside.

(b)   propagation of the action potential depends on the flow of current along the axoplasm.

(c)   the resting potential moves away from the potassium equilibrium potential if the membrane permeability to potassium rises.

(d)   the resting potential decreases in magnitude if the sodium permeability of the membrane rises.

(e)   the resting potential falls immediately to zero if the sodium extrusion mechanism is poisoned.

12.6 **The action potential in nerve:**
(a)   is initiated by a depolarization of the membrane.
(b)   is a change in membrane potential towards the equilibrium potential for sodium ions.
(c)   involves a decrease in the membrane permeability to potassium ions.
(d)   is associated with an increase in the electrical resistance of the membrane.
(e)   is propagated along the axon by means of the release of acetylcholine.

12.7 **Concerning the nerve fibres of higher mammals:**
(a)   the resting potential is within 20 mV of the potassium equilibrium potential.
(b)   the rising phase of the action potential is largely due to influx of sodium ions.
(c)   the duration of the rising phase of the action potential is 8–10 msec.
(d)   the peak of the action potential is within 20 mV of the chloride equilibrium potential.
(e)   the falling phase of the action potential is largely due to increased activity of the sodium pump.

12.8 **With reference to conduction along nerve axons:**
(a)   conduction velocity in a particular axon is related to the strength of the stimulus.
(b)   in myelinated axons the action potential is generated only at the nodes of Ranvier.
(c)   if a stimulus is applied half-way along a motor axon, the action potential will travel only in the direction towards the muscle it supplies.
(d)   conduction velocity in somatic motor nerve fibres is in the range 1–10 m/sec.
(e)   the smaller the diameter of the axon, the greater is the conduction velocity.

12.9 **In a nerve fibre:**
(a)   at rest, the concentration of potassium ions in the axoplasm exceeds that in the interstitial fluid.
(b)   at the peak of the action potential, the internal concentration of sodium ions is very nearly the same as when the nerve is at rest.
(c)   the rising phase of the action potential is due to transient inhibition of the sodium pump.
(d)   during the rising phase of the action potential, there is an increase in efflux of potassium ions.
(e)   if metabolic activity is blocked, the action potential mechanism is immediately blocked.

12.10   With reference to the action potential in nerve:
(a)   the membrane potential reverses polarity.
(b)   the process is initiated by hyperpolarization of the cell membrane.
(c)   the peak of the action potential is a few millivolts more positive than the sodium equilibrium potential.
(d)   the increase in membrane permeability to potassium precedes the increase in membrane permeability to sodium.
(e)   the increase in sodium permeability during the action potential depends on depolarization of the membrane.

Nerve fibre types

12.11   A cutaneous nerve contains:
(a)   sensory nerve fibres.
(b)   nerve fibres up to 20 μm in diameter.
(c)   parasympathetic nerve fibres.
(d)   motor nerve fibres to skeletal muscle.
(e)   motor nerve fibres to smooth muscle.

12.12   Concerning nerve fibres:
(a)   unmyelinated axons are thicker than myelinated axons.
(b)   several unmyelinated fibres are enclosed together in a single Schwann cell sheath.
(c)   a single myelinated fibre is enclosed in a single Schwann cell sheath.
(d)   unmyelinated nerve fibres have nodes of Ranvier.
(e)   conduction of the nerve impulse in myelinated fibres is saltatory.

12.13   With reference to the medial popliteal nerve (a mixed peripheral nerve) in a normal human:
(a)   the largest nerve fibres have a diameter of about 20 μm.
(b)   the largest nerve fibres are efferent fibres.
   When an electrical stimulus is applied percutaneously to the nerve:
(c)   with a threshold stimulus, the smaller nerve fibres will be preferentially stimulated.
(d)   the M response recorded from electrodes over the gastrocnemius muscle is generated by action potentials in the extrafusal muscle fibres.
(e)   the H response recorded from electrodes over the gastrocnemius muscle is generated by action potentials in the intrafusal muscle fibres.

12.14 **In the sciatic nerve:**
(a) there are both myelinated and non-myelinated nerve fibres.
(b) the largest-diameter nerve fibres supply the skin.
(c) joint position sense is carried by small diameter fibres.
(d) pain and temperature sensations are carried by the same nerve fibres.
(e) motor nerve fibres to intrafusal muscle fibres are on average of greater diameter than those to extrafusal fibres.

Division of nerve

12.15 **Immediately after complete division of a mixed peripheral nerve:**
(a) the denervated muscles exhibit the characteristic features of an 'upper motoneurone lesion'.
(b) there is insensibility in an area of skin.
(c) the denervated area of skin will be cooler than the surrounding area.
(d) the sweat glands in the denervated skin will respond to an increase in temperature in the hypothalamus.
(e) the cut nerve fibres of the central stump are capable of regenerating along the nerve sheath.

12.16 **Two weeks after section of a cutaneous nerve, the denervated skin is studied with the subject in a warm environment. Will the following be observed?**
(a) insensible perspiration.
(b) cold skin.
(c) sweating.
(d) wheal formation (swelling) when the skin is damaged.
(e) flaring of the skin when it is damaged.

12.17 **After regeneration of a sectioned mixed peripheral nerve, by comparison with normal (i.e. before the nerve was cut):**
(a) even if only a proportion of the motor nerve fibres originally functional have regenerated, the tension produced by the muscle may be undiminished.
(b) re-innervated extrafusal muscle fibres may be hypertrophied.
(c) after re-innervation, the number of muscle fibres in a motor unit may be greater.
(d) the twitch tension produced by an individual muscle fibre may be greater.
(e) each muscle fibre responds repetitively to a single nerve impulse.

12.18 After section of a mixed peripheral nerve:
(a) there will be wasting of muscle fibres.
(b) regenerating nerve tips advance at about 1 cm per day.
(c) the subject is aware of sensation when the skin over the regenerating tips of axons is tapped lightly.
(d) the conduction velocity of regenerating fibres is greater than in unsevered nerve.
(e) a firm touch to the skin at the time when sensory endings are being re-innervated frequently causes the sensation of pain.

Nerve: general

12.19 An increase in impulse frequency in efferent fibres of the vagus nerves causes:
(a) decrease in the secretion of gastric juice.
(b) slowing in the frequency of the heart beat.
(c) dilatation of the bronchi.
(d) increased contraction of the smooth muscle in the small intestine.
(e) vasoconstriction of the blood vessels in the abdominal organs.

12.20 Are the following statements about block of conduction in nerve fibres correct?
(a) very small diameter fibres are more susceptible to block by hypoxia than large fibres.
(b) larger diameter is associated with greater susceptibility to block by physical pressure.
(c) larger diameter is associated with greater susceptibility to block by local anaesthetics.
(d) a fall in the concentration of calcium ions in the surrounding fluid may produce nerve block.
(e) hyperpolarization of nerve fibres by the application of an electrical current may produce nerve block.

Neuromuscular transmission

12.21 At the skeletal neuromuscular junction:
(a) most of the acetylcholine released when a nerve impulse invades the motor nerve terminal diffuses into the bloodstream.
(b) acetylcholine released at one endplate depolarizes the endplates of neighbouring muscle fibres.
(c) increase in the release of acetylcholine results in an increase in the twitch tension produced by the muscle fibre.
(d) attachment of acetylcholine to its postsynaptic receptors results in the opening of ion channels in the membrane.
(e) acetylcholine applied at any point along the muscle fibre causes the muscle fibre to contract.

12.22 **Concerning transmission at the skeletal neuromuscular junction:**
(a)   if the hydrolysis of acetylcholine is prevented, acetylcholine applied to the endplate may cause paralysis.
(b)   if a muscle is denervated, the endplate becomes hypersensitive to acetylcholine.
(c)   if a muscle is denervated, the region of the muscle fibre exhibiting sensitivity to applied acetylcholine spreads to regions previously insensitive.
(d)   if the action potential mechanism is blocked in nerve and muscle by a specific poison (such as tetrodotoxin), acetylcholine applied to the endplate will still cause the occurrence of an endplate potential.
(e)   if the action potential mechanism is blocked in nerve and muscle by a specific poison, acetylcholine applied to the endplate will cause the fibre to twitch.

12.23 **Concerning neuromuscular transmission in humans:**
(a)   calcium entry into the presynaptic terminal is an essential step in the release of transmitter following an action potential in the motor nerve.
(b)   succinylcholine causes a depolarization of the postsynaptic membrane.
(c)   blockade of transmission by curare is by competitive inhibition of the receptors on the postsynaptic membrane.
(d)   the blockade of transmission by curare can be antagonized by an anticholinesterase.
(e)   spontaneous release of transmitter occurs in the absence of action potentials in the motor nerve.

12.24 **Concerning nerve and skeletal muscle:**
(a)   curare abolishes the muscular contraction in response to electrical stimulation of the motor nerve supplying the muscle.
(b)   curare abolishes the muscular contraction in response to an electrical stimulus applied directly to a muscle.
(c)   tetrodotoxin (an agent that blocks voltage-sensitive sodium channels) abolishes the muscular contraction in response to electrical stimulation of the motor nerve supplying the muscle.
(d)   tetrodotoxin abolishes the muscular contraction in response to an electrical stimulus applied directly to a muscle.
(e)   tetrodotoxin abolishes miniature endplate potentials.

12.25 Concerning motor nerve terminals:
(a) as an action potential approaches the nerve terminals, its conduction speed decreases.
(b) an agent that blocks calcium channels in the nerve membrane prevents conduction of the action potential in nerve.
A brief electric pulse is applied via an intracellular microelectrode into a motor nerve terminal.
(c) if the pulse takes the membrane potential to +45 mV, neurotransmitter is released.
(d) if the pulse takes the membrane potential to the equilibrium potential for calcium ions (+120 mV), neurotransmitter is released.
(e) the release of neurotransmitter by a depolarizing pulse is blocked by agents that block calcium channels.

Skeletal muscle

12.26 Concerning skeletal muscle in an adult human:
(a) when a fibre shortens, the length of the I band decreases.
(b) when a fibre shortens, the length of the A band decreases.
(c) when a fibre shortens, its diameter increases.
(d) the force of contraction is directly proportional to the rate of shortening.
(e) each fibre is supplied by branches of several motor nerve fibres.

12.27 Concerning ionized calcium [Ca²⁺] and muscle:
(a) the concentration of $[Ca^{2+}]$ in extracellular fluid is about 1 mmol per litre.
(b) the concentration of $[Ca^{2+}]$ in intracellular fluid in resting muscle is about 0.1 mmol per litre.
(c) myosin-ATPase is inactive when the intracellular calcium concentration is at the level found in resting muscle fibres.
(d) an increase in intracellular concentration is an essential link in excitation–contraction coupling.
(e) an action potential in the muscle fibre causes an increase of about 10-fold in intracellular concentration.

12.28 Concerning activation of skeletal muscle:
(a) the activation of myosin-ATPase in excitation-contraction coupling is by an increase in intracellular magnesium concentration.
(b) the increase in intracellular calcium concentration produced by an action potential is mainly due to influx of calcium across the muscle fibre membrane.
(c) the duration of the twitch depends on the rate of reabsorption of Ca^{2+} by the sarcoplasmic reticulum.
(d) the fall in calcium concentration after myosin activation is due to active pumping of calcium ions out of the myoplasm.
(e) after activation, the return of calcium concentration to normal is due to movement into the cisternae (sarcoplasmic reticulum).

12.29 **Concerning skeletal muscle:**
(a) the nuclei lie in the centre of the muscle fibres.
(b) each muscle fibre has a single nucleus
(c) the transverse tubular system is in continuity with the extracellular space.
(d) the transverse tubules enter muscle fibres randomly along their length.
(e) the cisternae are in continuity with the extracellular space.

12.30 **In skeletal muscle:**
(a) when the muscle is relaxed, myosin heads are detached from thin (actin) filaments.
(b) myosin heads are continually hydrolysing ATP.
(c) contraction is initiated by a rise in intracellular ATP concentration.
(d) contraction is produced by a configurational change of myosin heads with respect to the thick filaments from which they arise.
(e) during each muscle fibre twitch, each myosin head attaches to and detaches from the thin filament several times.

12.31 **In skeletal muscle:**
(a) during active contraction, the muscle fibre becomes hotter.
(b) if the muscle is passively stretched during a contraction, it produces less tension than that of an isometric contraction.
(c) if the muscle shortens during a contraction, it produces less tension than that of an isometric contraction.
(d) during a tetanic contraction, more ATP is utilized by fast than by slow skeletal muscle fibres generating the same force.
(e) attachment of ATP to the myosin heads is essential for the dissociation of the actomyosin complex.

12.32 **Concerning skeletal muscle:**
(a) during a voluntary contraction, a skeletal muscle shortens typically to 50% of its resting length.
(b) transverse tubules store calcium.
(c) the function of transverse tubules is to carry action potentials to the depths of the muscle fibre.
(d) depolarization of the transverse tubules causes hyperpolarization of the membranes of the cisternae.
(e) modulation of the increase in calcium concentration is a physiological mechanism for modulating the contractility.

12.33   With reference to motor units in skeletal muscle in a human adult:

(a)   the number of muscle fibres in a motor unit is greater for a muscle involved in producing strong coarse movements than in one involved in finely-controlled movements.

(b)   a single muscle fibre is usually innervated by branches from several motor axons.

(c)   an action potential in a nerve axon will normally lead to excitation of every muscle fibre making up that motor unit.

(d)   the strength of muscle contraction is increased by recruitment of more motor units.

(e)   during the tendon jerk reflex, active motor units produce fused tetanic contractions.

12.34   Figure 12.34 shows the relationship between active isometric tension and initial length in a skeletal muscle fibre.

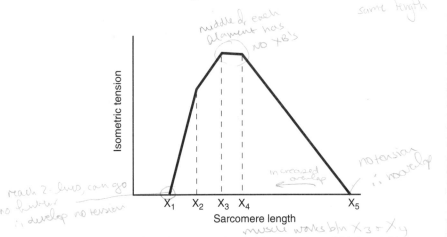

(a)   at sarcomere length X_5, there is complete overlap of thick and thin filaments.

(b)   sarcomere length X_5 corresponds to the maximum length of the muscle in the body.

(c)   between sarcomere lengths X_5 and X_4, there is partial overlap between thick and thin filaments.

(d)   the constancy of tension between sarcomere lengths X_3 and X_4 reflects the fact that in the middle of each thick filament cross-bridges are particularly abundant.

(e)   at sarcomere length X_1, the tips of the thick filaments reach the Z lines.

12.35 A skeletal muscle is set up under after-load isotonic conditions (Figure 12.35). When the muscle is stimulated to shorten maximally, could the following three curves represent the physiological relationships?

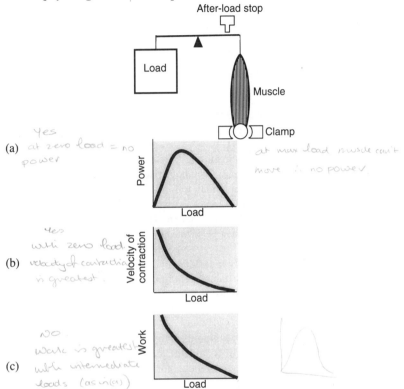

After-load stop

Load

Muscle

Clamp

(a) *Yes*
at zero load = no power

at max load muscle can't move ∴ no power

(b) *Yes*
with zero load velocity of contraction is greatest.

(c) *No*
Work is greatest with intermediate loads (as in (a))

The muscle was then set up for isometric recording. Could the following two curves represent the physiological relationships?

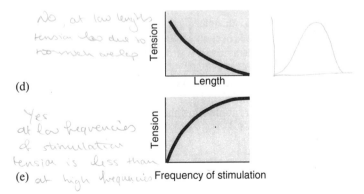

(d) *No, at low lengths tension less due to too much overlap*

(e) *Yes at low frequencies of stimulation tension is less than at high frequencies*

12.36 A record of a single skeletal muscle twitch is shown in Figure 12.36. Are the following statements true?

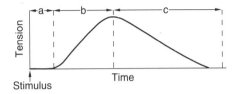

(a)   this is an isotonic contraction.
(b)   calcium is released from the sarcoplasmic reticulum during period a.
(c)   during the period c the muscle fibre membrane is refractory so that a second action potential cannot arise.
(d)   the muscle action potential follows the same time course as the mechanical record.
(e)   the prolonged contraction that results from repetitive stimulation would rise to a higher peak tension than the twitch.

12.37 Concerning skeletal muscle:
(a)   in skeletal muscle, a stain for choline esterase will specifically stain the endings of the sensory nerve fibres.
(b)   the average length of a sarcomere in a human skeletal muscle is 2.5 μm.
   Are the following statements true about the events leading up to the contraction of a skeletal muscle fibre?
(c)   during the propagation of the action potential in the nerve there is a net entry of K^+ ions into the axon.
(d)   before the release of transmitter, Ca^{2+} ions enter the nerve endings.
(e) Ca^{2+} from the extracellular fluid enters the muscle fibre through its surface membrane during the action potential.

12.38 Concerning skeletal muscle:
(a)   when a muscle fibre is excited via its motor nerve, action potentials travel away from each other towards the ends of the muscle fibre.
(b)   in a twitch, the action potential and the mechanical response follow approximately the same time course.
(c)   a rise in temperature increases the duration of the muscle twitch.
(d)   a rise in temperature diminishes the twitch:tetanus tension ratio.
(e)   a rise in temperature of 3°C has a negligible effect on the tetanic tension.

Cardiac muscle

12.39 Concerning the heart:
(a) cardiac muscle has a system of transverse tubules.
(b) when activated by direct electrical stimulation, the rate of increase in tension is similar in skeletal and in cardiac muscle.
(c) modulation of the increase in internal calcium ion concentration is a physiological mechanism for modulating the twitch tension in a cardiac muscle fibre.
(d) over the course of a period of minutes or longer, the cardiac output equals the venous return.
(e) in the cardiac cycles immediately following the administration of adrenaline, the cardiac output exceeds the venous return.

12.40 Regarding ventricular cardiac muscle:
(a) the upstroke of the action potential is mainly due to inflow of sodium ions.
(b) the long duration of the action potential is mainly due to a persistent increase in the permeability of the membrane to sodium ions.
(c) the duration of the absolute refractory period is the same as that in skeletal muscle.
(d) action potentials elicited during the relative refractory period are of shorter duration.
(e) on sympathetic stimulation the duration of the plateau phase of the cardiac action potential is shortened.

12.41 Concerning the heart:
(a) the duration of ventricular contraction is at least 10 times longer than the duration of the cardiac action potential.
(b) during sympathetic stimulation, the ventricle sucks in blood from the atrium during diastole.
(c) the rate of depolarization of the pacemaker cells during diastole is diminished by sympathetic stimulation.
(d) in the pacemaker cells, the action potential is mainly due to influx of sodium ions.
(e) in Purkinje cells, the action potential is mainly due to influx of sodium ions.

Smooth muscle

12.42 In relation to muscular activity in the gut:
(a) activity of the vagus nerves has relatively little influence on stomach motility.
(b) the oesophageal phase of swallowing is under vagal control.
(c) ingestion of sizeable volumes of fluid into the stomach increases intragastric pressure markedly.
(d) whenever a peristaltic wave propels chyme towards the pylorus, most of this chyme passes out of the stomach.
(e) secretion of secretin by the duodenum inhibits gastric motility.

12.43 **An agent that causes an increase in contraction of all smooth muscle in the body would lead to:**
(a)   an increase in resistance to air flow in the bronchioles.
(b)   an increase in venous capacity.
(c)   an increase in the total peripheral vascular resistance.
(d)   an increase in pressure in the stomach.
(e)   accommodation of the eye for near vision.

12.44 **Concerning smooth muscle in the gut:**
(a)   it may show spontaneous rhythmic activity.
(b)   it can contract to one-tenth of its original length and continue to exert tension.
(c)   it may be stimulated to contract by chemicals circulating in the blood.
(d)   it may be stimulated to contract by neural activity.
(e)   its contraction may be inhibited by neural activity.

12.45 **Intestinal smooth muscle:**
(a)   is innervated by the terminals of nerves whose cell bodies lie in the spinal chord.
(b)   has a sensory innervation.
(c)   contains actin and myosin.
(d)   conducts action potentials from cell to cell.
(e)   may contract in response to chemicals reaching it via the blood.

12.46 **Concerning smooth muscle:**
(a)   smooth muscle is found in the skin.
(b)   calcium is required for its contraction.
(c)   the entry of sodium ions is the main charge carrier for the upstroke of the action potential.
An agent that causes an increase in contraction of all vascular smooth muscle would lead to:
(d)   an increase in central venous pressure.
(e)   an increase in arterial blood pressure.

12.47 **Concerning intra-ocular smooth muscle and its control:**
(a)   the pathway of the pupillary light reflex traverses the lateral geniculate nucleus.
(b)   the ciliary muscle in the eye contracts spontaneously in the absence of nerve stimulation.
(c)   dilatation of the pupil is effected both by neural and humoral mechanisms.
(d)   constriction of the pupil is effected both by neural and by humoral mechanisms.
(e)   contraction of the ciliary muscle causes the lens to become thinner.

Muscle in general

12.48 **Are the following common to all three types of muscle (skeletal, cardiac and smooth)?**
(a) they undergo summation and tetanus when rapidly stimulated.
(b) they show striations under the light microscope.
(c) action potentials are generated when their membranes are depolarized.
(d) the interaction of actin, myosin and ATP is responsible for generation of force by the muscle cells.
(e) an increase in Ca^{++} concentration inside the cell is necessary for contraction.

12.49 **With reference to the several types of muscle:**
(a) skeletal muscle fibres have intercalated discs.
(b) cardiac muscle fibres have cross-striations.
(c) smooth muscle fibres have transverse tubules.
(d) in all three types of muscle, the contractile machinery is organized into an orderly array of thick and thin filaments.
(e) muscle spindles are found in cardiac muscle.

ANSWERS

12.1
(a) Yes. This is the definition of the equilibrium potential.
(b) Yes. If the membrane is permeable to only one ion, there will be net movement of this ion across the membrane until the voltage difference exactly balances the concentration difference.
(c) No. It would be zero if the concentrations on the two sides of the membrane were equal.
(d) No. Equilibrium potential is defined as the potential that would be observed assuming the membrane were permeable. A state of impermeability to the ion does not influence the equilibrium potential.
(e) No. $E_{Na^+} = 55\,mV$
$E_{K^+} = -90\,mV$ approximately.

12.2
(a) Yes.
(b) No. The equilibrium potential of a given ion across a membrane is directly proportional to the ratio of concentrations of the ion across the membrane.
(c) No. The resting potential depends on the equilibrium potentials of all permeant species weighted according to the permeabilities and the concentrations of these ions.

(d)   No. If the membrane were equally permeable to all ions, the membrane potential would depend on the permeabilities and concentrations of all the ions.

(e)   No. Two ions with the same charge will only have the same equilibrium potential if their concentration ratios across the membrane happen to be identical.

12.3

(a)   Yes.

(b)   No. If membrane channels allowing a particular ion to pass open, and the membrane potential is at the equilibrium potential for that ion, then there is no net movement across the membrane of the ion.

(c)   Yes.

(d)   Yes. Molecules carry no charge and are therefore uninfluenced by an electric field.

(e)   No. Membrane current is carried by ions.

12.4

(a)   Yes. The axon at rest is in a steady state; for each ion, the rate of influx equals the rate of efflux.

(b)   Yes. Whenever the membrane potential is changing, there is a net flow of current which charges the membrane capacitance.

(c)   No. Whenever the membrane potential is constant, there is no net flow of current across the membrane.

(d)   No. Although the net flow of charge is zero, there is a net exit of potassium ions balanced principally by a net entry of sodium ions.

(e)   Yes. During the downstroke of the action potential, the membrane conductance for potassium is higher than in the axon at rest. This is called the 'delayed rectifier' and contributes to the rapidity with which the membrane potential is restored to normal in readiness for conducting a subsequent impulse.

12.5

(a)   No. At rest, the inside of the nerve fibre is negative to the outside.

(b)   Yes. The local circuit mechanism of propagation of the action potential depends on the flow of current along the axoplasm.

(c)   No. If the membrane permeability to potassium rises, the resting potential moves towards, not away from, the potassium equilibrium potential.

(d)   Yes. A rise in the sodium permeability of the membrane results in a move of the resting potential towards the sodium equilibrium potential, i.e. the membrane potential decreases.

(e)   No. The resting potential is little affected in the short term if the sodium extrusion mechanism is poisoned. The absolute permeability of the membrane is so low that it takes many hours for the concentration gradients to dissipate if the sodium extrusion mechanism is poisoned.

12.6

(a)   Yes. The permeability of the nerve membrane is voltage dependent; depolarization causes sodium gates to open.

(b)   Yes. Because the gates that open are specific for sodium ions.

(c)   No. The permeability to potassium increases after the peak of the action potential.

(d)   No. The opening of ionic gates constitutes a reduction in membrane resistance.

(e)   No. Acetylcholine release is not an essential step in propagation of the action potential.

12.7

(a)   Yes.

(b)   Yes.

(c)   No. It is less than 0.5 msec.

(d)   No. The resting potential is usually within 20 mV of the chloride equilibrium potential; the voltage of the peak of the action potential is within 20 mV of the sodium equilibrium potential.

(e)   No. The downstroke of the action potential is due largely to passive efflux of potassium ions down their electrochemical gradient.

12.8

(a)   No. The conduction velocity is independent of the stimulus strength.

(b)   Yes.

(c)   No. The action potential so elicited would travel in both directions.

(d)   No. 15 to 70 m/sec would be an appropriate range.

(e)   No. The smaller the diameter of an axon, the slower it conducts.

12.9

(a)   Yes. The high concentration of potassium ions in the axoplasm compared with that in the interstitial fluid is the origin of the resting potential.

(b)   Yes. The sodium that crosses the membrane charges the membrane capacitance; the amount of sodium is so small that its effect on the internal concentration of sodium ions is negligible. At the peak of the action potential, the internal concentration of sodium ions is to a very close approximation the same as when the nerve is at rest.

(c)   No. The rising phase of the action potential is due to inward movement of sodium ions down their electrochemical gradient. Transient inhibition of the sodium pump would be without significant effect on the membrane potential.

(d)   Yes. During the rising phase of the action potential, the membrane potential moves away from the potassium equilibrium potential so, although at this phase there is no change in potassium permeability, there is an increase in efflux of potassium ions because of the increased driving force.

(e)   No. If metabolic activity is blocked, the action potential mechanism is unaffected in the short term because it depends on ions moving down their respective electrochemical gradients.

12.10

(a)   Yes. At rest the membrane potential is negative and during the action potential it reverses.

(b)   No. The process is initiated by depolarization of the cell membrane.

(c)   No. The peak of the action potential is close to the sodium equilibrium potential; this proximity to the sodium equilibrium potential is because, at this time, the membrane is more permeable to sodium than to other ions. The peak of the action potential is, however, less positive than the sodium equilibrium potential because the equilibrium potentials of other permeant ions are less positive than the sodium equilibrium potential.

(d)   No. The increase in membrane permeability to potassium occurs after the increase in membrane permeability to sodium.

(e)   Yes. The increase in sodium permeability during the action potential depends on depolarization of the membrane.

12.11

(a)   Yes.

(b)   No. Only in nerves to skeletal muscles are there nerve fibres up to 20 μm in diameter. In cutaneous nerves the thickest fibres are around 12 μm in diameter.

(c)   No. The parasympathetic nervous system does not project to the skin.

(d)   No. A cutaneous nerve supplies the skin, not motor nerve fibres to skeletal muscle.

(e)   Yes. The sympathetic nerve fibres innervating, for instance, blood vessels in the skin, run in the cutaneous nerve.

12.12

(a)   No. Unmyelinated fibres are thinner (0.5–1 μm) than myelinated fibres (2.5–20 μm).

(b)   Yes. Whereas each myelinated nerve fibre has its own separate Schwann cell sheath, several unmyelinated fibres are enclosed together in a single Schwann cell sheath.

(c)   Yes.

(d)   No. Myelinated nerve fibres exhibit nodes of Ranvier; unmyelinated fibres do not.

(e)   Yes. Conduction of the nerve impulse in myelinated fibres is from node to node, i.e. saltatory.

12.13

(a)   Yes. These are the group 1A afferent fibres.

(b)   No. The efferent fibres are smaller than the group 1A afferents.

(c)   No. The larger nerve fibres are preferentially simulated.

(d)   Yes.

(e)   No. The M and H responses are both generated by extrafusal muscle fibres. The M is the response to direct stimulation of efferent nerve fibres. The H is the reflex response to the stimulation of afferent nerve fibres.

12.14

(a)   Yes. There are, for instance, both myelinated and non-myelinated sensory nerve fibres.

(b)   No. The largest-diameter nerve fibres supply skeletal muscle spindles.

(c)   No. Joint position sense is carried by group 1B fibres, which are large diameter fibres.

(d)   No. Pain and temperature sensations are carried by separate nerve fibres.

(e)   No. Motor nerve fibres to intrafusal muscle fibres are of smaller diameter than those to extrafusal fibres.

12.15

(a)   No. There is a flaccid paralysis as it is a 'lower motoneurone lesion'.

(b)   Yes.

(c)   No. It will be warmer due to interruption of the sympathetic vasoconstrictor nerve fibres.

(d)   No. The sweat glands are also denervated.

(e)   Yes.

12.16

(a)   Yes. Insensible perspiration is seepage of fluid through the skin, a physical process independent of nerve supply.

(b)   No. The skin will be warm because the sympathetic nerve supply is interrupted, allowing dilatation of blood vessels.

(c)   No. There will be no sweating because sweating depends on the sympathetic nerve supply to the skin.

(d)   Yes.

(e)   No. Flaring is an 'axon reflex'; by two weeks the sensory nerve fibres subserving this reflex will have degenerated.

12.17

(a)   Yes. The mechanisms are explained in (b) and (c).

(b)   Yes. Re-innervated fibres hypertrophy and each re-innervated fibre provides a greater twitch tension than normal.

(c)   Yes. Normally the number of muscle fibres in a motor unit is limited by competition among motor nerve endings to innervate muscle fibres. When, after section, the number of innervating motor nerve fibres is sub-normal, each can innervate a larger number of muscle fibres so the number of muscle fibres comprising a motor unit is increased.

(d)   Yes. See (b).

(e)   No. The response to a single action potential in the motor nerve is a single muscle twitch, as normal.

12.18

(a)   Yes. Denervation results in wasting of muscle fibres.

(b)   No. Regenerating nerve tips advance at about 1 mm per day, not 1 cm per day.

(c)   Yes. The regenerating tips show an abnormal mechanosensitivity, so the subject is aware of sensation when the skin over the re-generating tips of axons is tapped lightly. This provides the doctor caring for the patient with a useful index of regeneration.

(d)   No. The conduction velocity of regenerating fibres is less than in unsevered nerve, about one-fifth the normal speed. With time, the conduction velocity increases but never exceeds about half the normal conduction velocity.

(e)   Yes. At the time when sensory endings are being reinnervated, sensation starts to return but, since the pattern of afferent impulses is initially unlike the pattern before severance of the nerve, the central nervous system tends to interpret the input as pain. So a firm touch to the skin frequently causes the sensation of pain.

12.19

(a)   No. An increase in impulse frequency in efferent fibres of the vagus nerves causes a marked increase in the secretion of gastric juice.

(b)   Yes.

(c)   No. Vagal activity causes constriction of the bronchi.

(d)   Yes.

(e)   No. Vagal activity causes increased motility and secretory activity and consequently vasodilatation of the blood vessels in the abdomen.

12.20

(a)   Yes. The surface:volume ratio is greater for small diameter fibres than for large. The amount of metabolic activity required of a nerve to maintain the concentration gradients of ions is thus greater for small fibres than for large, so the small fibres are more susceptible to block by hypoxia than large fibres.

(b)   Yes.

(c)   No. Local anaesthetics block small diameter fibres before large.

(d)   No. A fall in the concentration of calcium ions in the surrounding fluid renders the fibres more excitable.

(e)   Yes. Hyperpolarization of nerve fibres stabilizes the membrane and may produce nerve block.

12.21

(a)   No. The arrival of a nerve impulse at the motor nerve terminal leads to release of acetylcholine into the synaptic cleft but the acetylcholine is so rapidly hydrolysed by acetylcholine esterase that the amount diffusing into the blood is negligible.

(b)   No. The effect of released acetylcholine is strictly confined to the endplate at which it is released; the mechanism is described in (a).

(c)   No. More than sufficient acetylcholine is released to bring the muscle fibre to its threshold for conducting an action potential, so increase in the release of acetylcholine does not result in an increase in the twitch tension produced by the muscle fibre.

(d)   Yes. The opening of ion channels in the membrane is the mechanism whereby acetylcholine has its effects at this junction.

(e)   No. The postsynaptic receptors for acetylcholine are confined to the endplate region of the muscle fibre. Therefore, acetylcholine only causes the muscle fibre to contract if applied at the endplate region.

12.22

(a)   Yes. If the hydrolysis of acetylcholine is prevented and acetylcholine is applied to the endplate, this will result in depolarization block and hence muscular paralysis.

(b)   Yes.

(c)   Yes. This induction (up-regulation) of new receptor sites for neurotransmitter is a feature of denervation.

(d)   Yes. The channels opened by acetylcholine are different in their properties from action potential channels, so that acetylcholine applied to the endplate will still cause the occurrence of an endplate potential even if the action potential mechanism is blocked.

(e)   No. In skeletal muscle, contraction depends on the occurrence of an action potential in a muscle fibre. If the action potential mechanism is blocked, acetylcholine applied to the endplate will not cause the fibre to twitch.

12.23

(a)   Yes.

(b)   Yes. It causes a depolarization block of neuromuscular transmission of short duration.

(c)   Yes.

(d)   Yes. Physostigmine reverses the blockade of curare in this way.

(e)   Yes. Packets of acetylcholine are released spontaneously from the nerve terminals and produce miniature endplate potentials.

12.24

(a)   Yes. Curare blocks transmission at the skeletal neuromuscular junction.

(b)   No. Curare does not interfere with the action potential mechanism and so does not block the contraction of muscle induced by direct electrical stimulation.

(c)   Yes. Since tetrodotoxin blocks voltage-sensitive sodium channels, it blocks the action potential mechanism and therefore blocks nervous conduction.

(d)   Yes. Since tetrodotoxin blocks voltage-sensitive sodium channels, it blocks the conduction mechanism in skeletal muscle fibres.

(e)   No. Miniature endplate potentials are due to the spontaneous release of neurotransmitter chemical; they occur in the absence of action potentials in the motor nerve terminal and so tetrodotoxin does not abolish them.

12.25

(a)   Yes. As an action potential approaches the motor nerve terminal, the nerve fibre narrows and finally becomes unmyelinated. As a result, the conduction speed of the action potential decreases.

(b)   No. In mammalian peripheral nerve, the action potential mechanism depends on voltage-dependent sodium channels, not on calcium channels.

(c)   Yes.

(d)   No. If the pulse takes the membrane potential to the equilibrium potential for calcium ions ($+120\,\text{mV}$), there is no driving force for calcium ions. Although the calcium channels are opened by the pulse, there is no net entry of calcium, which is an essential step in neurotransmitter release.

(e)   Yes. Calcium entry is an essential step in neurotransmitter release.

12.26

(a)   Yes. The I band (isotropic, or non-birefringent) band corresponds to the region where there are thin (actin) filaments only. As a muscle fibre shortens, the overlap between thick and thin filaments increases, so the length of the A band decreases.

(b)   No. The A band (anisotropic, birefringent) corresponds to the thick (myosin) filaments. During muscle shortening, these filaments slide over the thin filaments with no change in length.

(c)   Yes. Since there is little movement of water across the cell membrane as a muscle contracts, the muscle volume is essentially constant, so shortening must be accompanied by thickening.

(d)   No. The force of contraction is inversely related to the rate of shortening.

(e)   No. Each muscle fibre is controlled by a single motor nerve.

12.27

(a)   Yes. 1 mmol per litre is a typical value for the concentration of $[Ca^{2+}]$ in extracellular fluid.

(b)   No. The concentration of $[Ca^{2+}]$ in intracellular fluid in resting muscle is about 10^{-4} mmol per litre.

(c)   Yes.

(d)   Yes.

(e)   No. An action potential in the muscle fibre causes an increase of about 100-fold in intracellular concentration.

12.28

(a)   No. The activation of myosin-ATPase in excitation–contraction coupling is by an increase in intracellular calcium concentration.

(b)   No. Most of the Ca^{2+} released into the cytoplasm of a skeletal muscle fibre by an action potential comes from the cisternae.

(c)   Yes.

(d)   Yes. See (e).

(e)   Yes. The fall in calcium concentration after myosin activation is due to active pumping of calcium ions out of the myoplasm into the cisternae.

12.29

(a)   No. The nuclei lie peripherally.

(b)   No. Each muscle fibre has many nuclei.

(c)   Yes. If a muscle is immersed in ferritin (a protein containing iron) and subsequently examined, the ferritin is found to have filled the transverse tubular system, indicating that it is in continuity with the extracellular space.

(d)   No. The transverse tubules enter the muscle fibre only along certain 'lines', the Z-line in the frog and the I/A boundary in the mammal.

(e)   No. In the experiment described in (c), the ferritin is not found in the cisternae, indicating that they are not in continuity with the extracellular space.

12.30

(a)   No. When the muscle is relaxed, myosin heads are attached to thin filaments but the necks are extended so no tension is exerted.

(b)   No. With the muscle relaxed, the intracellular concentration of calcium is so low that the ATPase is inactive.

(c)   No. Contraction is initiated by a rise in intracellular calcium concentration.

(d)   Yes. Contraction is due to a flexing of the neck joining the head to the thick filament.

(e)   Yes. Myosin heads run along the thin filament like legs running along a tight rope.

12.31

(a)   Yes. In addition to the energy used in production of tension and shortening, energy is released in the form of heat. This represents inefficiency in energy-releasing mechanisms.

(b)   Yes. If a muscle is passively stretched during a contraction, it is analogous to pulling the carpet away from under the feet when someone is running. The myosin heads slip and this reduces the tension developed.

(c)   Yes. If a muscle shortens during a contraction, each myosin head exerts less tension than it does during an isometric con- traction.

(d)   Yes. A fast muscle achieves its speed by having a very quick cycle time for attachment and detachment of myosin heads to actin filaments. Each cycle requires the same amount of energy expenditure. When tension is to be maintained, as in a tetanic contraction, a high rate of cycling utilizes more ATP than is the case for slow skeletal muscle fibres generating the same force.

(e)   Yes.

12.32

(a) No. During a contraction in the body, a skeletal muscle shortens by a maximum of 15% of its resting length.

(b) No. The cisternae, not the transverse tubules, store calcium.

(c) Yes. The spread of electrical activity along the transverse tubules is an important component of the mechanism for rapid activation of muscle fibres.

(d) No. Depolarization of the transverse tubules causes depolarization of the membranes of the cisternae.

(e) No. In skeletal muscle, the increase in calcium concentration is in excess of that needed to cause total activation of myosin ATPase; modulation of the increase in calcium concentration is not a physiological mechanism for modulating the twitch tension.

12.33

(a) Yes. For a muscle involved in producing strong coarse movements, motor units consist of a large number of fibres so that activity in relatively few motor nerve fibres gives a strong contraction. For a muscle involved in finely-controlled movements, the nervous system operates via a large number of motor units each with few muscle fibres; this allows fine control of the movement.

(b) No. A single muscle fibre is innervated by one motor axon.

(c) Yes.

(d) Yes. The recruitment of motor units is one of the ways in which the central nervous system can increase the strength of muscle contraction.

(e) No. The motor component of the tendon jerk reflex is a muscular twitch.

12.34

(a) No. At sarcomere length X_5, there is no overlap of thick and thin filaments and hence the lack of any active tension.

(b) No. In the body, muscle operates in the region X_3 to X_4.

(c) Yes. Tension development depends on the extent of overlap between thick and thin filaments. As we move from X_5 towards X_4, the degree of overlap increases and this accounts for the progressive rise in tension in moving from X_5 towards X_4.

(d) No. The constancy of tension between sarcomere lengths X_3 and X_4 reflects the fact that the middle of each thick filament lacks cross-bridges.

(e) Yes. When the tips of the thick filaments reach the Z lines they can slide no further over the thin filaments and hence can develop no tension; this corresponds to sarcomere length X_1.

12.35

(a)   Yes. With zero load, the muscle develops no power. With excessive loads the muscle cannot move the load and so develops no power. The power is maximum at intermediate loads.

(b)   Yes. With zero load the velocity of contraction is greatest. As the load increases, the velocity progressively declines and reaches zero when the load is so great that it cannot be moved.

(c)   No. As in (a), the work is greatest for intermediate loads and falls to zero for zero load and for excessive loads that the muscle cannot move.

(d)   No. At low lengths, the tension developed is very low because of excessive overlap of thick and thin filaments. As the length increases, the tension rises to a maximum and thereafter, as the length is increased so that cross-bridges on thick filaments cannot attach to thin filaments, the tension falls again.

(e)   Yes. At low frequencies of stimulation, the tension is less than at high frequencies because at low frequencies, there is insufficient time for the contractile component to stretch the series elastic component.

12.36

(a)   No. The y-axis shows that the tension rises; in an isotonic contraction the tension does not change ('isotonic' means 'the same tension').

(b)   Yes.

(c)   No. Towards the end of period c, a second stimulus to the muscle would produce a second response. This is a point of contrast with cardiac muscle, in which the refractory period lasts until the end of contraction, this being a mechanism to prevent tetanization of cardiac muscle.

(d)   No. The muscle action potential follows a much more rapid time course than the mechanical record.

(e)   Yes. Repetitive stimulation allows the contractile element to take up the slack provided by the series elastic component, and so the prolonged contraction that results from repetitive stimulation rises to a higher peak tension than the twitch.

12.37

(a)   No. Choline esterase is the enzyme needed for synthesis of acetylcholine and is concentrated in the endings of motor nerve fibres. A stain for choline esterase will therefore specifically stain the endings of the motor nerve fibres.

(b)   Yes.

(c)   No. During the propagation of the action potential in the nerve there is a net entry of Na^+ ions into the axon.

(d)   Yes. This entry of Ca^{2+} ions into the nerve endings is an essential step in the release of transmitter.

(e)   Yes. There is some entry of Ca^{2+} through the surface membrane and this triggers a much larger release of intracellular Ca^{2+} from intracellular stores.

12.38

(a)   Yes. The action potential is initiated at the endplate, which lies near the middle of the muscle fibre. Thence the action potential spreads in opposite directions towards the two poles of the fibre.

(b)   No. In a twitch, the action potential lasts a small fraction of the duration of the mechanical response.

(c)   No. A rise in temperature increases the rate of dissociation of calcium from actomyosin and this decreases the duration of the muscle twitch.

(d)   No. A rise in temperature, by decreasing the duration of the contraction, also decreases its tension since there is less time for the contractile component to stretch the series elastic component; the tetanic tension is unaltered so the rise in temperature increases the twitch:tetanus tension ratio.

(e)   Yes.

12.39

(a)   No. Transverse tubules are found only in skeletal muscle and provide a mechanism for very rapid activation.

(b)   No. Skeletal muscle contracts much more quickly, hence the need for the transverse tubule system in skeletal muscle but not in cardiac muscle.

(c)   Yes. In cardiac muscle, the increase in calcium concentration does not cause total activation of myosin ATPase; modulation of the increase in calcium concentration is a physiological mechanism for modulating the force of contraction.

(d)   Yes. This must be so otherwise the heart would progressively overfill or empty. In the short term, the pulmonary vascular capacity may alter, allowing a transient difference between the outputs of the two ventricles and hence a transient difference between cardiac output and venous return.

(e)   Yes. By increasing cardiac contractility and heart rate, adrenaline increases the stroke volume over a few cycles, pumping more blood out from the great veins than enters them. After a few cycles, a new steady state is reached, with cardiac output once again equalling venous return.

12.40

(a)   Yes.

(b)   No. The long duration of the action potential is mainly due to a persistent increase in the permeability of the membrane to calcium ions.

(c)   No. In cardiac muscle, the duration of the absolute refractory period is greatly in excess of that in skeletal muscle. This is associated with the fact that, when functioning is physiological, skeletal muscle can be tetanized whereas cardiac muscle cannot.

(d)   Yes.

(e)   Yes. The shortening of the duration of the plateau phase of the cardiac action potential on sympathetic stimulation accompanies the increase in heart rate.

12.41

(a)   No. For the heart, the duration of the cardiac action potential is almost as long as that of ventricular contraction.

(b)   Yes. During sympathetic stimulation of an excised animal heart, at each beat the wall of the atrium is drawn into the mitral orifice during each diastole, proving that the pressure in the atrium is negative to atmospheric at this stage. Thus the ventricle sucks in blood from the atrium during diastole.

(c)   No. The rate of depolarization of the pacemaker cells is increased by sympathetic stimulation.

(d)   No. In the pacemaker cells, the action potential is mainly due to influx of calcium ions.

(e)   Yes.

12.42

(a)   No. Activity of the vagus nerves potently increases stomach motility.

(b)   Yes.

(c)   No. Ingestion of sizeable volumes of fluid into the stomach results in receptive relaxation and there is little change in intragastric pressure.

(d)   No. When a peristaltic wave propels chyme towards the pylorus, most of this chyme is churned back into the stomach and only a small proportion passes out of the stomach.

(e)   Yes.

12.43

(a) Yes. Contraction of bronchial smooth muscle will narrow the bronchioles, so there will be an increase in resistance to air flow in the bronchioles.

(b) No. Contraction of venular smooth muscle will reduce the venous capacity.

(c) Yes. Contraction of arteriolar smooth muscle throughout the body will cause an increase in the total peripheral vascular resistance.

(d) Yes. Contraction of smooth muscle in the stomach wall will cause an increase in pressure in the stomach.

(e) Yes. Contraction of the ciliary muscle takes the strain off the suspensory ligament and the lens becomes fat, i.e. the eye is accommodated for near vision.

12.44

(a) Yes.

(b) Yes. In this respect it is unlike striated muscle in which tension falls off rapidly with reduction in initial length.

(c) Yes. For instance circulating catecholamines cause the smooth muscle sphincters of the bowel to contract.

(d) Yes.

(e) Yes. Many smooth muscles have a double innervation, sympathetic and parasympathetic, the effects of which are often in opposite directions.

12.45

(a) No. The innervation of smooth muscle is by autonomic nerve fibres and these have a peripheral synaptic relay.

(b) No. Unlike skeletal muscle, smooth muscle has no sensory innervation.

(c) Yes. All types of muscle contain actin and myosin, although these are not arranged so regularly in smooth as in cardiac or skeletal muscle.

(d) Yes. Intestinal smooth muscle is so-called 'single-unit' smooth muscle, with cytoplasmic connections between cells. It conducts action potentials from cell to cell.

(e) Yes. Like other 'single-unit' smooth muscles, it may contract in response to chemicals reaching it via the blood.

12.46

(a) Yes. Smooth muscle is found in the skin, for instance in arteriolar walls and in the erector pili muscles.

(b) Yes. Calcium is required for the contraction of all types of muscle.

(c) No. In smooth muscle, the entry of calcium ions is the main charge carrier for the upstroke of the action potential.

(d) Yes. An agent that causes an increase in contraction of all vascular smooth muscle would lead to an increase in central venous pressure by venoconstriction.

(e)   Yes. An agent that causes an increase in contraction of all vascular smooth muscle would lead to an increase in arterial blood pressure by arteriolar constriction.

12.47
(a)   No. The pathway is via the retino-tectal projection which branches from the optic nerve before that nerve reaches the lateral geniculate nucleus.
(b)   No. The ciliary muscle in the eye relies on neural stimuli for its contraction.
(c)   Yes. Dilatation of the pupil is effected both by activity of sympathetic neurones and by circulating catecholamines.
(d)   No. Constriction of the pupil is effected only via its parasympathetic innervation.
(e)   No. Contraction of the ciliary muscle results in relaxation of the suspensory ligament, so its contraction causes the lens to become thicker.

12.48
(a)   No. This is a property only of skeletal muscle.
(b)   No. Smooth muscle has no striations.
(c)   Yes.
(d)   Yes.
(e)   Yes.

12.49
(a)   No. Cardiac muscle fibres, but not skeletal muscle fibres, have intercalated discs.
(b)   Yes. Cardiac muscle fibres have cross-striations, although these are not so clear as in skeletal muscle.
(c)   No. Only skeletal muscle fibres have transverse tubules.
(d)   No. In smooth muscle fibres, the contractile machinery is not organized into an orderly array of thick and thin filaments.
(e)   No. Muscle spindles are found in skeletal muscle, not in cardiac or smooth muscles.

13 Motor control, balance

Motor control	13.1–13.12
Balance	13.13–13.19

QUESTIONS

Motor control

13.1 In mammalian muscle spindles:
(a) the receptors are modified muscle cells. ∧⃒
(b) the receptors are in the polar regions of the spindle. –
(c) the receptors connect with the spinal cord via non-medullated nerve fibres. ⋏
(d) the axons from primary ('annulo-spiral') endings have greater diameter than those from secondary ('flower-spray') endings. ⋏⃒
(e) when intrafusal muscle fibres are activated via the gamma motor nerves, their central ('equatorial') regions contract actively. ⋏⃒

13.2 With reference to the muscle spindle:
(a) the primary sensory ending is stimulated by shortening of the extrafusal fibres around the muscle spindle. ?
(b) the primary sensory ending in a given muscle is stimulated when an antagonist muscle shortens.
(c) the primary sensory ending is stimulated by contraction of the intrafusal muscle fibres. ⊣
(d) the contractile component of the spindle is smooth muscle. ∾
(e) the motoneurones supplying the intrafusal muscle fibres are smaller than those supplying the extrafusal fibres. ⊣ ?

13.3 Figure 13.3 shows the activity of afferent nerve fibres X, Y and Z from three different proprioceptors in response to increased tension produced, firstly, by passive muscle stretch, and, secondly, a twitch produced by activation of alpha, but not gamma, motor nerve fibres.

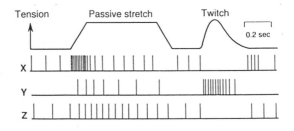

(a)   Y is the nerve fibre from a Golgi tendon organ receptor.
(b)   X is the nerve fibre from a muscle spindle secondary sensory ending.
(c)   Z is the nerve fibre from a muscle spindle primary sensory ending.
(d)   the receptor attached to fibre X has a greater dynamic sensitivity than that attached to Z.
(e)   the diameter of nerve fibre X is greater than that of nerve fibre Z.

13.4   With further reference to Figure 13.3:
(a)   the diameter of nerve fibre X is typically $7 \, \mu m$.
(b)   muscle vibration at 50 Hz would elicit more frequent action potentials in X than in Y or Z.
(c)   activity in Y inhibits the alpha motoneurones supplying the muscle.
(d)   activity in X inhibits the alpha motoneurones supplying the antagonist muscle.
(e)   nerve fibre Z has monosynaptic connections with the alpha motoneurones supplying the muscle.

13.5   The following occur during the production of muscle contraction via the indirect (gamma) pathway:
(a)   increase in discharge of gamma motoneurones.
(b)   relaxation of the polar regions of the intrafusal muscle fibres.
(c)   stretching of equatorial region of intrafusal fibres.
(d)   decrease in discharge of muscle spindle afferent axons.
(e)   increased discharge of alpha motoneurones.

13.6   Concerning the muscle spindle receptors and afferent nerves in an adult human:
(a)   the response of a primary ending shows a larger dynamic component during stretch than does that of a secondary ending.
(b)   when a primary ending is activated, the action potentials in the afferent nerve fibre are initiated in the sensory terminals themselves.
(c)   the afferent arising from the primary ending may connect directly (i.e. monosynaptically) with alpha motoneurones.
(d)   the afferent arising from the secondary ending may connect directly (i.e. monosynaptically) with alpha motoneurones.
(e)   the primary ending acts as the principal receptor in the tendon jerk reflex.

13.7 **With reference to motor units in skeletal extrafusal muscle in an adult mammal:**

(a) from the point of view of neural control, a motor unit is the functional unit in a muscle.

(b) the number of muscle fibres in a motor unit is about the same in all muscles.

(c) one way in which the strength of contraction of a muscle is increased is by recruitment of more motor units.

(d) steady tension during voluntary movements results from the fact that active motor units always produce fused tetanic contractions.

(e) an action potential in a nerve axon will normally excite every muscle fibre making up that motor unit.

13.8 **In an anaesthetized animal, electrical stimuli were applied percutaneously below the level of the knee to the nerve supplying the gastrocnemius muscle. The records show the electromyogram recorded from skin electrodes overlying the gastrocnemius muscle.**

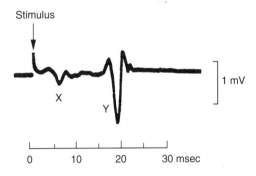

(a) The electrical activity recorded is due to the extracellular voltage field generated by membrane current in the motor nerve terminals.

(b) administration of strychnine (which blocks inhibition in the spinal cord) will cause an increase in the size of wave Y.

(c) administration of a neuromuscular blocking agent while maintaining ventilation artificially will abolish both waves X and Y.

(d) decerebration will cause an increase in the size of wave Y.

(e) administration of anticholinesterase will cause a prolongation of wave X.

13.9   Concerning skeletal muscle in an adult human:
(a)   a single extrafusal muscle fibre is usually innervated via two or more endplates.
(b)   a single intrafusal muscle fibre is usually innervated via two or more endplates.
(c)   a single gamma motor nerve fibre usually innervates muscle fibres in several spindles.
(d)   when an intrafusal muscle fibre contracts, the middle of the fibre is stretched.
(e)   if the nerve to a muscle is cut and the muscle is stretched, the muscle contracts.

13.10   Concerning skeletal muscle in the adult human:
(a)   the gastrocnemius muscle usually has a single muscle spindle.
(b)   muscles involved in the performance of fine movement have a greater density of muscle spindles than those involved in course movements.
(c)   in the motor nerve supplying a typical skeletal muscle, there are about 10 times as many fibres innervating the extrafusal muscle fibres as there are innervating intrafusal fibres.
(d)   most of the nerve fibres innervating intrafusal muscle fibres send branches to extrafusal fibres.
(e)   typically the gamma efferent nerve fibres end in direct association with the sensory terminals.

13.11   Concerning skeletal muscle in an adult human:
(a)   more than two-thirds of all myelinated axons in nerve innervate muscle spindles.
(b)   the intrafusal muscle fibres are innervated by alpha motoneurones.
(c)   the intrafusal muscle fibres are thicker than the extrafusal fibres.
(d)   at the neuromuscular junction of intrafusal muscle fibres, the neurotransmitter chemical is glutamate.
(e)   when the endplate of an extrafusal muscle fibre is depolarized to threshold, this triggers contraction of the whole length of the fibre.

13.12   Concerning skeletal muscle:
(a)   a single muscle fibre is usually innervated by branches from several motor axons.
(b)   a single group IA afferent nerve fibre innervates receptors in several spindles.
(c)   during a voluntary contraction, there is a pause in the discharge of spindle afferents.
(d)   *in vivo*, gamma activation causes contraction of intrafusal muscle fibres.
(e)   *in vivo*, gamma activation causes contraction of extrafusal muscle fibres.

Balance

13.13 **Consider a normal subject sitting in a Barany chair, with head held upright and stationary with respect to the body:**

(a)   when the chair is rotated, the semicircular canals most involved in sensing this rotation are the lateral ones.

(b)   at the start of a rotation at a constant angular velocity, the slow component of the nystagmus the subject exhibits will be in the opposite direction from that of the rotation.

(c)   if the subject closes his eyes and the rotation continues at a constant angular velocity for half a minute, the subject will continue to be aware of the rotation.

(d)   if the chair is abruptly stopped, there is a nystagmus with slow component in the same direction as the previous rotation.

(e)   when rotation stops, and the subject stands, he tends to fall forward.

13.14 **If cold water is introduced into the external auditory meatus of a subject lying supine, to elicit vestibulo-ocular reflexes:**

(a)   reflex eye movements will be generated in a normal subject within 2 sec.

(b)   the reflex eye movements produced in a normal subject are due to direct transmission of mechanical forces from the external meatus to the semicircular canals.

(c)   the slow phase of nystagmus in a normal subject will be towards the side that is cooled.

(d)   a slow deviation of the visual axis occurring without the fast phase indicates midbrain damage.

(e)   caloric testing of this type can result in eye movements, even in unconscious patients.

13.15 **A person stands on the deck of a rolling boat. Receptors contributing to the postural adjustments necessary for remaining upright include:**

(a)   pressure receptors in the skin of the soles of the feet.

(b)   proprioceptors in the muscles of the legs.

(c)   receptors in the capsules of the joints between the upper cervical vertebrae.

(d)   hair cells in the otolith organs of the vestibules.

(e)   hair cells in the semicircular canals.

13.16 If in a quadruped the neck is flexed while the trunk remains stationary:

(a) the pattern of activity in vestibular receptors remains the same.

(b) the resultant vestibular reflexes would include an increase in extensor tonus in the hindlimbs.

(c) the resultant neck reflexes would include an increase in extensor tonus in the hindlimbs.

(d) together, the vestibular and neck reflexes would produce a greater change in extensor tonus in the hindlimbs than either of the reflexes alone.

(e) the tonus in the superior rectus muscles in the orbits would increase.

13.17 Concerning balance and caloric testing:

(a) when a subject is rotated with eyes open on a Barany chair at a constant angular velocity for 1 min, the eyes rotate relative to the head throughout the entire period.

(b) stimulation of receptors in the posterior semicircular canal will induce eye movements in the horizontal plane.

(c) cold water injected into the external auditory meatus flows into the vestibular apparatus and bends the cilia of the hair cells.

(d) for a person at zero gravity (in parabolic flight), rotation of the head is accompanied by reflex eye movements.

(e) for a person at zero gravity (in parabolic flight), lack of deviation of the visual axis with caloric testing indicates defective labyrinthine function.

13.18 Concerning righting reflexes:

(a) the receptors responsible for neck reflexes are uniformly distributed in the intervertebral muscles throughout the cervical region.

(b) the vestibular receptors signal the geometric relationship of the trunk to the head.

(c) when a person voluntarily moves the head on the trunk, the vestibular and neck reflexes tend to cancel each other.

(d) when in a standing subject the body is tilted laterally from the vertical, there is reflex extension of the downhill leg.

(e) a passenger in an aeroplane performing a properly-banked turn receives vestibular input indicating the direction of down-ness to be towards the centre of the earth.

13.19 **A normal subject is rotated in a rotating chair in a clockwise direction at constant angular velocity for one minute:**

(a) with the eyes open at the start of the rotation, visual and vestibular input exert opposing influences on eye movements.

(b) with the eyes open towards the end of the rotation the vestibular input has declined relative to the visual input.

(c) immediately after the end of the rotation, if the eyes are open, visual and vestibular input exert opposing influences on eye movements.

(d) if the eyes have been closed during the rotation, when the rotation ceases the eye movements will be more pronounced if the eyes remain closed than if they are opened.

(e) in a labyrinthine-defective subject who has been rotated with eyes closed, when the rotation ceases there will be reflex eye movements.

ANSWERS

13.1

(a) No. The receptors are the endings of sensory nerve fibres; these wind around the modified muscle cells.

(b) No. The receptors wind around the equatorial regions of the spindles.

(c) No. The receptors connect with the spinal cord via medullated nerve fibres.

(d) Yes.

(e) No. When intrafusal muscle fibres are activated via the gamma motor nerves, their polar regions contract actively.

13.2

(a) No. Shortening of the extrafusal fibres around the muscle spindle takes the tension off the intrafusal fibres and any resting discharge in the primary sensory ending is reduced or abolished.

(b) Yes. Shortening of the antagonist muscle stretches the prime mover, and the primary sensory ending in a muscle spindle is stimulated.

(c) Yes. Contraction of the intrafusal muscle fibres stretches the equatorial sensory region and stimulates the primary sensory ending.

(d) No. It is striped muscle, the fibres of which are thinner than extrafusal muscle fibres.

(e) Yes. The motoneurones supplying the intrafusal muscle fibres are gamma motoneurones, smaller than the alpha motoneurones that supply the extrafusal fibres.

13.3

(a) Yes.

(b) No. Secondary spindle receptors show a response that is proportional to stretch, not to the rate of change of stretch.

(c)   No. Z shows a response that is proportional to passive stretch, not to the rate of change of stretch; the discharge ceases when extrafusal fibres contract during the twitch. This static type of response is characteristic of secondary, not primary receptors.

(d)   Yes. This is shown by the high discharge rate during the onset of stretching.

(e)   Yes. X is a group IA afferent, while Z is a Group II afferent.

13.4

(a)   No. X is a Group IA afferent, which typically has a diameter of 20 μm.

(b)   Yes. Vibration of a muscle at 50 Hz selectively activates primary endings.

(c)   Yes. Tendon organ stimulation elicits reflex inhibition of the muscle to which the tendon is attached; this is a protective reflex preventing excessive muscular contraction with the accompanying risk of rupture of muscle fibres and avulsion of the tendon from the bone.

(d)   Yes. This is reciprocal innervation causing inhibition of motoneurones to antagonist muscles accompanying excitation of the muscle containing the spindle from which the sensory ending arises.

(e)   No. Z is a group II afferent and does not make monosynaptic connections with motoneurones.

13.5

(a)   Yes.

(b)   No. Increased action potential activity of fusimotor efferents causes the intrafusal muscle fibres to contract.

(c)   Yes.

(d)   No. Stretching of the equatorial region of the spindle fibres increases the discharge of muscle spindle afferent axons.

(e)   Yes. This is the final link in the chain.

13.6

(a)   Yes.

(b)   No. Action potentials are initiated at the first node of Ranvier of the afferent nerve fibre.

(c)   Yes. When activated by a tap to the patella tendon, the afferent arising from the primary ending connects monosynaptically with alpha motoneurones of its motoneurone pool to initiate the tendon jerk reflex.

(d)   No. The afferent arising from the secondary ending always operates via interneurones; it never connects monosynaptically with alpha motoneurones.

(e)   Yes. With its high dynamic sensitivity, the primary ending is the main sensor when the tendon is tapped and so acts as the principal receptor in the tendon jerk reflex.

13.7

(a) Yes. Since an action potential in the motor nerve fibre causes all muscle fibres in the motor unit to contract, from the point of view of neural control, a motor unit is the functional unit in a muscle.

(b) No. In large muscles subserving strong coarse movements (e.g. gastrocnemius), a motor unit comprises several hundred muscle fibres. In small muscles used for finely-controlled movements (e.g. the extrinsic ocular muscles), the motor unit may comprise about four muscle fibres.

(c) Yes. Recruitment of more motor units increases the strength of muscle contraction.

(d) No. Asynchrony in activity in different motor units produces a smooth movement even although each motor unit alone may contribute an unfused contraction.

(e) Yes.

13.8

(a) No. It is due to extracellular current generated by the muscle fibres.

(b) Yes. The excitability of spinal motoneurones is increased and spinal reflexes are exaggerated.

(c) Yes. Muscular activity due to activation via motor nerve fibres is blocked.

(d) Yes. Antigravity reflexes are exaggerated.

(e) Yes. Acetylcholine will persist at the endplate and cause repetitive firing of muscle fibres.

13.9

(a) No. A single extrafusal muscle fibre is usually innervated by a single endplate.

(b) Yes. A single intrafusal muscle fibre receives motor innervation at each pole.

(c) Yes. A single gamma motor nerve fibre usually divides into branches to innervate muscle fibres in several spindles. In each spindle, all the branches of a gamma fibre usually innervate intrafusal fibres of a given type, e.g. the dynamic nuclear bag fibres in several spindles.

(d) Yes. The stretching of the middle of the intrafusal muscle fibre when the polar regions contract initiates nerve impulses in the spindle afferents.

(e) No. The contraction of a muscle when it is stretched is reflex and therefore depends on its innervation.

13.10

(a)   No. There are more than 100 spindles in a muscle of this size.

(b)   Yes.

(c)   No. Alpha and gamma efferent axons are usually about equal in number; alpha may exceed gamma, but never by a factor of 10.

(d)   No. Most efferent nerve fibres go to one or the other type of muscle fibres, not to both.

(e)   No. They innervate the endplates of intrafusal muscle fibres at the poles. The stretch receptors coil around the equatorial region of these muscle fibres.

13.11

(a)   Yes. The sensory and motor innervation of spindles is so intense that, together, these nerve fibres constitute more than two-thirds of all myelinated axons in the nerve.

(b)   No. The intrafusal muscle fibres are innervated by gamma motoneurones.

(c)   No. The intrafusal muscle fibres are thinner than the extrafusal fibres.

(d)   No. At the neuromuscular junction of intrafusal muscle fibres, the neurotransmitter chemical is acetylcholine, as for other striated muscle fibres.

(e)   Yes. In the case of the intrafusal fibre, excitation at an endplate only activates the pole on the same side of the equator as the endplate. By contrast, when the endplate of an extrafusal muscle fibre is depolarized to threshold, this triggers contraction of the whole length of the fibre.

13.12

(a)   No. A single muscle fibre is innervated by a single motor axon.

(b)   No. A single group IA afferent nerve fibre innervates receptors in only one spindle.

(c)   No. A voluntary contraction is produced by coactivation of alpha and gamma motoneurones, with an increase, no pause, in discharge of spindle afferents.

(d)   Yes. Gamma motor fibres innervate intrafusal fibres, so their activation causes contraction of those intrafusal muscle fibres.

(e)   Yes. *In vivo*, gamma activation causes contraction of intrafusal fibres and hence a reflex contraction of extrafusal muscle fibres.

13.13

(a)   Yes. The plane of these canals is closest to the plane of rotation.

(b)   Yes. Such a movement of the eyes tends to stabilize the visual image.

(c)   No. The frictional forces in the semicircular canals are such that, after half a minute of rotation at a constant angular velocity, there is no movement of the endolymph relative to the walls of the canals and hence no sense of rotation.

(d)   Yes. The inertia of the endolymph gives the subject the impression of a rotation in the opposite sense from the rotation that has just stopped. Hence the appropriate direction for the slow component of the nystagmus is in the same direction as the previous rotation.

(e)   No. He tends to fall sideways because the world seems to be rotating from left to right or right to left.

13.14

(a)   No. It takes 20 sec or more for eye movements to be generated.

(b)   No. It is the cooling of the endolymph and the resulting convection currents that stimulate the receptors in the semicircular canals.

(c)   Yes. The cold endolymph is dense and so tends to fall. This is the same movement as produced by a rotation of the nose away from the side of injection. To stabilize the visual image, this would require a lateral deviation of the gaze towards the side of the injection.

(d)   No. This indicates damage to higher centres.

(e)   Yes. Caloric testing yields eye movements in an unconscious patient whose brain-stem is functioning.

13.15

(a)   Yes.

(b)   Yes.

(c)   Yes. These are activated as the head moves on the trunk and initiates neck reflexes.

(d)   Yes. These are sensitive to linear acceleration.

(e)   Yes. These signal rotational movement.

13.16

(a)   No. The orientation of the head in space alters and this changes the pattern of stimulation of the otolith receptors.

(b)   No. The forelimbs extend.

(c)   Yes. For the neck reflexes, the change in tonus in limb musculature is such as to push the trunk back into line with the head.

(d)   No. The two tend to cancel. This is probably why a human or other animal is free to move the head on the trunk without initiating inappropriate postural reflexes.

(e)   Yes. This is a reflex with sensors in the semicircular canals and helps to stabilize the retinal image.

13.17

(a)   Yes. The mechanics of the inner ear are such that after about 20 sec of uniform angular rotation, the signal from the labyrinth has declined effectively to zero. However, with the eyes open, the nystagmus continues due to visual input.

(b)   No. The posterior semicircular canal is approximately in the vertical plane, so stimulation will induce eye movements in the vertical plane.

(c)   No. Cold water injected into the external auditory meatus cools the surrounding tissues and induces convection currents in the endolymph; it is these convection currents that simulate head rotation and elicit reflex eye movements. The water cannot reach the vestibular apparatus.

(d)   Yes. For a person at zero gravity (in parabolic flight), the inertia of endolymph is unaltered and so rotation of the head results in movement of endolymph relative to the membraneous labyrinth. Rotation of the head is therefore accompanied by reflex eye movements.

(e)   No. At zero gravity, caloric testing elicits no reflex deviation of the visual axis; the mechanism of this artificial reflex in the normal gravitational field depends on the fall or rise of endolymph as a result of changes in its density. This fall or rise depends on gravity.

13.18

(a)   No. The receptors responsible for neck reflexes are found mainly in muscles between the skull and C1, and between C1 and C2.

(b)   No. The proprioceptors in the upper cervical region signal the geometric relationship of the trunk to the head.

(c)   Yes.

(d)   Yes.

(e)   No. A passenger in an aeroplane performing a properly-banked turn receives vestibular input indicating the direction of down-ness to be the result of two forces, one being gravitational (towards the centre of the earth) and the other being the force required to accelerate the body in the direction of the turn, i.e. towards the centre of curvature of the flight path.

13.19

(a)   No. With the eyes open at the start of the rotation, visual and vestibular input both signal the rotation and cooperate in their reflex effects.

(b)   Yes.

(c)   Yes. Immediately after the end of the rotation, if the eyes are open, the visual input signals that the head is stationary while the vestibular input signals a reversal in the direction of rotation.

(d)   Yes. If the eyes have been closed during the rotation, when the rotation ceases, if the eyes remain closed the vestibular input produces pronounced reflex eye movements; with the eyes open, the central nervous system is informed of the lack of rotation of the head so the reflex eye movements are less pronounced.

(e)   No. Reflex eye movements when the rotation ceases depend entirely on labyrinthine input. So in a labyrinthine-defective subject who has been rotated with eyes closed, there will be no eye movements.

14 Central nervous system

QUESTIONS

Spinal cord, synapses, spinal reflexes

14.1 A somatic lower motoneurone in the human spinal cord:
(a) usually innervates only one muscle fibre.
(b) lies on the same side of the body as the muscle it innervates.
(c) lies on the same side of the body as the muscle spindle receptors that cause its monosynaptic activation.
(d) has synapses on its cell body.
(e) has synapses on its dendrites.

14.2 An alpha motoneurone in the human spinal cord:
(a) receives synaptic inputs only from interneurones.
(b) innervates several muscle fibres.
(c) may innervate fibres in more than one muscle.
(d) has a myelinated axon.
(e) innervates smooth muscle fibres.

14.3 Concerning the spinal cord:
(a) each spinal segment has two dorsal roots.
(b) the motoneurones are located in the dorsal root ganglia.
(c) the grey matter of the spinal cord lies outside the white matter.
(d) the grey appearance of grey matter is due to myelin sheaths.
(e) in the lumbar region, the nerve roots ascend from their segment of origin to the level where they emerge from the vertebral column.

14.4   With respect to spinal reflexes:
(a)   the response may involve the contraction of more than one muscle.
(b)   if a painful stimulus is applied to one leg, the reflex effects may involve motoneurones on both sides of the cord.
(c)   reflexes may be elicited if the dorsal roots are cut.
(d)   every reflex involves at least one synapse in the spinal cord.
(e)   every reflex involves a synapse in a dorsal root ganglion.

14.5   With reference to reflexes and spinal cord mechanisms:
(a)   the delay introduced by each synapse on a reflex pathway is around 10 msec.
(b)   when the Achilles tendon is struck, the reflex response time and the subject's reaction time are approximately equal.
(c)   there are inhibitory alpha motoneurones.
(d)   axon collaterals from alpha motoneurones project directly up to the motor region of the cerebral cortex.
(e)   axon collaterals whose activity has inhibitory effects on the firing of their own neurones constitute one form of negative feedback.

14.6   Concerning the knee jerk reflex in the human:
(a)   the contraction of the quadriceps femoris muscle that occurs in the knee jerk reflex is a response to stimulation of muscle spindle receptors.
(b)   the afferent nerve fibres involved in the reflex arc are myelinated fibres.
(c)   it has a shorter reflex response time than a flexor withdrawal reflex.
(d)   antagonist muscles relax before the reflex contraction occurs.
(e)   if afferents from Golgi tendon organs (group IB afferents) are activated, they increase the amplitude of the tendon jerk reflex.

14.7   Concerning tendon jerk reflexes in a normal human:
(a)   most of the delay between the tap and the onset of EMG (electromyograph) activity is attributable to conduction along the afferent and efferent nerve fibres.
(b)   for the patellar reflex, the reflex time is within 1 msec of that for the jaw jerk reflex.
(c)   it is enhanced if the gamma motoneurones in the motor nerve are blocked.
(d)   the muscle goes into a long tetanic contraction.
(e)   the mechanical contraction of the muscle follows the same time course as the EMG.

14.8   Concerning the knee jerk reflex in a normal adult human:
(a)   the reflex response time is about 1 msec.
(b)   the motoneurones whose activity leads to reflex contraction of the quadriceps muscle lie in a separate motoneurone pool from those activated during a voluntary contraction of the muscle.
(c)   the reflex is monosynaptic.
(d)   the associated inhibition of motoneurones supplying antagonist muscles is monosynaptic.
(e)   the amplitude of the reflex contraction can be voluntarily influenced by the subject.

Spinal cord

14.9   The dorsal (or posterior) columns:
(a)   consist largely of second-order neurones.
(b)   carry most of the central afferent fibres that subserve temperature sensation.
(c)   carry fibres mainly from receptors on the ipselateral side of the body.
(d)   carries fibres, most of which terminate on cells in the gracile and cuneate nuclei.
(e)   are major input pathways to the cerebellum.

14.10   The lateral spinothalamic tracts:
(a)   consist largely of second-order neurones.
(b)   carry most of the central afferent fibres that subserve temperature sensation.
(c)   carry fibres mainly from receptors on the ipsilateral side of the body.
(d)   carry fibres, most of which terminate on cells in the thalamus.
(d)   are major input pathways to the cerebellum.

14.11   Joint position sense in the left arm is impaired if there is damage to:
(a)   the dorsal column on the left in the upper cervical region.
(b)   the thalamus on the left.
(c)   the post-central gyrus of the right cerebral hemisphere.
(d)   the cerebellum.
(e)   the superior colliculi.

14.12   Features of viral infection of the anterior horn cells of the spinal cord include:
(a)   muscular paralysis.
(b)   muscular spasticity.
(c)   wasting of muscles.
(d)   respiratory paralysis.
(e)   clouding of consciousness.

Spinal transection

14.13   An hour after an uncomplicated transection of the spinal cord at the level of C8 in an adult human:
(a)   there is profuse sweating of the skin of the trunk.
(b)   there is a spastic paralysis in the limbs.
(c)   the bladder is atonic.
(d)   the patient is unconscious.
(e)   the blood pressure is elevated.

14.14   Long-term consequences of uncomplicated transection of the spinal cord at the level of C8 include:
(a)   loss of tendon jerks in the legs.
(b)   loss of abdominal reflexes.
(c)   loss of the cremasteric reflex.
(d)   plantar flexion when the sole of the foot is firmly stroked.
(e)   loss of the normal shivering reflex in the legs in response to a cold environment.

14.15   Long-term consequences of uncomplicated transection of the spinal cord at the level of C8 in an adult man include:
(a)   loss of reflex emptying of the bladder.
(b)   reflex fall in blood pressure as the bladder fills.
(c)   loss of reflex erection of the penis.
(d)   orthostatic hypotension.
(e)   lack of sweating below the level of the lesion.

14.16   In a subject with a complete spinal transection at the C8 segmental level:
(a)   there is diaphragmatic breathing.
(b)   the intercostal muscles contract in time with the respiratory cycle.
(c)   the chest wall is sucked in during inspiration.
(d)   the subject is able to speak.
(e)   the cough reflex is absent.

14.17   The long-term consequences of hemisection of the spinal cord at the level of T8 include:
(a)   an ipselateral extensor plantar response (Babinski positive).
(b)   ipselateral spasticity below the level of the lesion.
(c)   loss of temperature sense in the ipsilateral leg.
(d)   loss of position sense in the ipsilateral leg.
(e)   loss of crude touch sense in the ipsilateral leg.

Higher centres

14.18 The Purkinje cells of the cerebellar cortex have axons which:
(a) constitute the main efferent pathway from the cerebellar cortex.
(b) may terminate in the spinal cord.
(c) may terminate in the cerebellar nuclei.
(d) may terminate in excitatory synapses.
(e) influence mainly ipsilateral movements.

14.19 In each case, does a lesion in the structure mentioned below left give rise to the condition mentioned below right?
(a) cerebral cortex tremor at rest.
(b) cerebellum tremor appearing as an accompaniment of voluntary movement.
(c) cauda equina dorsiflexion in Babinski's test.
(d) medulla nasal regurgitation during swallowing.
(e) pyramidal tract exaggerated knee-jerks

14.20 Damage to the basal ganglia usually causes in limb musculature:
(a) spasticity.
(b) interference with voluntary movement.
(c) involuntary movements.
(d) intention tremor.
(e) disorder of posture.

14.21 With respect to brain structure and function:
(a) if a patient becomes anoxic, the cerebral cortex suffers irreversible damage before the brain-stem.
(b) disturbance of consciousness can result from damage confined to the brain-stem.
(c) the sleep centres lie in the basal ganglia.
(d) in the cerebral cortex of a normal subject, the two hemispheres are of approximately equal importance in speech.
(e) a lesion of the cortical motor area for speech (Broca's area) usually results in excessive talking.

14.22 If the cerebral cortex is irrevocably damaged by a period of anoxia but the patient is still breathing spontaneously:
(a) the limbs will withdraw from a painful stimulus.
(b) the pupils will be unresponsive to light.
(c) the patient may speak.
(d) the limbs will have normal muscle tone.
(e) the eyes may be open and the eyeballs moving.

14.23 The hypothalamus contains cells which are specifically sensitive to:
(a) arterial blood pressure.
(b) thyroid-stimulating hormone (TSH) concentration.
(c) hydrogen ion concentration.
(d) partial pressure of oxygen.
(e) plasma volume.

14.24 The hypothalamus:
(a) is about the same size as the lentiform nucleus.
(b) lies in the mesencephalon.
(c) contains neurones specifically sensitive to a rise in temperature.
(d) contains neurones specifically sensitive to a rise in osmolarity of the extracellular fluid.
(e) projects profusely to the limbic system.

14.25 Concerning the nerve supply to the human skin:
(a) the promotion of heat loss from the skin involves increased activity in some sympathetic nerve fibres and decreased activity in others.
(b) the cold clammy skin of a patient in haemorrhagic shock is due to intense activity in all the sympathetic nerve fibres to the skin.
(c) the sympathetic postganglionic fibres supplying sweat glands are cholinergic.
(d) the forearm skin receives a parasympathetic nerve supply.
(e) the synapse between sympathetic preganglionic and postganglionic fibres lies in the dermis.

14.26 Atropine blocks the action of acetylcholine at parasympathetic postganglionic nerve endings. Its local application to the eye causes:
(a) dilatation of the pupil.
(b) impaired ability to focus on nearby objects.
(c) difficulty in looking upwards.
(d) some impairment of fluid drainage from the anterior chamber.
(e) everything to appear dimmer than normal to the subject.

14.27 Interruption of the cervical sympathetic trunk results in ipsilateral:
(a) ptosis.
(b) pupillary dilatation.
(c) exophthalmos.
(d) vasodilatation in the skin of the face.
(e) paralysis of lachryimation.

14.28 Concerning neural control of breathing:
(a) respiratory movements depend on bursts of action potentials in the motor nerves innervating the respiratory muscles.
(b) neuromuscular blockade prevents spontaneous respiration.
(c) the respiratory muscles are skeletal muscles.
(d) if the function of the medulla oblongata fails, spontaneous respiration ceases.
(e) if cerebral cortical function fails, spontaneous respiration ceases.

14.29 Concerning respiration and vocalization (making a vocal sound):
(a) spontaneous respiratory movements still occur in a subject who has suffered a complete transection of the midbrain.
(b) spontaneous respiratory movements occur in a subject who has suffered a complete transection of the spinal cord at the second cervical segmental level.
(c) a subject with no cortical function may vocalize.
(d) a subject with no brain-stem function may vocalize.
(e) a subject with a complete transection of the midbrain may be able to speak.

14.30 Concerning the brain:
(a) if the brain-stem is not functioning, the subject asphyxiates unless artificially ventilated.
(b) if the corpus callosum is cut, the subject can still name objects presented in the right part of the visual field.
(c) if the brain-stem is not functioning, the heart may continue to beat indefinitely, in an artificially ventilated subject.
(d) if the cerebral cortex is not functioning, the heart may continue to beat for years.
(e) if the cerebral cortex is not functioning, the subject may speak.

14.31 In a human adult with loss of function of the left cerebral hemisphere, there is likely to be:
(a) normal speech.
(b) a paralysis of voluntary movement on the right side of the body.
(c) an involuntary tremor on the right side of the body.
(d) blindness in the left peripheral visual field.
(e) loss of sensation on the left side of the body.

14.32   Are the following associations appropriate?

(a)	occipital cortex	consensual light reflex.
(b)	presynaptic inhibition	increased rate of calcium entry into the presynaptic nerve terminal.
(c)	postsynaptic inhibition	reduced sensitivity of receptors on the postsynaptic membrane.
(d)	surround (lateral) inhibition	mechanism which enhances two-point discrimination.
(e)	right-sided hemisection of the upper thoracic spinal cord	loss of temperature sensation in the right leg.

Pain

14.33   Concerning pain:
(a)   nociceptive receptors are encapsulated.
(b)   when local anaesthetic is injected into a peripheral nerve, the sensation of pain is enhanced before it is blocked.
(c)   endorphins enhance nociception.
(d)   the central pathways project via the lateral spinothalamic tracts.
(e)   the central pathways project via the grey matter of the spinal cord.

14.34   Concerning pain:
(a)   on the nociceptive pathway, there is a synaptic relay in the grey matter of the spinal cord.
(b)   the sensation of pain is enhanced by concomitant activity in large afferent nerve fibres.
(c)   the sensation of pain is enhanced by electrical stimulation of the dorsal columns at a site above the segmental level of the pain.
(d)   nociceptive endings project in peripheral nerves via small medullated nerve fibres.
(e)   nociceptive endings project in peripheral nerves via unmedullated nerve fibres.

14.35   Concerning pain:
(a)   'fast pain' is mediated by unmyelinated nerve fibres.
(b)   'slow pain' is more likely to become persistent than 'fast pain'.
(c)   persistent pain is a common consequence of avulsion of peripheral nerves.
(d)   during an elective amputation, local anaesthetic injected into the limb nerves as an adjunct to general anaesthesia reduces the incidence of 'phantom limb'.
(e)   viral infections of anterior horn cells of the cord cause neuralgia more frequently than viral infections of posterior horn cells.

Sleep

14.36 Concerning sleep:
(a)   a person is more disoriented after deprivation of paradoxical sleep (REM sleep) than after deprivation of an equal amount of orthodox sleep.
(b)   after deprivation of paradoxical sleep for two nights a person adapts and, when allowed to sleep undisturbed, the amount of paradoxical sleep is initially less than normal.
(c)   during sleep there is an increase in release of acetylcholine in the cerebral cortex.
(d)   after a complete disconnection of the higher centres from the brain-stem at the upper midbrain level, the cortex is permanently in the sleeping state.
(e)   during orthodox sleep, the electroencephalogram (EEG) is isopotential.

Cerebral environment

14.37 Concerning the blood flow to the brain and intracranial pressure:
(a)   in normal brain the blood flow is directly proportional to the mean arterial blood pressure in the range 60–160 mmHg.
(b)   cerebral ischaemia results in the formation of cerebral oedema.
(c)   lowering the packed cell volume with an accompanying lowering of the haemoglobin concentration to 110 g Hb per litre of blood will result in a reduction of oxygen supply to the brain.
(d)   as an intracranial mass expands, the rate of rise of intracranial pressure progressively declines.
(e)   a rise in intracranial pressure results in a reflex fall in the mean systemic arterial blood pressure.

14.38 Concerning the brain:
(a)   a rise in arterial PCO_2 leads to a rise in intracranial pressure.
(b)   calcium channel blocking agents cause the cerebral vessels to go into spasm.
(c)   calcium channel blocking agents protect central neurones against excitotoxic damage.
(d)   n-methyl-d-aspartate (NMDA) administration protects central neurones against excitotoxic damage.
(e)   GABA is an excitotoxin.

14.39   Concerning the central nervous system:
(a)   glial cells are filled with cerebrospinal fluid.
(b)   on its transit from the blood plasma to the neurones of the brain, oxygen must cross the blood-brain barrier.
(c)   axons from pyramidal cells in the motor region of the cerebral cortex project directly and without synaptic relay to the skeletal muscle fibres whose activity they influence.
(d)   nerve fibres from a cutaneous receptor project directly and without synaptic relay to the somatosensory region of the cerebral cortex.
(e)   if a part of the central nervous system is destroyed by disease, it is replaced by division of nerve cells in neighbouring regions of brain tissue.

Nervous system in general

14.40   Concerning the nervous system:
(a)   the motor command for a voluntary movement is initiated in the cerebral cortex.
(b)   destruction of the cerebellum is without effect on voluntary movement.
(c)   destruction of the basal ganglia is without effect on voluntary movement.
(d)   increase in the strength of a stimulus to receptors in the skin leads to an increase in the amplitude of action potentials passing along the sensory nerve fibres.
(e)   increase in the strength of a stimulus to nociceptors in the skin leads to an increase in frequency of impulses in fibres of the spinothalamic tracts.

Cerebrospinal fluid

14.41   Cerebrospinal fluid (CSF):
(a)   is more acid than blood plasma.
(b)   would be formed at a greater rate if the plasma became hyper tonic.
(c)   is formed by simple ultrafiltration of plasma.
(d)   contains less protein than plasma.
(e)   is absorbed into the venous sinuses.

14.42 Concerning the cerebrospinal fluid (CSF):
(a) about half of it is formed at the choroid plexuses.
(b) it is in free ionic communication with the extracellular fluid compartment of the central nervous system.
(c) it contains potassium at a lower concentration than in blood plasma.
(d) ventilation is stimulated if its pH is decreased.
(e) in metabolic acid-base disturbances, the [H$^+$] of the CSF is readily changed in parallel with changes in plasma [H$^+$].

14.43 Concerning the cerebrospinal fluid (CSF):
(a) its osmolarity is about half that of plasma.
(b) its specific gravity is about half that of brain.
(c) it has a volume of about 150 ml.
(d) it is formed at the rate of about 700 ml in 24 hours.
(e) it circulates through the cerebral ventricles.

14.44 The blood-brain barrier in the human adult:
(a) separates the cerebrospinal fluid from the interstitial fluid of the brain.
(b) exists only at the choroid plexus.
(c) restricts the entry of ions into the brain.
(d) restricts the entry of lipid soluble compounds into the brain.
(e) allows the concentration of glucose in the CSF to equilibrate with that of plasma.

ANSWERS

14.1
(a) No. It usually innervates a group of muscle fibres called the motor unit.
(b) Yes.
(c) Yes.
(d) Yes.
(e) Yes.

14.2
(a) No. An alpha motoneurone receives synaptic inputs from primary afferent nerve fibres and from corticospinal neurones in addition to input from interneurones.
(b) Yes. Each motor nerve fibre innervates several muscle fibres, this being the motor unit.
(c) No. An alpha motoneurone only innervates fibres in a single muscle.
(d) Yes.
(e) No. An alpha motoneurone innervates skeletal, not smooth, muscle fibres.

14.3

(a)   Yes. Each spinal segment has a dorsal root on each side.

(b)   No. The motoneurones are located in the anterior horns of the grey matter of the cord.

(c)   No. The grey matter of the spinal cord lies inside the white matter.

(d)   No. The grey appearance of grey matter is due to the cell bodies of neurones; myelin sheaths appear white.

(e)   No. The lumbar and sacral regions of the spinal cord are higher in the vertebral canal than the corresponding vertebrae; the nerve roots descend several segments before they emerge from the vertebral column.

14.4

(a)   Yes. A reflex response is a movement and this usually involves the contraction of more than one muscle.

(b)   Yes. A painful stimulus applied to one leg causes reflex withdrawal of the stimulated limb and a crossed extensor reflex contra-laterally.

(c)   No. If the dorsal roots are cut the reflexes can no longer be elicited.

(d)   Yes.

(e)   No. There are no synapses in the dorsal root ganglion.

14.5

(a)   No. The delay introduced by each synapse is around 0.8 msec.

(b)   No. When the Achilles tendon is struck, the reflex response time is much shorter (typically 30 msec) than the subject's reaction time (at least 100 msec); the reflex pathway is directly via the cord whereas the reaction time involves paths via the cerebral cortex.

(c)   No. All alpha motoneurones are excitatory.

(d)   No. There are no axon collaterals from alpha motoneurones that project directly up to the motor region of the cerebral cortex.

(e)   Yes.

14.6

(a)   Yes.

(b)   Yes.

(c)   Yes. Because the tendon jerk is monosynaptic, it has a shorter reflex response time than a withdrawal reflex, which is polysynaptic.

(d)   No. Inhibition of antagonist muscles is disynaptic and hence its delay is longer than that of the reflex contraction.

(e)   No. Afferents from Golgi tendon organs inhibit the motoneurone pool of the muscle whose tendon is tapped. So when they are activated, they decrease the amplitude of the tendon jerk reflex.

14.7

(a)   Yes. The reflex is monosynaptic; the time taken for the activity to traverse the spinal cord is around 1 msec and most of the remainder of the time delay between stimulus and response is attributable to conduction along the afferent and efferent nerve fibres.

(b)   No. The peripheral pathway for the patellar reflex is several times as long as for the jaw jerk reflex. So the reflex time is several times as long.

(c)   No. The tendon jerk reflex may be slightly reduced if the gamma motoneurones in the motor nerve are blocked because of removal of ongoing excitation of spindle receptors by fusimotor tone.

(d)   No. The tendon jerk is very brief; it is not a long tetanic contraction.

(e)   No. The mechanical contraction of the muscle follows a much slower time course than the EMG.

14.8

(a)   No. 30 msec would be a correct answer.

(b)   No. Influences from many different sources, including reflex and volitional, converge on a motoneurone.

(c)   Yes. The tendon jerks are the only monosynaptic reflexes in the body.

(d)   No. The orthodromic inhibitory pathway is disynaptic.

(e)   Yes.

14.9

(a)   No. They consist of first-order neurones.

(b)   No. They carry central afferent fibres subserving fine tactile discrimination, pressure and vibration.

(c)   Yes.

(d)   Yes.

(e)   Yes. The dorsal columns carry fibres conveying proprioceptive information and are an important input pathway to the cerebellum.

14.10

(a)   Yes.

(b)   Yes.

(c)   No. The lateral spinothalamic tract is crossed.

(d)   Yes.

(e)   No. The cerebellum receives mainly proprioceptive input.

14.11

(a)   Yes. The dorsal column contains the fibres responsible for joint position sense and the fibres ascend uncrossed. So joint position sense in the left arm is impaired if there is damage to the dorsal column on the left in the upper cervical region.

(b)   No. The ascending paths decussate (cross the midline) in the hind-brain and the thalamic relay is contralateral to the peripheral inner-vation. So joint position sense in the left arm is not impaired if there is damage to the thalamus on the left.

(c)   Yes. The post-central gyrus is in the somatosensory receiving area of the cortex and it is connected with the contralateral periphery. So joint position sense in the left arm is impaired if there is damage to the post central gyrus of the right cerebral hemisphere.

(d)   No. The cerebellum is not involved in perception.

(e)   No. The superior colliculi are concerned with vision, not with somaesthetic senses.

14.12

(a)   Yes. Muscular paralysis is due to denervation of the muscles.

(b)   No. Muscular spasticity is a feature of an upper motoneurone lesion; interference with the anterior horn cells is a lower motoneurone lesion.

(c)   Yes. As a result of disuse, muscles tend to waste.

(d)   Yes. Respiratory paralysis occurs due to denervation of the respiratory muscles (diaphragm and intercostal muscles) when the cervical and thoracic segments, respectively, are involved.

(e)   No. Consciousness depends on the interaction of the brain-stem and the cerebral cortex. Damage to anterior horn cells does not interfere with consciousness.

14.13

(a)   No. Like somatic spinal reflexes, autonomic spinal reflexes are paralysed at this stage.

(b)   No. There is a flaccid paralysis below the level of the transection.

(c)   Yes.

(d)   No. Consciousness is not impaired.

(e)   No. The blood pressure is usually depressed because the influence from the vasomotor centre has been disconnected, and because of the temporary cessation of all spinal cord activity.

14.14

(a)   No. Tendon jerks are increased below the level of the transection.

(b)   Yes. Abdominal reflexes depend on the integrity of the corticospinal projection.

(c)   Yes. The cremasteric reflex depends on the integrity of the cortico-spinal projection.

(d)   No. Below the level of a spinal transection, the response to stroking the sole of the foot is dorsiflexion.

(e)   Yes. In spinal man, shivering never occurs in musculature below the level of the lesion.

14.15

(a)   No. Micturition is a spinal reflex. The subject will have an 'automatic bladder'.

(b)   No. As the bladder fills, the blood pressure rises; this is unlike the intact human in whom the blood pressure is stabilized by reflexes mediated via higher centres.

(c)   No. This occurs as a component of the mass reflex.

(d)   Yes. Raising the subject from the horizontal to the sitting position results in a fall in blood pressure because there can be no reflex adjustment via the brain-stem (except a vagally-mediated increase in heart rate).

(e)   No. Many subjects sweat profusely as a result of uncontrolled spinal sympathetic output; this condition may be hard to control.

14.16

(a)   Yes. The innervation of the diaphragm is via the phrenic nerve, arising from the cord at segmental levels C3, 4 and 5. So in a subject with a complete spinal transection at the C8 segmental level, there is diaphragmatic respiration.

(b)   No. The innervation of the intercostal muscles is from the thoracic segments of the cord. So in a subject with a complete spinal transection at the eighth cervical segmental level, the intercostal muscles do not contract in time with the respiratory cycle.

(c)   Yes. Because of the combination of descent of the diaphragm on inspiration with lack of synchronous contraction of intercostal muscles, the chest wall is sucked in during inspiration.

(d)   Yes.

(e)   No. The cough reflex depends on nerve pathways above the level of transection, so the cough reflex is present. The cough itself may, however, be weaker than normal because intercostal muscles and abdominal muscles cannot assist in producing the brisk expiratory effort.

14.17

(a)   Yes.

(b)   Yes.

(c)   No. Temperature afferents travel in the lateral spinothalamic tracts, which are crossed.

(d)   Yes.

(e)   No. Crude touch from each leg travels up the cord bilaterally in both the anterior spinothalamic tracts; crude touch sensation is impaired, not lost, on both sides.

14.18
(a)   Yes.
(b)   No. They end in the cerebellar nuclei.
(c)   Yes.
(d)   No. They terminate in inhibitory synapses.
(e)   Yes.

14.19
(a)   No. Tremor at rest is characteristic of lesions of the basal ganglia.
(b)   Yes.
(c)   No. A lesion of the cauda equina abolishes the Babinski response.
(d)   Yes.
(e)   Yes.

14.20
(a)   Yes.
(b)   Yes.
(c)   Yes. Involuntary movements are often regarded as the hallmark of disease of the basal ganglia.
(d)   No. Intention tremor is a sign of cerebellar disease.
(e)   Yes.

14.21
(a)   Yes.
(b)   Yes.
(c)   No. They lie in the midbrain reticular formation.
(d)   No. In most subjects, the speech areas are in the left hemisphere.
(e)   No. A lesion of Broca's area usually results in a reduction in talking and 'telegram' speech. Excessive talking is characteristic of a lesion of Wernicke's area.

14.22
(a)   Yes. This reaction is a spinal reflex.
(b)   No. The pupils will respond to light because the brain-stem is intact.
(c)   No. Not without the cerebral cortex.
(d)   No. The limbs will be spastic.
(e)   Yes.

14.23
(a)   No. These are in the carotid sinuses and aortic arch.
(b)   Yes. TSH inhibits thyrotrophin-releasing hormone-secreting cells.
(c)   No. These are in the medulla.
(d)   No. These are in the peripheral chemoreceptors.
(e)   No. These are in the atria.

14.24

(a) No. The hypothalamus is much smaller than the lentiform nucleus.
(b) No. The hypothalamus lies in the diencephalon.
(c) Yes.
(d) Yes.
(e) Yes. The limbic system receives its input about the internal environment mainly from the hypothalamus.

14.25

(a) Yes. Increased activity in fibres to sweat glands is accompanied by decreased activity in fibres to the arterioles supplying the superficial plexus of skin blood vessels.
(b) Yes.
(c) Yes.
(d) No. The autonomic innervation is purely sympathetic.
(e) No. The synapse lies in a paravertebral ganglion or in a collateral ganglion distant from the skin itself.

14.26

(a) Yes. Because of paralysis of the constrictor pupillae muscle.
(b) Yes. Because of paralysis of the ciliary muscle.
(c) No. There is no effect on extrinsic ocular muscles.
(d) Yes. The canal of Schlemm tends to be held open by contraction of the ciliary muscle.
(e) No. Everything tends to appear brighter because of the dilated pupil.

14.27

(a) Yes.
(b) No. The dilator pupillae muscle, supplied by the cervical sympathetic, is paralysed.
(c) No. Enophthalmos would be correct.
(d) Yes. Due to paralysis of the vasoconstrictor nerve supply.
(e) No. Lachrymation is under the control of the parasympathetic nervous system.

14.28

(a) Yes. The respiratory cycle is neurally generated.
(b) Yes. Neuromuscular transmission is an essential step in the activation of the respiratory muscles, as for all skeletal muscles.
(c) Yes.
(d) Yes. The involuntary breathing pattern is generated in the medulla, and any overriding voluntary command for respiratory muscles traverses it. So if the function of the medulla oblongata fails, spontaneous respiration ceases.

(e)   No. The cerebral cortex is not essential for respiratory movements, although commands for voluntary changes in pattern are initiated there.

14.29
(a)   Yes. The bulk of the respiratory neurones lies in the medulla and pons. So spontaneous respiratory movements could occur in a subject who has suffered a complete transection of the midbrain.
(b)   No. The neural pathway for control of the respiratory muscles, both the diaphragm and the intercostals, traverses the cord at the second cervical segmental level. A complete transection at the level of C2 disconnects this pathway for the diaphragm (segmental innervation C3 to C5) and for the intercostals (thoracic segments). So spontaneous respiratory movements are absent in a subject who has suffered a complete transection of the spinal cord at the second cervical segmental level.
(c)   Yes. A subject with no cortical function may vocalize, although the sounds contain no meaning; they are entirely reflex.
(d)   No. A subject with no brain-stem function makes no spontaneous movements; such a subject will not vocalize.
(e)   No. Speech depends on commands from the cerebral cortex traversing the midbrain en route for the cord. So a subject with a complete transection of the midbrain cannot speak.

14.30
(a)   Yes. The respiratory centres lie in the brain-stem, so if the brain-stem is not functioning, the subject asphyxiates unless artificially ventilated.
(b)   Yes. The right part of the visual field projects to the left hemisphere which houses the speech centres. So if the corpus callosum is cut, the subject can name objects presented in the right part of the visual field.
(c)   No. If the brain-stem is not functioning, the heart ceases to beat after a few days or weeks at most. The reason for this failure is not understood.
(d)   Yes. Spontaneous beating of the heart does not depend on cortical function.
(e)   No. The cortex houses the speech centres, so if the cerebral cortex is not functioning, the subject cannot speak.

14.31
(a)   No. The speech centres are in the left hemisphere in almost all people.
(b)   Yes. The left cerebral hemisphere projects to the right side of the spinal cord, so interruption of function of the left cerebral hemisphere results in a paralysis of voluntary movement on the right side of the body.
(c)   No. An involuntary tremor is not a feature of hemispheric lesions.

(d)   No. Loss of function of the left cerebral hemisphere results in blindness in the right peripheral visual field.

(e)   No. The left cerebral hemisphere receives input from the right side of the spinal cord, so interruption of function of the left cerebral hemisphere results in loss of sensation on the right, not on the left side of the body.

14.32

(a)   No. The pathway for the consensual light reflex (constriction of the pupil when a light is shone in the opposite eye) does not traverse the visual cortex.

(b)   No. In presynaptic inhibition, the excursion (amplitude) of the action potential in the presynaptic terminal is reduced and consequently there is a reduction, not an increase, in calcium entry into the presynaptic terminal.

(c)   No. Postsynaptic inhibition is due to the opening of chloride channels in the postsynaptic membrane; there is no reduction in sensitivity of postsynaptic receptors.

(d)   Yes.

(e)   No. Temperature sensation is carried in the lateral spinothalamic tracts, the fibres of which have crossed in the spinal cord.

14.33

(a)   No. Nociceptive receptors are free nerve endings.

(b)   No. When local anaesthetic is injected into a peripheral nerve, the small diameter nerve fibres (nociceptive fibres) are blocked first. The sensation of pain is not enhanced before it is blocked.

(c)   No. Endorphins reduce nociception.

(d)   Yes. The lateral spinothalamic tracts are the principal path for the transmission of 'first', or fast pain.

(e)   Yes. The projection via the grey matter of the spinal cord is the principal path for the transmission of 'second' or slow pain.

14.34

(a)   Yes. There is a synaptic relay in the grey matter of the spinal cord and this is an important site for modulation of the nociceptive signal on its journey to the higher centres.

(b)   No. Activity in large afferent nerve fibres depresses synaptic transmission along nociceptive pathways, so the sensation of pain is reduced by concomitant activity in large afferent nerve fibres.

(c)   No. Stimulation of the dorsal columns reduces nociception, probably via antidromically-conducted impulses travelling down from the site of stimulation and depressing synaptic transmission along nociceptive pathways. Consequently, the sensation of pain is reduced by electrical stimulation of the dorsal columns.

(d)   Yes. Nociceptive endings project in peripheral nerves via small medullated nerve fibres; this is the pathway responsible for 'fast pain'.

(e)   Yes. Nociceptive endings project in peripheral nerves via unmedullated nerve fibres; this is the pathway responsible for 'second pain'.

14.35

(a)   No. 'Fast pain' is mediated by fine myelinated nerve fibres.

(b)   Yes.

(c)   Yes.

(d)   Yes. The mechanism is that, even under general anaesthesia, the inescapable trauma to peripheral nerves during amputation sets up nerve impulses and, if these have access to the cord, they tend to set up persistent central 'pain' circuits; local anaesthesia of the limb nerves blocks the pathway and so reduces the incidence of 'phantom limb'.

(e)   No. Viral infections of posterior horn cells and homologous cells in the brain-stem (e.g. herpes zoster) carry the well-recognized danger of leading to neuralgia, such as trigeminal neuralgia. Viral infections of anterior horn cells, e.g. poliomyelitis, do not. So viral infections of posterior horn cells of the cord cause neuralgia more frequently than viral infections of anterior horn cells.

14.36

(a)   Yes. Paradoxical sleep is very important for our well-being and deprivation rapidly leads to disorientation. The mechanism of this effect is unknown.

(b)   No. After deprivation of paradoxical sleep for two nights, a person, when allowed to sleep undisturbed, has a much larger proportion of paradoxical sleep to catch up with the previous deprivation.

(c)   No. Release of acetylcholine into the cortex is the mechanism whereby the ascending reticular formation keeps the cortex awake; during sleep there is a decrease in release of acetylcholine in the cerebral cortex.

(d)   No. After a complete disconnection of the higher centres from the brain-stem at the upper midbrain level, the cortex is permanently in the waking state; sleep is an active process mediated by ascending influences from the midbrain, pons and medulla.

(e)   No. During orthodox sleep, the EEG exhibits low frequency oscillations of high voltage. The EEG is isopotential only when cortical function is lost entirely.

14.37

(a)   No. Over this range, the brain exhibits autoregulation of its blood flow, i.e. the flow is almost unchanged by changes in the mean arterial blood pressure.

(b)   Yes. Ischaemia damages the capillary endothelium with a resultant formation of oedema.

(c)   No. The lowering of the packed cell volume results in a lowering of the viscosity of blood. The blood flow therefore increases and this more than offsets the reduced oxygen carrying power of the blood.

(d)   No. The opposite. Over a certain range, an increase in volume in the brain displaces CSF and blood from the skull contents and the pressure rise is relatively modest. As the mass expands further, the intracranial pressure rises ever more rapidly.

(e)   No. The reflex effect of increased intracranial pressure is a proportional rise in mean systemic arterial blood pressure, assisting perfusion of the cerebral tissues.

14.38

(a)   Yes. Due to dilatation of the cerebral vessels.

(b)   No. Calcium channel blocking agents cause smooth muscle to relax and so promote perfusion of cerebral vessels.

(c)   Yes. Excitotoxic damage is mediated by calcium entry into neurones, so calcium channel blocking agents help to protect.

(d)   No. NMDA opens membrane channels that allow calcium to enter; NMDA is an excitotoxin.

(e)   No. GABA is the principal inhibitory neurotransmitter in the higher centres.

14.39

(a)   No. Glial cells, like all other cells, are filled with intracellular fluid; cerebrospinal fluid is the extracellular fluid of the brain.

(b)   Yes. Oxygen readily crosses the blood-brain barrier.

(c)   No. Axons from pyramidal cells in the motor region of the cerebral cortex influencing skeletal muscle fibres do so by synaptic influences on the motoneurones in the spinal cord; there is no direct, non-synaptic pathway from the cortex to skeletal muscle fibres.

(d)   No. Nerve fibres from a cutaneous receptor project via the central afferent pathways to the cortex; on the specific pathways there are two synaptic relays. There are no pathways that run directly and without synaptic relay from somaesthetic receptors to the somato-sensory region of the cerebral cortex.

(e)   No. In adult humans, central neurones are postmitotic and are not replaced by precursor cells; if a part of the central nervous system is destroyed by disease, it cannot be replaced by division of nerve cells in neighbouring regions of brain tissue.

14.40

(a)   Yes.
(b)   No. Destruction of the cerebellum results in intention tremor.
(c)   No. Destruction of the basal ganglia results in paucity or complete paralysis of voluntary movement.
(d)   No. Increase in the strength of a stimulus to receptors in the skin leads to an increase in the frequency of impulses, not their amplitude.
(e)   Yes.

14.41

(a)   Yes. Normal CSF pH is about 7.32.
(b)   No. Although formation is not only by passive processes, a hypertonic plasma would diminish the rate of extravasation of fluid; water would tend to move from CSF to plasma.
(c)   No. Active processes are involved.
(d)   Yes. CSF contains less protein than even the small amount in other extracellular, extravascular fluids.
(e)   Yes. Absorption is via the arachnoid villi.

14.42

(a)   Yes. Probably about 50% of the CSF is formed at the choroid plexuses; it also escapes in an actively controlled manner from all CNS capillaries into the interstitium and subarachnoid space (across the blood-brain barrier).
(b)   Yes. The whole of the cerebral ventricles and subarachnoid space together with the extracellular fluid are without barriers to diffusion; CSF is an extension of the interstitial fluid of the central nervous system.
(c)   Yes. Potassium concentration is regulated at the blood-brain barrier: cerebral extracellular and CSF $[K^+]$ is just over half that in plasma.
(d)   Yes. The chemosensitive areas near the ventral surface of the medulla are stimulated by the acidity of CSF.
(e)   No. The blood-brain barrier is relatively impermeable to $[H^+]$.

14.43

(a)   No. The osmolarity of CSF is close to that of plasma.
(b)   No. Its specific gravity is just slightly less than brain (the specific gravity of CSF is 1.01, that of brain is 1.04).
(c)   Yes.
(d)   Yes.
(e)   Yes.

14.44

(a)   No. The blood-brain barrier separates the plasma from the cerebrospinal fluid and the interstitial fluid of the brain; the latter two are in continuity with each other.

(b)   No. The blood-brain barrier exists throughout the vasculature of the brain, not only at the choroid plexus.

(c)   Yes.

(d)   No. Lipid soluble compounds can dissolve in the membranes of the cerebral endothelial cells and thus bypass the blood-brain barrier.

(e)   No. The concentration of glucose in the CSF is only 80% of its concentration in the plasma.

15 Autonomic nervous system

QUESTIONS

15.1 Concerning the autonomic nervous system:
(a)   parasympathetic nerve fibres usually have a synaptic relay close to or in the structure that they innervate.
(b)   the sympathetic nerve supply to the hand arises from the thoracic cord.
(c)   most of the cell bodies of sympathetic nerve fibres leaving the spinal cord lie in the dorsal root ganglia.
(d)   the preganglionic sympathetic nerve fibres are thicker than the postganglionic ones.
(e)   at the synapse between pre- and postganglionic sympathetic nerves, the transmitter is acetylcholine.

15.2 Are these the locations of cell bodies from which preganglionic autonomic nerve fibres arise?
(a)   parasympathetic, in the hypothalamus.
(b)   parasympathetic, in the medulla oblongata.
(c)   parasympathetic, in cervical segments of the spinal cord.
(d)   sympathetic, in thoracic segments of the spinal cord.
(e)   parasympathetic, in the lumbar segments of the spinal cord.

15.3 Concerning the autonomic nervous system:
(a)   the skin receives parasympathetic nerve fibres.
(b)   the sympathetic nerve supply for the whole body arises from the thoracolumbar region of the spinal cord.
(c)   preganglionic sympathetic nerve fibres leave the spinal cord with the segmental anterior roots.
(d)   the postganglionic sympathetic nerve fibres are unmyelinated.
(e)   sympathetic ganglia contain synapses.

15.4 Concerning autonomic control of the alimentary canal:
(a)   the parasympathetic supply to the whole of the large intestine is through the vagus nerves.
(b)   acetylcholine is the transmitter for 'receptive relaxation' in the stomach.
(c)   increased sympathetic activity increases the frequency of the basic electrical rhythm.
(d)   the gall bladder is contracted by vagal activity.
(e)   contraction of the internal anal sphincter is mediated by noradrenaline.

15.5   Stimulation of the sympathetic nervous supply to the lungs:
(a)   is without effect on the blood vessels.
(b)   relaxes the bronchial smooth muscle.
(c)   constricts the openings of the alveoli.
(d)   assists the matching of ventilation and perfusion in exercise.
(e)   increases the diffusion coefficient of oxygen.

15.6   With reference to the sympathetic supply to the skin:
(a)   skin temperature increases if the sympathetic nerve supply is interrupted.
(b)   the increase in skin blood flow in exercise is due to sympathetic overactivity.
(c)   sympathetic fibres carry afferent information from temperature receptors.
(d)   the ganglionic relay is in the dermis.
(e)   sweating is mediated by sympathetic efferents.

15.7   With reference to the cardiovascular system:
(a)   the vagus carries afferent impulses from the carotid bodies.
(b)   the efferent pathway for reflex adjustment of heart rate is both vagal and sympathetic.
(c)   the muscle layers of veins contain noradrenergic nerve endings.
(d)   increased vagal activity leads to lengthening of diastole.
(e)   increased sympathetic activity shortens the duration of the P–R interval of the ECG.

15.8   Concerning the autonomic nervous system:
(a)   preganglionic sympathetic fibres are mostly shorter than preganglionic vagal fibres.
(b)   the sympathetic nerve fibres supplying the feet have their cell bodies in the spinal cord.
(c)   all pre- to postganglionic transmission is by acetylcholine.
(d)   preganglionic parasympathetic fibres to the abdominal viscera have cell bodies in the thoracic region of the spinal cord.
(e)   preganglionic sympathetic fibres are myelinated.

15.9   Are the following correctly included in the effects of an increase in sympathetic activity?
(a)   increase in gastric motility.
(b)   constriction of hepatic arterioles.
(c)   increase in the ratio of glucagon to insulin secretion by the pancreatic islets.
(d)   promotion of liver glycogenolysis.
(e)   release of acetylcholine from nerve endings in the adrenal medulla.

15.10 **Are the following correctly listed as effects of parasympathetic activity?**

(a) dilatation of the pupils of the eyes.

(b) increased ventricular contractility in the heart.

(c) inhibition of inspiratory activity.

(d) urge to defaecate.

(e) relaxation of the pylorus.

15.11 **Are the following correctly listed as effects of parasympathetic activity?**

(a) salivation.

(b) gastrin secretion.

(c) pancreatic secretion with high bicarbonate content.

(d) contraction of the sphincter of Oddi.

(e) contraction of the urinary bladder.

15.12 **With reference to the innervation and activation of smooth muscle:**

(a) autonomic nerve endings form motor endplates on visceral muscle.

(b) one sympathetic postganglionic nerve fibre may activate many smooth muscle cells.

(c) smooth muscle requires calcium ions to enter the cells for contraction to occur.

(d) a single cell may have receptors for different transmitter substances.

(e) intestinal smooth muscle is arranged in two layers, with circular muscle nearer the lumen.

15.13 **Increased activity in the efferent fibres of the vagus nerve supplying the mammalian heart:**

(a) can produce cardiac arrest.

(b) causes an increased sodium permeability in pacemaker cells.

(c) causes depolarization of cells of the sino-atrial (SA) node.

(d) speeds conduction through the atrioventricular (AV) node.

(e) is effective after previous treatment of the heart with atropine.

ANSWERS

15.1

(a) Yes.

(b) Yes.

(c) No. Their cell bodies lie in the lateral horn of the grey matter of the spinal cord.

(d) Yes.

(e) Yes.

15.2

(a)   No. The hypothalamus is the highest centre of autonomic control, but it exerts its effects by neurones that impinge on the autonomic preganglionic neurones, none of which lie in the hypothalamus itself.

(b)   Yes. This is the site of origin of fibres that travel in the vagus nerves: the cranial division of the parasympathetic system.

(c)   No. No autonomic fibres arise from the cervical segments.

(d)   Yes. The sympathetic cell bodies are in the lateral horns of the grey matter that extend from the second thoracic to the second lumbar segment.

(e)   No. The cells for this lower division of the parasympathetic outflow are in the sacral segments.

15.3

(a)   No. The skin receives no parasympathetic nerve supply.

(b)   Yes. The sympathetic outflow from the spinal cord is from the second thoracic to second lumbar segments.

(c)   Yes. Preganglionic sympathetic nerve fibres leave the spinal cord with the segmental anterior roots and then separate as white rami communicans.

(d)   Yes. The postganglionic sympathetic nerve fibres are unmyelinated, which gives them their grey appearance.

(e)   Yes. Sympathetic ganglia are the site for the peripheral synapse on the sympathetic projection from the spinal cord to the target organ.

15.4

(a)   No. The parasympathetic supply to part of the colon and to the rectum is from the sacral parasympathetic outflow.

(b)   No. This is vagally mediated, but is not cholinergic. Nitric oxide is involved.

(c)   No. The basic electrical rhythm frequency is independent of autonomic influences.

(d)   Yes. Both hormonal and neural factors influence gall bladder contraction.

(e)   Yes. Contraction of the internal anal sphincter is mediated by noradrenaline, this being a sympathetic effect.

15.5

(a)   No. Although variations in vascular diameter are mainly passive, allowing distension as flow increases, sympathetic stimulation tends to stiffen the walls of vessels so that they do not over-distend.

(b)   Yes.

(c)   No. Openings of alveoli are not actively constricted or dilated.

(d)   Yes. As described in (a), the sympathetic effect is to tend to stiffen the walls of vessels so that they do not over-distend at the bases; such over-distension would exacerbate $\dot{V}_A/Q$ mismatching.

(e)   No. This is a physicochemical property.

15.6

(a)   Yes. Normal sympathetic 'tone' maintains a degree of arteriolar constriction. If this is abolished there is increased skin blood flow and a warm area in the distribution of the interrupted nerve supply.

(b)   No. Sympathetic activity causes arteriolar constriction; a reduction in sympathetic activity to cutaneous blood vessels causes an increase in blood flow.

(c)   No. Afferent information from temperature receptors is carried in somatic, not sympathetic, nerves.

(d)   No. The ganglionic relays are in the ganglia of the sympathetic chain, close to the vertebral column.

(e)   Yes. These are cholinergic in humans.

15.7

(a)   No. Afferents from the aortic bodies and aortic arch baroreceptors travel along with the vagus. Carotid body and carotid sinus afferents travel in the sinus nerve, which joins the glossopharyngeal nerve.

(b)   Yes.

(c)   Yes. Sympathetic venoconstrictor influences are important in the adjustment of venous capacity.

(d)   Yes. By their influence on the sino-atrial node, vagal efferents slow the heart by prolonging the interval between pacemaker discharges.

(e)   Yes. Sympathetic activity increases the rate of conduction through the atria and so reduces the P–R interval of the ECG.

15.8

(a)   Yes. Sympathetic preganglionic fibres relay relatively close to their emergence from the spinal cord. Parasympathetic relays are near or in the walls of the tissues or organs supplied.

(b)   No. The sympathetic nerve fibres supplying the feet have their cell bodies in the sympathetic ganglia, not in the spinal cord.

(c)   Yes.

(d)   No. Preganglionic sympathetic, not parasympathetic, fibres have cell bodies in the thoracic region of the spinal cord.

(e)   Yes. Hence the term 'white rami'.

15.9

(a) No. Sympathetic influences in general quieten the gut.

(b) Yes. 'Splanchnic' constriction, which occurs in response, for example, to a fall in arterial blood pressure by the baroreceptor reflex, includes the hepatic vascular bed.

(c) Yes. Glucagon tends to release glucose, and insulin tends to store it. Sympathetic activity is called for in 'fight or flight', in which glucose is mobilized in readiness for skeletal muscular activity.

(d) Yes. Increase in catecholamines promotes breakdown of liver glycogen, thence greater availability of glucose for muscular activity.

(e) Yes. The neuro-endocrine 'synapses' in the adrenal medulla are analogous to those in sympathetic ganglia. The preganglionic fibres terminate on adrenaline-secreting cells.

15.10

(a) No. Sympathetic activity dilates the pupil.

(b) No. This is a sympathetic effect.

(c) No. Vagal afferents from stretch receptors can inhibit inspiratory activity, but these are not part of the parasympathetic system.

(d) Yes.

(e) Yes.

15.11

(a) Yes. Salivary secretion is entirely under neural, mainly para-sympathetic, control.

(b) Yes.

(c) No. The neural or cephalic phase of pancreatic secretion is character-ized by a high enzyme content. High bicarbonate results from hormonal stimulation when acid chyme enters the duodenum.

(d) No. Parasympathetic activity causes relaxation of the sphincter of Oddi allowing bile and pancreatic juice to enter the duodenum.

(e) Yes. Sacral parasympathetic efferents stimulate contraction of the urinary bladder.

15.12

(a) No. Motor endplates only occur on skeletal muscle fibres.

(b) Yes.

(c) Yes. In smooth muscle, calcium entry is an essential step in excitation-contraction coupling. In some smooth muscle there is some internal calcium available for release from the sarcoplasmic reticulum, but this is not the main mechanism. This is a point of contrast with skeletal muscle.

(d) Yes.

(e) Yes.

15.13

(a)   Yes. Vagal activity, if sufficiently intense, can produce cardiac arrest.

(b)   No. Vagal activity causes an increased potassium permeability in pacemaker cells.

(c)   No. Vagal activity stabilizes the cells of the sino-atrial (SA) node.

(d)   No. Vagal activity slows conduction through the atrioventricular (AV) node.

(e)   No. Atropine blocks cholinergic transmission at parasympathetic neuro-effector junctions. So vagal activity is ineffective after previous treatment of the heart with atropine.

16 Formation and excretion of urine

QUESTIONS

Kidney

16.1 Concerning the kidneys and their function:
(a) the colloid osmotic pressure of blood in the glomerulus favours the formation of glomerular filtrate.
(b) the hydrostatic pressure of ultrafiltrate in Bowman's capsule favours the formation of glomerular filtrate.
(c) the wall of the thick segment of the ascending limb of the loop of Henle is impermeable to water.
(d) in water diuresis, the osmolarity of the extracellular fluid of the renal medulla is less than in the non-diuretic situation.
(e) in water diuresis, the permeability of the collecting duct is increased by comparison with the non-diuretic situation.

16.2 In a healthy human in anti-diuresis:
(a) the wall of the descending limb of the loop of Henle is readily permeable to water.
(b) the wall of the ascending limb of the loop of Henle, as it joins the distal convoluted tubule, is impermeable to water.
(c) as erythrocytes travel along the descending limbs of the vasa recta to the tip of the renal papilla, they lose at least a half of their intracellular water.
(d) as tubular fluid flows along successive sections of the nephron, its volume progressively decreases.
(e) as tubular fluid flows along successive sections of the nephron, its osmolarity progressively increases.

16.3 Concerning urea:
(a) it is the principal end-product of nitrogen metabolism.
(b) in a normal person it is mostly produced in the liver.
(c) in a normal person its plasma concentration is around 8 mmol per litre.
(d) in renal failure the rise in plasma urea concentration is due to deficient renal tubular secretion of urea.
(e) a normal person on a high protein diet can excrete a more concentrated urine than a person on a low protein diet.

16.4 Concerning renal function, the glomerular filtration rate (GFR) is increased by:
(a) constriction of the afferent arterioles.
(b) constriction of the efferent arterioles.
(c) increase in the concentration of plasma proteins.
(d) increase in the capsular pressure.
(e) a fall in the concentration of anti-diuretic hormone in the blood.

16.5 Concerning renal function in a healthy human adult:
(a) the glomerular filtration rate is typically 700 ml per min.
(b) the renal plasma flow is typically 1.2 litres per min.
(c) most of the water filtered at the glomerulus is subsequently reabsorbed.
(d) the glomerular filtrate contains glucose at about the same concentration as that in plasma.
(e) the glomerular filtrate contains globulin at about the same concentration as that in plasma.

16.6 Concerning the proximal convoluted tubule of a nephron:
(a) about two-thirds of the fluid filtered at the glomerulus is reabsorbed in the proximal convoluted tubule.
(b) the reabsorbed fluid is isosmotic with plasma.
(c) water is actively pumped from tubular fluid to renal interstitial fluid.
(d) the wall of the proximal convoluted tubule is permeable to water.
(e) hydrogen ions are pumped out of the tubular fluid in the proximal convoluted tubule.

16.7 In the renal tubular fluid, secreted hydrogen ions are buffered by:
(a) monohydrogen phosphate ions (HPO_4^{2-}).
(b) urea.
(c) chloride ions.
(d) ammonia.
(e) sodium ions.

16.8 **Concerning the kidneys and renal function:**
(a) the energy required for filtration of fluid in the glomeruli is generated by the heart.
(b) the mean blood pressure in glomerular capillaries is about the same as in capillaries in skeletal muscle.
(c) the energy required for the osmotic gradient in the interstitium of the renal medulla is provided by the pumping of ions across the wall of the thick part of the ascending limb of the loop of Henle.
(d) the colloid osmotic pressure of the plasma increases by about 20% as it passes along a glomerular capillary bed.
(e) the rate of filtration of glomerular fluid increases along the length of the glomerular capillary.

16.9 **In a normal human who has a diuresis due to drinking a large volume of water:**
(a) the osmolarity of the urine is less than 300 mosmol per litre.
(b) the renal venous blood has a higher osmolarity than the renal arterial blood.
(c) the glomerular filtration rate may be 50% above that in the non-diuretic situation.
(d) vigorous muscular exercise will enhance the diuresis.
(e) within an hour, the subject excretes a larger percentage of the fluid load than if he drinks isosmotic saline.

16.10 **Concerning normal renal function:**
(a) the maximum concentration of urine that the human kidney can produce is four times that of plasma.
(b) about half the osmolarity of concentrated urine is due to urea.
(c) a human can survive by drinking sea water instead of fresh water (sea water has three times the osmolarity of the plasma).
(d) the lowest concentration of urine that the human kidney can produce is equal to the osmolarity of plasma.
(e) in diuresis, the urine contains all the water that is filtered at the glomerulus.

16.11 **Do the following substances have a renal tubular transport maximum?**
(a) para-amino hippuric acid (PAH).
(b) glucose.
(c) inulin.
(d) phosphate.
(e) alanine.

16.12 For the following substances, is the rate of urinary excretion linearly dependent on its plasma concentration?
(a) glucose.
(b) inulin.
(c) creatinine.
(d) para-amino hippuric acid (PAH).
(e) water.

16.13 Concerning the kidney:
(a) at a given moment for a given subject, the renal clearance of all chemicals is the same.
(b) in a person excreting concentrated urine, the osmolarity of renal venous plasma is less than that of renal arterial plasma.
(c) the concentration of creatinine is greater in renal venous plasma than in renal arterial plasma.
(d) in a subject secreting acid urine, the concentration of hydrogen ions is greater in renal venous plasma than in renal arterial plasma.
(e) in a subject secreting acid urine, the concentration of ammonium ions is greater in renal venous plasma than in renal arterial plasma.

16.14 Concerning renal function:
(a) if there is intravascular haemolysis, haemoglobin appears in the glomerular filtrate.
(b) the lining of the bladder is freely permeable to water.
(c) bicarbonate readily diffuses across the renal tubular epithelium.
(d) the renal plasma flow may be estimated from the clearance of para-amino hippuric acid (PAH).
(e) the osmolarity of tubular fluid as it enters the distal convoluted tubule is equal to that of the plasma.

16.15 Concerning the kidney:
(a) inulin clearance is used to estimate the renal plasma flow.
(b) inulin is an endogenous chemical.
(c) creatinine clearance can be used to estimate the glomerular filtration rate (GFR).
(d) creatinine is an endogenous chemical.
(e) the plasma concentration of creatinine is used clinically to estimate the glomerular filtration rate (GFR).

16.16 **A healthy human in anti-diuresis has received an injection of inulin. Would the following statements be true?**

(a) the concentration of inulin in the glomerular filtrate is equal to that in plasma.

(b) the concentration of inulin in the tubular fluid increases progressively all the way along the nephron.

(c) the concentration of inulin in the urine is at least 100 times that in the plasma.

(d) the concentration of inulin in the interstitial fluid of the renal medulla is equal to that in plasma.

(e) when inulin is injected for measurement of clearance, the concentration of inulin in renal venous plasma is negligible.

16.17 **Concerning investigation of renal function:**

(a) the use of clearance rate is an application of the law of conservation of matter.

(b) in measuring the renal clearance of a chemical, it is necessary to measure the concentration of the substance in renal venous plasma.

(c) when inulin is injected for clearance measurements, the concentration of inulin in renal venous plasma is approximately 20% of that in arterial plasma.

(d) when para-amino hippuric acid (PAH) is injected for clearance measurements, the concentration of PAH in renal venous plasma is negligible.

(e) if the glomerular filtration rate is reduced as a result of renal disease, the plasma creatinine concentration falls.

16.18 **Normal renal tubular function includes:**

(a) formation of ammonia.

(b) formation of the renal medullary osmotic gradient.

(c) reabsorption of all the glucose in the glomerular filtrate.

(d) active transport of urea.

(e) formation of bicarbonate.

16.19 **In the kidney:**

(a) half of the plasma flowing to the glomerular capillaries is filtered into the tubules.

(b) all of the sodium that passes into the glomerular filtrate is normally reabsorbed in the proximal tubule.

(c) acidaemia results in increased ammonia synthesis in tubular cells.

(d) the countercurrent mechanism results in the tubular fluid, when it leaves the loop of Henle, having a higher osmolarity than plasma.

(e) the excretion of an excessive water intake is assisted by decreased permeability to water of the collecting ducts.

16.20 **At the renal glomeruli, in normal physiological conditions:**
(a) fluid in the Bowman's capsule has the same electrolyte concentrations as plasma.
(b) blood in the efferent arterioles is more viscous than blood in the afferent arterioles.
(c) the hydrostatic pressure in the capillaries varies as the arterial blood pressure varies.
(d) the hydrostatic pressure in the capillaries is higher than in capillaries elsewhere, in a supine subject.
(e) the glucose concentration in the plasma leaving the glomerulus is virtually the same as that in the plasma entering the glomerulus.

16.21 **The following measurements were made on a subject:**

Plasma glucose concentration	**18.0 mmol/litre**
Urinary excretion of glucose	**0.18 mmol/min**
Glomerular filtration rate	**125 ml/min**
Urine flow	**2 ml/min**

Does this information allow the following conclusions to be drawn?
(a) the urine flow indicates that a diuresis is occurring.
(b) the urine concentration of glucose is 75 mmol/litre.
(c) the renal clearance of glucose is 10 ml/min.
(d) the Tm (transport maximum) for glucose is 2.0–2.1 mmol/min.
(e) the data indicate that glucose is actively secreted into the urine.

16.22 **In relation to renal function:**
(a) the renal plasma clearance of a substance is expressed as a volume of plasma per minute.
(b) if a substance not metabolized by the kidney is present in renal arterial blood but not in renal venous blood, it must be secreted by the renal tubules.
(c) if a substance not metabolized by the kidney is present in renal arterial blood but not in renal venous blood, its clearance is equal to the glomerular filtration rate.
(d) it is possible for the osmolarity of the urine to exceed the osmolarity of the interstitial fluid in the tip of the renal medullary papillae.
(e) correction of an increase in extracellular fluid volume includes an increase in secretion of aldosterone.

16.23 **With respect to plasma clearance and renal function:**
(a) the clearance of a substance can exceed the subject's glomerular filtration rate (GFR) only if the substance is secreted into the tubular fluid.
(b) if a substance is secreted into the urine, its clearance must exceed that of the subject's glomerular filtration rate.

(c)   the renal clearance for glucose in a normal subject is usually less than 1 ml per min.

(d)   if the plasma glucose concentration rises to three times normal (as a result, for instance, of glucose injected intravenously), the glucose clearance will rise.

(e)   if the plasma bicarbonate concentration doubles, the renal clearance of bicarbonate will rise.

16.24   If the concentration of a substance A in the plasma is Pa (mg per ml) and in the urine is Ua (mg per ml), and the volume of urine produced per minute is V (ml), are the following statements correct?

(a)   the rate of excretion of substance A is Ua × V (mg per min).

(b)   the quantity Ua × V/Pa is the minimum volume of plasma from which the kidneys could have obtained the amount of A excreted per minute.

(c)   if A is filtered at the glomerulus and neither secreted nor absorbed in the renal tubules, then Ua × V/Pa is the volume of plasma that flows through the renal circulation in one minute.

(d)   If A is inulin then Va × V/Pa is the volume of glomerular filtrate produced per minute.

(e)   if the ratio Ua/Pa exceeds the ratio Ub/Pb for a substance B which is only filtered, then A must be secreted by the renal tubules.

16.25   The following data concerning the renal handling of sodium and potassium are from a normal subject.

	Na^+ (mmol)	K^+ (mmol)
Amount per 24 hours:		
filtered in glomeruli	26 000	900
reabsorbed	25 850	900
secreted	0	100

In this subject:

(a)   the amount of sodium appearing in the urine is less than 5% of the filtered load.

(b)   the amount of potassium appearing in the urine is less than 5% of the filtered load.

(c)   the urinary loss of sodium exceeds that of potassium by a factor in excess of 10.

Concerning plasma electrolyte concentrations in general:

(d)   the concentration of sodium in plasma exceeds that of potassium by more than 10-fold.

(e)   the principal plasma anion is bicarbonate.

16.26   With regard to the mechanisms leading to the concentration of urine:

(a)   the urine entering the descending limb of the loop of Henle is approximately isotonic with arterial plasma.

(b)   the descending limb of the loop of Henle is freely permeable to electrolytes.

(c)   tubular fluid in the thin segment of the ascending limb is approximately isotonic with arterial plasma.

(d)   the thick portion of the ascending limb pumps electrolytes into the tubular fluid from the extracellular fluid.

(e)   the concentration of urea in the extracellular fluid of the renal medulla is greater than in that of the renal cortex.

16.27   With reference to the renal tubules:

(a)   at the tip of the loop of Henle in the renal medulla, the osmolarity of the tubular contents is several times that of the glomerular filtrate.

(b)   an increase in the filtered load of phosphate results in an increase in the glucose Tm (transport maximum).

(c)   the concentration of creatinine in the tubular fluid increases with distance along the tubule.

(d)   most of the water filtered at the glomerulus is reabsorbed in the distal convoluted tubules and collecting ducts.

(e)   the permeability of the collecting tubule to water is under the control of aldosterone.

16.28   In a normal subject excreting acid urine:

(a)   hydrogen ion movement from the tubular cytoplasm to the luminal fluid in the collecting ducts is down the electrochemical gradient for hydrogen ions.

(b)   the minimum urinary pH that can be attained is about 6.

(c)   the rate of hydrogen ion secretion in the proximal tubule is greater than that in the distal tubule.

(d)   a higher hydrogen ion concentration difference between tubular fluid and tubular cell cytoplasm is achieved in the proximal than in the distal tubule.

(e)   hydrogen ion secretion occurs largely in exchange for the reabsorption of chloride ions.

16.29   Concerning acid-base homeostasis and the kidney:

(a)   a strict vegetarian diet yields more acid than a mixed diet.

(b)   the ingestion of sodium lactate will result in an increase in renal excretion of bicarbonate.

(c)   urinary ammonia is largely derived from urea.

(d)   the ammonium ions in the tubular fluid originate from molecular ammonia transferred across the tubular epithelial cell membrane.

(e)   acidosis is likely to be accompanied by an increased concentration of ammonium ions in the urine.

16.30 For an adult human, the concentrations of a substance X in plasma and urine were found to be P_X and U_X respectively. The concentrations of inulin in the two fluids were P_I and U_I. Given the statement on the left, does the statement on the right necessarily follow?

(a) U_X/P_X is greater than U_I/P_I X is secreted into the urine.
(b) U_X/P_X = U_I/P_I X is not secreted into the urine.
(c) U_X/P_X is less than U_I/P_I X is reabsorbed from the urine.
(d) U_X = 0   X is not filtered.
(e) $U_X \times V/P_I$ = 40 ml/min   the subject's renal function is impaired.

16.31 At the tip of the loop of Henle in the papillary region of the renal medulla in a healthy person excreting concentrated urine:

(a) the osmolality of the tubular fluid is close to that of the peritubular fluid.
(b) the concentration of sodium chloride in tubular fluid is approximately the same as that of the peritubular fluid.
(c) the concentration of urea in tubular fluid is approximately the same as that of the peritubular fluid.
(d) there is net reabsorption of water.
(e) the tubular cells are actively reabsorbing solutes.

16.32 Which of the following provide proof that a substance X is added to the fluid in the renal tubule by the process of secretion?

(a) the concentration of X in the urine is greater than in the plasma.
(b) if inulin is infused, the concentration of X in the renal tubule increases to a greater extent than does the concentration of inulin.
(c) X is not filtered at all at the glomerulus but is found in significant concentration in the urine.
(d) the value for the plasma clearance of X is sometimes found to exceed the glomerular filtration rate.
(e) micropuncture experiments indicate that the concentration of X increases progressively as the tubular fluid passes distally.

16.33 An increased rate of renal tubular secretion of hydrogen ions:

(a) leads to a rise in the bicarbonate content of the blood.
(b) may lead to an increased excretion of ammonium ions.
(c) may be caused by respiratory acidosis.
(d) can be caused by inhibition of carbonic anhydrase in the kidneys.
(e) can cause the pH of the urine to fall as low as 2.2.

16.34 In a diuresis established in an experimental animal by overloading it with water:

(a) there is a reduction in the rate of water reabsorption in the proximal tubule.

(b)   a four-fold increase in the rate of excretion of water is accompanied by a four-fold increase in the rate of excretion of Na+.

(c)   activation of the sympathetic nervous system reduces the diuresis.

(d)   loss of 20% of the blood volume reduces the diuresis.

(e)   injection of hypertonic saline into the common carotid artery reduces the diuresis.

16.35 Concerning the kidney:

(a)   the proximal convoluted tubule cells contain a higher density of mitochondria than the distal tubule cells.

(b)   the distal tubule cells contain a higher concentration of mitochondria than the epithelial cells of the glomeruli.

(c)   the cells of Bowman's capsule are thinner than those of the proximal tubule.

(d)   reabsorption occurs at Bowman's capsule.

(e)   the Bowman's capsule consists of endothelial cells.

16.36 In the human kidney:

(a)   the proximal convoluted tubule is continuous with Bowman's capsule.

(b)   the proximal convoluted tubule has a brush border.

(c)   the descending limb of the loop of Henle has a brush border.

(d)   the nephrons with glomeruli that lie adjacent to the renal capsule have tubular loops that penetrate only a short way into the medulla.

(e)   the nephrons with juxtamedullary glomeruli have tubular loops that penetrate the medulla to near the tip of the renal papilla.

16.37 Concerning the human kidney:

(a)   the distal convoluted tubules of many nephrons join to form a single collecting duct.

(b)   all collecting ducts run through the medulla to the renal pelvis.

(c)   about 14% of glomeruli are juxtamedullary glomeruli.

(d)   in the medulla, tubular loops become wider in their route from the cortex to near the tip of the renal papilla.

(e)   in the medulla, the collecting ducts are wider near the tip of the renal papilla than close to the cortex.

16.38 Renal tubular secretion:

(a)   is the term applied to active transport in either direction across the tubular cells.

(b)   necessarily requires metabolic energy.

(c)   occurs in the glomeruli.

(d)   occurs in the descending limb of the loop of Henle.

(e)   occurs in the collecting ducts.

16.39 **Compared with the blood in the afferent arterioles, the blood in the efferent arterioles has a higher:**
(a) viscosity.
(b) haematocrit (packed cell volume).
(c) mean cell volume.
(d) plasma glucose concentration.
(e) plasma protein concentration.

16.40 **Concerning the juxtaglomerular apparatus:**
(a) the juxtaglomerular cells are modified smooth muscle cells.
(b) the juxtaglomerular cells lie in the wall of the afferent arteriole.
(c) the macula densa cells form part of the wall of the distal convoluted tubules.
(d) a rise in luminal pressure in the distal tubule causes the afferent arteriole to dilate.
(e) the juxtaglomerular apparatus is the source of renin.

16.41 **The vasa recta of the kidney:**
(a) have a well defined layer of smooth muscle.
(b) are larger than the capillaries in muscle.
(c) are supplied by blood that has previously passed through glomerular capillaries.
(d) travel perpendicular to the limbs of the loop of Henle.
(e) altogether carry about 10% of the renal blood flow.

16.42 **Concerning fenestrations in glomerular capillaries:**
(a) the fenestrations occur in podocytes.
(b) fluid passing through fenestrations is being actively secreted.
(c) each fenestration houses many pores.
(d) fenestrations allow the passage of more fluid (per square mm of capillary wall) than occurs in non-fenestrated capillaries.
(e) fenestrations separate plasma and the intracellular fluid of the endothelial cells.

16.43 **Concerning renal function:**
(a) the glomerular filtrate passes through the epithelial cells covering the glomerular capillaries.
(b) the osmolarity of the glomerular filtrate is reduced if the kidneys are cooled.
(c) erythrocytes are present in the glomerular filtrate.
(d) the obligatory loss of fluid in the urine of a 70 kg man is around 200 ml per 24 h.
(e) if the subject were to lose the ability to concentrate urine, the osmolarity of the urine would be about 30 mosmol per litre.

16.44   In a normal adult human excreting urine with a pH of 5.5:
(a)   the presence of ammonium ions in urine allows excretion of more hydrogen ions than would otherwise be possible.
(b)   the amount of titratable acid is determined only by the pH of the urine.
(c)   the bicarbonate concentration of the urine might exceed 24 mmol per litre.
(d)   the acidification of the urine requires energy derived from metabolism.
(e)   the acidification of the urine depends on the countercurrent multiplier system.

16.45   In a normal adult human excreting urine with a pH of 8.0:
(a)   the alkalinity of the urine could be due to eating a meaty diet.
(b)   the bicarbonate concentration of the urine exceeds 24 mmol per litre.
(c)   the kidney is capable of producing urine 1 pH unit more alkaline.
(d)   the fluid filtered in the renal glomeruli has a pH of 8.
(e)   a urine with this pH is a likely consequence of an obstructive respiratory disorder.

16.46   Concerning the kidney, can the total amount of the following substances leaving the kidney in renal venous blood exceed the total amount entering in renal arterial blood?
(a)   water.
(b)   bicarbonate.
(c)   creatinine.
(d)   ammonium ions.
(e)   sodium ions.

16.47   Measurements on a non-toxic substance X gave the following results:

Amount entering kidney in renal arterial blood	**2 units per min**
Amount leaving kidney in renal venous blood	**0 units per min**
Amount leaving kidney in urine	**2 units per min**

From this information, it can be concluded that:
(a)   X must be freely filtered in the renal glomeruli.
(b)   X must be actively secreted into the tubular fluid in the cortical region of the nephrons.
(c)   the walls of the tubular loop of Henle must be impermeable to X.
(d)   X must be being generated in the kidney.
(e)   in the blood, X must be firmly attached to the plasma proteins.

16.48   Concerning the kidney:
(a)   collecting ducts open at the tips of the papillae.
(b)   there are about 10 papillae in each kidney in the human.

(c)   renal reabsorption of non-polar chemicals occurs primarily in the cortex.

(d)   renal reabsorption of inorganic electrolytes occurs both in the cortex and in the medulla.

(e)   the vasa recta are supplied by efferent arterioles of renal corpuscles close to the medulla (the juxtamedullary corpuscles).

16.49 With reference to the structure and function of the kidney:

(a)   fenestrations are present in the vasa recta.

(b)   the permeability of the walls of capillaries in the glomerulus is about the same as that of the capillaries in the convoluted tubules.

(c)   in the kidney, mitochondria are more numerous in the cells of the distal than of the proximal convoluted tubule.

(d)   the blood supply to the kidney comes via the sinusoids of the adrenal cortex.

(e)   an erythrocyte traversing the kidney passes through two separate capillaries.

16.50 Concerning the kidney:

(a)   renal clearance of bicarbonate may be 20 times higher in a vegetarian than in a subject on a mixed diet.

(b)   blockage of one ureter by a renal stone leads to an increase in glomerular filtration rate in the kidney connected to that ureter.

(c)   drug interactions are less likely to occur between drugs that are eliminated from the body in the urine than between drugs inactivated in the liver.

(d)   aldosterone controls 70% of the renal tubular reabsorption of sodium.

(e)   the renal tubular reabsorption of water is enhanced by an increase in the amount of solute in the tubular fluid.

Ureter and bladder

16.51 Concerning the ureters:

(a)   they exhibit peristalsis.

(b)   the epithelial lining is several cells thick.

(c)   they contain nociceptive nerve endings.

(d)   they contain sensory endings which can initiate a reflex reduction of glomerular filtration.

(e)   they contain a sphincter of skeletal muscle fibres.

16.52 Concerning the urinary bladder of an adult human:

(a)   if fluid is injected via a urethral catheter, in the normal person the initial rise in pressure subsequently falls to some extent.

(b)   if fluid is injected via a catheter in a subject suffering from spinal shock immediately after a spinal transection, the bladder responds purely passively to distension.

(c)   doubling the volume from 200 ml to 400 ml will more than double the intravesicular pressure.

(d)   at a volume of 400 ml, in a normal person the intravesicular pressure exhibits transient rises.

(e)   parasympathetic stimulation causes the bladder to contract.

16.53 Concerning the bladder:

(a)   concentration of the urine occurs here.

(b)   the lining epithelium is keratinized.

(c)   the lining epithelium is readily damaged by hypertonic solution.

(d)   the epithelium has a brush border.

(e)   the muscle in the bladder wall is striated.

Calculations, interpretation of numerical and graphic data

16.54 A subject was deprived of water for a few hours, starting at time zero. Urine was collected at hourly intervals and the following data were obtained.

Time (hours)	Urine osmolarity (mosmol/litre)	Urine flow (ml/hr)
−1	72	520
0	70	530
1	76	505
2	95	210
3	185	110
4	550	30

From this data, it may be concluded that:

(a)   at time zero, the urine is isosmotic with plasma.

(b)   the subject may be suffering from diabetes insipidus.

(c)   at four hours, the concentration of urine is the maximum that the normal kidney can produce.

(d)   the data are compatible with a normal subject who has been drinking large amounts of fluid before the test period.

(e)   the subject may be suffering from renal failure.

16.55 The following data were derived from a patient.

Arterial blood:	PCO_2 = 25 mmHg
	PO_2 = 120 mmHg
	pH = 7.2, $[H^+]$ = 60 nmol per litre
Urine analysis:	NH_4^+ = 105 mmol/day
	Titratable acidity = 65 mmol/day

From this information, it may be concluded that:

(a)   the subject has a metabolic acidosis.

(b)   the subject is hyperventilating.

(c)   the subject is excreting an acid urine.

(d)   the subject's plasma bicarbonate concentration is around 30 mmol per litre.

(e)   the subject is in renal failure.

16.56 **With further reference to the patient in the previous question:**
(a) the rate of renal hydrogen ion excretion was 170 mmol/day.
(b) the peripheral chemoreceptors were being stimulated.
(c) the central chemoreceptors were the main mediators of the hyperventilation.
(d) from the rate of ammonium excretion, it can be concluded that the subject had an acid-base disturbance of long-standing.
(e) administration of ammonium chloride would improve the patient's condition.

16.57 **Figure 16.57 shows the changes in osmolarity ratio (osmolarity of tubular fluid relative to that of plasma) along a nephron with a long loop of Henle.**

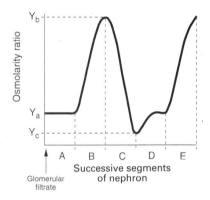

(a) the value of Y_a is 1.
(b) at the junction between segments A and B, the total flow of tubular fluid is about one-third of the glomerular filtration rate.
(c) the rise in osmolarity along segment B is due to water being actively pumped out of the tubular fluid.
(d) the fall in osmolarity along segment C is due to electrolyte being pumped out of the tubular fluid.
(e) the value of Y_c is about 1/3.

16.58 **With further reference to Figure 16.57:**
(a) segment C corresponds to the ascending limb of the loop of Henle.
(b) the osmolarity of blood perfusing the tissue corresponding to the junction between B and C is the same as that of renal arterial plasma.
(c) the osmolarity of blood perfusing tissues corresponding to the junction between D and E is less than that of renal arterial plasma.
(d) Y_b can reach a value of 10.
(e) segment E represents the rise in osmolarity occurring in the collecting ducts.

16.59 On the left is shown a relationship between the concentration of a chemical in plasma and the rate of urinary excretion of that chemical. In each case, you are to decide whether this relationship is appropriate for the chemical on the right.

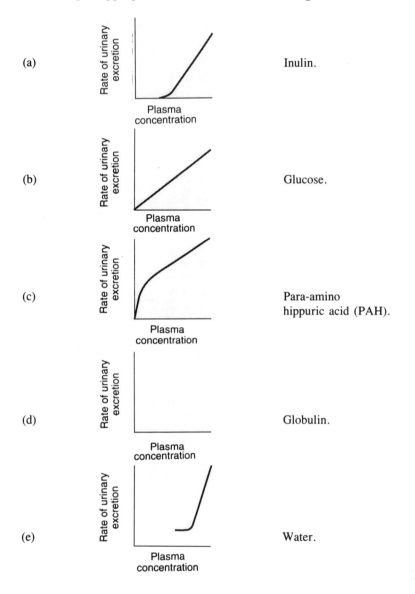

(a) Inulin.

(b) Glucose.

(c) Para-amino hippuric acid (PAH).

(d) Globulin.

(e) Water.

16.60 On the left is shown a relationship between the concentration of a chemical in plasma and its renal clearance. In each case, you are to decide whether this relationship is appropriate for the chemical on the right.

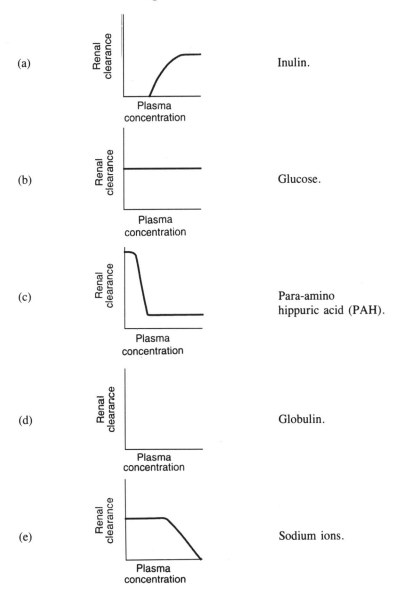

(a)   Inulin.

(b)   Glucose.

(c)   Para-amino hippuric acid (PAH).

(d)   Globulin.

(e)   Sodium ions.

16.61   Figure 16.61 shows the pH of renal tubular fluid as it passes along the renal tract for a healthy subject who has been given an acid load. Are the following statements true?

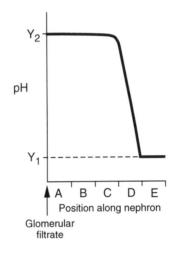

(a)   A typical value for Y_2 is pH $= 8.0$.
(b)   A typical value for Y_1 is pH $= 4.0$.
(c)   The amount of acid secreted (mmol H^+ per min) is greater in segment A than in segment D.
(d)   Segment D represents the collecting duct.
(e)   Segment E represents the ureter.

16.62   With further reference to Figure 16.61:
(a)   in segment A, hydrogen ions are being pumped against a high concentration gradient.
(b)   at the end of segment D, hydrogen ions are being pumped against a concentration gradient of around 10-fold.
(c)   concentration of hydrogen ions depends on a countercurrent mechanism.
(d)   the pH of the renal interstitial fluid at the end of segment D is below pH $= 7.0$.
(e)   if an inhibitor of carbonic anhydrase were administered, the level of Y_1 would fall lower.

16.63 Consider the data below.

	Inulin	PAH	Substance X
Plasma concentration (P) (mg/ml)	0.01	0.05	1.0
Urine concentration (U) (mg/ml)	0.4	10.0	15.0

Urine flow (V) = 2 ml/min

On the basis of these values:

(a) the glomerular filtration rate is 80 ml/min.
(b) the renal plasma flow is 700 ml/min.
(c) the renal clearance of X is 30 ml/min.
(d) given that X is freely filtered at the glomerulus, the filtration rate of X is 80 mg/min.
(e) the rate of reabsorption of X is 30 mg/min.

16.64 Consider the data below.

	Creatinine	PAH	Substance X
Plasma concentration (P) (mg/litre)	30	50	4.0
Urine concentration (U) (mg/litre)	1200	10 000	40

Urine flow (V) = 2 ml/min
PCV = 0.45

On the basis of these values:

(a) the best estimate of the glomerular filtration rate is 120 ml/min.
(b) the renal plasma flow is 500 ml/min.
(c) the renal blood flow is 730 ml/min (to 2 significant figures).
(d) given that substance X is freely filtered at the glomerulus, the filtered load of X is 240 mg/min.
(e) the fractional reabsorption of X is 0.75.

16.65 Figure 16.65 shows, for inulin and for glucose, the rate of renal excretion as a function of the plasma concentration. Data read from the graph are given below.

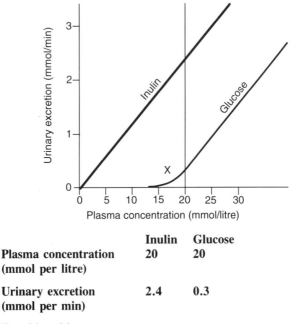

	Inulin	Glucose
Plasma concentration (mmol per litre)	20	20
Urinary excretion (mmol per min)	2.4	0.3

For this subject:

(a) the glomerular filtration rate is 120 ml per min.
(b) when the plasma concentration of glucose is 20 mmol per litre, the amount of glucose filtered is 2.1 mmol per min.
(c) the glucose Tm (transfer maximum) is 2.4 mmol per min.
(d) the relation for para-amino hippuric acid (PAH) would lie above that for inulin.
(e) administration of phlorizin, which competes with glucose for tubular reabsorption, would move the relation for glucose shown in figure 16.65 towards that for inulin.

16.66 With further reference to Figure 16.65 and processes involved:
(a) for glucose, the curvature of the graph in region X is partly due to variation in the glucose Tm for different nephrons.
(b) in a person with a reduced GFR but normal tubular function (as occurs in some elderly people), the plasma concentration of glucose at which the renal threshold for glucose excretion is exceeded is less than normal.

(c)   in most normal people, ingestion of 100 g glucose is without effect on the blood glucose concentration.

(d)   in a normal person, ingestion of 100 g glucose leads to a reduction in plasma insulin concentration.

(e)   in a normal person, ingestion of 100 g glucose is followed by a rise in plasma potassium concentration.

ANSWERS

16.1

(a)   No. The colloid osmotic pressure of blood in the glomerulus tends to pull fluid back into the glomerular capillary.

(b)   No. The hydrostatic pressure of ultrafiltrate in Bowman's capsule tends to counterbalance the driving force.

(c)   Yes. The wall of the thick segment of the ascending limb of the loop of Henle is involved in active pumping of electrolyte from tubular fluid to interstitium and is impermeable to water.

(d)   Yes. In water diuresis (i.e. after drinking a lot of water), the osmolarity gradient in the medulla is reduced, so the osmolarity of the extracellular fluid of the renal medulla is less than in the non-diuretic situation.

(e)   No. In water diuresis, the permeability of the collecting duct is decreased because anti-diuretic hormone secretion is inhibited. As a result of the reduced osmolarity of the medullary interstitium and reduced collecting duct permeability, water reabsorption is decreased.

16.2

(a)   Yes. A component of the countercurrent mechanism of concentration of urine is that the wall of the descending limb of the loop of Henle is readily permeable to water, allowing tubular fluid to lose water and approach the high osmolarity of the surrounding interstitium.

(b)   Yes. The wall of the ascending limb of the loop of Henle, as it joins the distal convoluted tubule, pumps electrolytes actively from tubular fluid to interstitium and establishes a concentration gradient between these fluids. Impermeabilty to water is essential to prevent the passive dissipation of this gradient by water flowing from tubular fluid to interstitial fluid.

(c)   Yes. As an erythrocyte travels along the descending limb of the vas rectum to the tip of the renal papilla, the osmolarity of the interstitial fluid increases by approximately four-fold; the plasma osmolarity increases almost as much, so the erythrocyte loses at least a half of its intracellular water.

(d)   Yes. At no site along the nephron is there a net movement of water from interstitium to tubular fluid, so as tubular fluid flows along the nephron, its volume stays constant or decreases.

(e)   No. As tubular fluid flows along the ascending limb of the loop of Henle, electrolyte is pumped from the tubular fluid to the interstitium; water does not follow, so the osmolarity of the tubular fluid decreases in this section of the nephron.

16.3

(a)   Yes.

(b)   Yes. In a normal human nitrogen-containing metabolites are converted to urea and this occurs only in the liver.

(c)   Yes.

(d)   No. The movement of urea across the tubular wall is passive. In renal failure the rise in plasma urea concentration is due to reduced glomerular filtration.

(e)   Yes. A normal person on a high protein diet can excrete a more concentrated urine than can one on a low protein diet because the body produces more urea and urea contributes to the countercurrent mechanism of producing concentrated urine.

16.4

(a)   No. Constriction of the afferent arterioles reduces the filtration pressure and so reduces the GFR.

(b)   Yes. Constriction of the efferent arterioles increases the filtration pressure and so increases the GFR.

(c)   No. Increase in the concentration of plasma proteins increases the force keeping fluid in the glomerular capillaries and so reduces the GFR.

(d)   No. If the capsular pressure is increased, this reduces the effective filtration force and so reduces the GFR.

(e)   No. Anti-diuretic hormone is without influence on glomerular filtration. It operates in the collecting ducts.

16.5

(a)   No. The glomerular filtration rate is typically 120 ml per min.

(b)   No. The renal plasma flow is typically 700 ml per min; 1.2 litres per min is a typical value for the blood flow.

(c)   Yes. 99% of the water filtered at the glomerulus is subsequently reabsorbed in a normally hydrated person.

(d)   Yes. Glucose, being a small molecule, is readily filtered at the glomerulus so the glomerular filtrate contains glucose at about the same concentration as that in plasma.

(e)   No. Globulin, being a large molecule, is not filtered at the glomerulus so the glomerular filtrate contains almost no globulin.

16.6

(a)   Yes.

(b)   Yes. Absorption is isosmotic.

(c)   No. Sodium is pumped from tubular cells to renal interstitial fluid and water follows passively.

(d)   Yes. This allows the water to flow passively out of the tubular fluid.

(e)   No. Hydrogen ions are pumped into the tubular fluid in the proximal convoluted tubule.

16.7

(a)   Yes. HPO_4^{2-} is a proton acceptor; when it takes up a hydrogen ion it becomes $H_2PO_4^{-}$.

(b)   No. Urea is a molecule and takes no part in acid-base reactions in the tubular fluid.

(c)   No. Chloride ions are the conjugate base of hydrochloric acid which is a very strong acid; they therefore take no part in acid-base reactions in the tubular fluid.

(d)   Yes. Ammonia is a base that combines with protons to form NH_4^{+}. It is produced by the renal tubule cells and provides powerful buffering of hydrogen ions.

(e)   No. Sodium ions take no part in acid-base reactions in the tubular fluid.

16.8

(a)   Yes. The filtration pressure is provided by the blood pressure in the glomerular capillaries and this pressure is generated by the heart.

(b)   No. The balance of resistances in the renal circulation, with the glomerular capillaries being drained by efferent arterioles, results in the glomerular capillary pressure being much higher than that in skeletal muscle capillaries.

(c)   Yes. This is the origin of the increased osmotic pressure on which the countercurrent mechanism is based.

(d)   Yes. About 20% of the plasma fluid is filtered in transit along the glomerular capillary bed and so the concentration of colloid increases by this factor.

(e)   No. Because of (d), the colloid osmotic pressure tending to restrain glomerular filtration rises progressively and the hydrostatic pressure falls a little. It is probable that filtration ceases before the blood reaches the efferent end of the glomerular capillary.

16.9

(a)   Yes. In water diuresis, the urine has an osmolarity close to zero.

(b)   Yes. The kidney is losing hypo-osmolar urine so the renal venous blood has a higher osmolarity than the renal arterial blood.

(c)   No. The glomerular filtration rate is not influenced by the state of diuresis or anti-diuresis.

(d)   No. With vigorous muscular exercise, the renal blood flow falls, the glomerular filtration rate is reduced and the diuresis abates.

(e)   Yes. Drinking water results in dilution of the extracellular fluid and hence inhibition of secretion of antidiuretic hormone. Drinking isosmotic saline does not cause as large an inhibiton of ADH secretion.

16.10

(a)   Yes.

(b)   Yes.

(c)   No. The human kidney can produce urine with a tonicity that is four times that of plasma, but half of the urinary osmolyte is urea. So although the kidney can produce urine with tonicity equal to that of sea water, it cannot produce urine with as high a concentration of sodium chloride. A human cannot survive by drinking sea water instead of fresh water.

(d)   No. The normal kidney can produce a urine that is almost solute-free.

(e)   No. If this were true, the output would be over 170 litres per day. Even in diuresis, at most the urine contains 10% of the water that is filtered at the glomerulus.

16.11

(a)   Yes. PAH is secreted into the urine by tubule cells and this mechanism can be saturated.

(b)   Yes. Glucose is reabsorbed by a tubular active transport mechanism; this mechanism can be saturated.

(c)   No. Inulin is not transported across the tubular wall.

(d)   Yes. There is a transport maximum (Tm) for phosphate reabsorption; this Tm is lowered by the action of parathormone.

(e)   Yes. Alanine is reabsorbed by a tubular active transport mechanism; this mechanism can be saturated.

16.12

(a)   No. Glucose is actively reabsorbed in the renal tubules; until its plasma concentration reaches a threshold none appears in the urine.

(b)   Yes. Since inulin is freely filtered at the glomerulus and does not move across the tubule wall, its rate of urinary excretion is linearly dependent on its plasma concentration.

(c)   Yes. Since, like inulin, creatinine is freely filtered at the glomerulus and does not move across the tubule wall, its rate of urinary excretion is linearly dependent on its plasma concentration.

(d)   No. PAH is actively secreted into the urine and this process has a transport maximum (Tm) value. So its rate of urinary excretion is not linearly dependent on its plasma concentration.

(e)   No. The rate of excretion of water varies over a range of several fold whereas the concentration of water in the blood varies very little. As the concentration of water in the blood falls (osmolarity rises), the urinary excretion falls to a constant low level of 'obligatory' excretion. Hence the relationship between the two cannot be linear.

16.13

(a)   No. For instance, for a typical normal subject the clearance for glucose is zero and that for inulin is equal to the glomerular filtration rate.

(b)   Yes. The osmolarity of renal venous plasma is less than that of renal arterial plasma because the kidney is extracting from the blood proportionally more solute than solvent.

(c)   No. The concentration of creatinine is less in renal venous plasma than in renal arterial plasma bcause the kidney is extracting from the blood proportionally more creatinine than water; creatinine is filtered and thereafter remains in the tubular fluid whereas water is filtered and then largely reabsorbed.

(d)   No. In a subject secreting acid urine, the concentration of hydrogen ions is less in renal venous plasma than in renal arterial plasma because the kidney is effectively extracting hydrogen ions from the renal blood.

(e)   Yes. In a subject secreting acid urine, the renal tubular cells produce ammonia and some spills over into the blood. As a result, the concentration of ammonium ions is greater in renal venous plasma than in renal arterial plasma.

16.14

(a)   Yes. The size of the haemoglobin molecule is smaller than the sieve size of the glomerulus. So if there is intravascular haemolysis, haemoglobin appears in the glomerular filtrate.

(b)   No. If the lining of the bladder were freely permeable to water, concentrated urine excreted by the kidney would become isosmotic while being stored in the bladder and the homeostatic role of the kidney would be jeopardized.

(c)   No. In common with other electrolytes, bicarbonate diffuses very slowly across the renal tubular epithelium. Its reabsorption depends on the tubular secretion of hydrogen ions.

(d)   Yes. PAH is freely filtered at the glomerulus, is secreted into the urine in the tubular regions and is not reabsorbed. The renal blood is thus completely cleared of PAH and the renal plasma flow may be estimated from the clearance of PAH.

(e)   No. Electrolyte is actively pumped from tubular fluid to interstitium in the ascending limb of the loop of Henle without accompanying water; the osmolarity of tubular fluid as it enters the distal convoluted tubule is less than that of the plasma; it is about one-third.

16.15

(a)   No. Inulin is freely filtered at the glomerulus and is neither secreted nor reabsorbed in the tubular system; its clearance is therefore used to estimate the glomerular filtration rate.

(b)   No. Inulin is a polysaccharide not normally present in the body; it must be infused intravenously in order to measure the glomerular filtration rate by the inulin method.

(c)   Yes. Like inulin, creatinine is freely filtered at the glomerulus and is neither secreted nor reabsorbed in the tubular system; its clearance is therefore used to estimate the GFR.

(d)   Yes. Creatinine is an endogenous chemical. It is formed in the body by a slow spontaneous transformation from creatine phosphate in muscle.

(e)   Yes. The rate at which creatinine is released from muscle is fairly constant when the subject is resting. Therefore, if the GFR falls, the plasma concentration of creatinine rises. The plasma concentration of creatinine is used clinically to estimate changes in glomerular filtration rate; this avoids the need for collecting 24 hr samples of urine.

16.16

(a)   Yes. Since the pore size of the glomerular filter is much larger than that of the inulin molecule, the concentration of inulin in the glomerular filtrate is equal to that in plasma.

(b)   Yes. Fluid is progressively reabsorbed the whole length of the nephron, so the concentration of inulin in the tubular fluid increases progressively all the way along the nephron.

(c)   Yes. Since the subject is in anti-diuresis, more than 99% of filtered fluid is reabsorbed, so the concentration of inulin in the urine is at least 100 times that in the plasma.

(d)   No. Inulin is distributed throughout the extracellular fluid because it passes across the capillary wall. Water is removed from the interstitium of the renal medulla by the countercurrent mechanism. This results in an increase in concentration of inulin; the concentration of inulin in the interstitial fluid of the renal medulla is about four times the plasma concentration.

(e)   No. Inulin is freely filtered at the glomerulus but is not transferred across the tubular walls. Inulin entering the efferent arterioles in the 80% of unfiltered plasma thus passes to the renal venous plasma.

16.17

(a)   Yes. The use of clearance relies on the assumption that the amount of a substance leaving the glomerular plasma equals the amount excreted in the urine over a given period of time. This assumption is the law of conservation of matter.

(b)   No. The renal clearance of a substance X is the amount of X excreted in the urine per min divided by the arterial plasma concentration of X. The real venous plasma concentration does not come into the calculation.

(c)   No. Glomerular filtration rate divided by renal plasma flow = 120/700 = 0.2. All filtered inulin is excreted whereas most filtered water is reabsorbed. So about 20% of inulin entering the renal artery is removed by the kidney; the remaining 80% leaves the kidney in the renal venous plasma. Thus its concentration in renal venous blood is about 80% of the arterial concentration.

(d)   Yes. The concentration of PAH in renal venous plasma is negligible because all PAH is removed from the plasma (by filtration at the glomerulus and secretion along the tubules) and is excreted in the urine.

(e)   No. It rises.

16.18

(a)   Yes. Variation in the amount of ammonia formed in and secreted by tubular cells allows adjustable excretion of H^+ in the form of ammonium salts in the urine.

(b)   No. The formation of the renal medullary osmotic gradient is the function of the loop of Henle.

(c)   Yes. Glucose is all reabsorbed in normal circumstances.

(d)   No. Urea is not secreted by tubular cells: it moves by diffusion: some re-enters the blood; some moves out of the nephron and in again, according to differences in gradients and in permeability along the nephron.

(e)   Yes. Bicarbonate is formed from CO_2 entering tubule cells both from filtrate and from plasma, catalysed by carbonic anhydrase; bicarbonate then diffuses into the blood.

16.19

(a)   No. Normally about one-fifth.

(b)   No. About 80% is reabsorbed here.

(c)   Yes. This allows greater loss of protons as ammonium ions.

(d)   No. The tubular fluid leaving the loop of Henle is hypotonic. It is the tubular fluid in the deepest part of the loop and the interstitial fluid around that part that become hypertonic.

(e)   Yes. There is an osmotic gradient tending to draw water into the interstices from the tubular fluid and thus to reabsorb it. The more permeable the tubule to water, the more readily is it reabsorbed.

16.20

(a)   Yes. Since electrolytes pass freely through into the glomerular filtrate, the concentrations are, for practical purposes, the same as in plasma. (There are small differences because of the difference in protein concentration.)

(b)   Yes. The haematocrit increases during passage through the glomerulus because some (about one-fifth) of the plasma volume is lost.

(c)   No. There is an important autoregulatory control mechanism which keeps glomerular capillary pressure, and renal blood flow, near constant during fluctuations of arterial blood pressure.

(d)   Yes. Pressure in other capillaries averages about 20mmHg unless there is a higher pressure due to gravity. In the glomeruli it is around 50 mmHg, providing an effective filtration pressure, sufficient to counteract the opposing osmotic force of 25 mmHg oncotic pressure, and the hydrostatic back pressure from the filtered fluid in the capsule.

(e)   Yes. About one-fifth of the plasma volume is filtered off; one-fifth of the glucose flowing in the plasma is therefore filtered off with the fluid. This does not materially change the concentration of glucose in the plasma, which continues out through the efferent arteriole.

16.21

(a)   Yes. The urine flow in a non-diuretic subject is about 1 ml/min.

(b)   No. Urinary concentration of glucose =

$$\frac{\text{amount of glucose per min}}{\text{volume of urine per min}} = \frac{0.18}{2} = 90\,\text{mmol/litre.}$$

(c)   Yes. Renal clearance of glucose = (U(glucose) × V)/P(glucose) = (0.18 mmol/min)/(18 mmol/litre) = 0.01 litres/min.

(d)   Yes. Tm for glucose = (mass of glucose filtered per min) − (mass of glucose excreted per min) = (18 × 0.125 mmol/min) − (0.18 mmol/min) = (2.25 − 0.18)mmol/min.

(e)   No. Such an inference can only be made if the clearance of a substance is in excess of the glomerular filtration rate.

16.22

(a)   Yes. The calculation is made as though a volume of plasma were completely cleared of the substance each minute.

(b)   Yes. If a substance is completely cleared from the plasma, it must be secreted into the urine, and such secretion occurs in the renal tubules.

(c)   No. The clearance of a substance entirely removed from the plasma is equal to the renal plasma flow.

(d)   No. The final concentration of the urine depends on the osmotic gradient moving water from the lumen of the distal nephron into papillary interstitial fluid.

(e)   No. Aldosterone secretion must decrease if an excess of extracellular fluid is to be corrected, so that less sodium and water are reabsorbed.

16.23

(a)   Yes.

(b)   No. The substance may also be reabsorbed. This is true, for instance, of potassium.

(c)   Yes. It is usually zero.

(d)   Yes. Glucose will appear in the urine because the Tm (transport maximum) is exceeded; the glucose clearance will rise above zero.

(e)   Yes. Bicarbonate behaves as though it has a Tm (transport maximum). At plasma levels below about 28 mmol per litre bicarbonate is almost completely reabsorbed. Above this plasma level, it spills over into the urine, with a consequent rise in its clearance.

16.24

(a)   Yes. Urine volume $\times$ urine concentration = excretion rate.

(b)   Yes. This is the formula for, and the definition of, 'plasma clearance'.

(c)   No. The clearance for a substance that is only filtered gives the glomerular filtration rate, which is about one-fifth of the plasma flow.

(d)   Yes. Inulin is filtered, but not absorbed or secreted, see (c).

(e)   Yes. This means that 'more plasma is cleared' of substance A than of substance B. B is not absorbed, so clearance of B must be equal to or greater than the glomerular filtration rate (GFR). So if clearance of A is greater, A must be secreted.

16.25

(a)   Yes. This is straightforward arithmetic: amount of sodium excreted = 26 000 − 25 850 = 150; 5% of 26 000 = 1300.

(b)   No. Amount in urine = 900 − 900 + 100 = 100. 5% of 900 = 45, so more than 10% of the filtered load is in the urine.

(c)   No. Urinary loss of K^+ is 100, and of Na^+ is 150, mmol/day.

(d)   Yes. The ratio $[Na^+]:[K^+]$ in plasma is approximately 30.

(e)   No. In plasma, the principal anion is Cl^-.

16.26

(a)   Yes. Water and solutes are reabsorbed isosmotically in the proximal convoluted tubule.

(b)   No. The descending limb of the loop of Henle is freely permeable only to water, not to electrolytes.

(c)   No. It is hypertonic.

(d)   No. Electrolyte (probably primarily chloride) is pumped in the opposite direction.

(e)   Yes. Urea contributes to medullary hypertonicity.

16.27

(a)   Yes. The countercurrent mechanism brings this about.

(b)   No. There is an inverse relation between glucose and phosphate reabsorption, so an increase in the filtered load of phosphate results in a decrease in the glucose Tm.

(c)   Yes. Because of water reabsorption.

(d)   No. By far the greatest part of the water is reabsorbed in the proximal tubule, although the final amount is further regulated by the degree of anti-diuretic hormone activity affecting the distal tubule.

(e)   No. The relevant hormone is anti-diuretic hormone.

16.28

(a)   No. The hydrogen ion concentration in such a subject is greater in the luminal fluid than in the tubular cell cytoplasm. So hydrogen ions are pumped against this concentration gradient; an energy-requiring pump mechanism is needed.

(b)   No. The minimum is about 4.5.

(c)   Yes.

(d)   No. The reverse is the case. There is a bigger difference because in the distal tubule almost all bicarbonate has been recaptured, urine buffers have taken up protons so the pH of the tubular fluid has fallen.

(e)   No. This is nonsense. Hydrogen and chloride ions carry opposite charges and so would move in the same direction to preserve electroneutrality. Hydrogen ions are secreted largely in exchange for sodium ions.

16.29

(a)   No. A strict vegetarian diet yields alkali whereas a mixed diet yields acid.

(b)   Yes. The lactate is metabolized so that effectively sodium hydroxide is released into the body. This metabolic alkalosis promotes renal excretion of bicarbonate.

(c)   No. Ammonia is formed from glutamine in the tubule cells.

(d)   Yes.

(e)   Yes. The major part of excess acid is excreted in the form of ammonium ions.

16.30

(a)   Yes. For any chemical, $U/P = C/V$, where C is the clearance of the chemical and V is the urinary volume per unit time. So for X, its clearance was greater than the inulin clearance, i.e. X must be secreted into the urine.

(b)   No. X may be being both secreted and reabsorbed.

(c)   No. X may not be freely filtered at the glomerulus.

(d)   No. X may be freely filtered and subsequently completed reabsorbed e.g. para-amino hippuric acid.

(e)   Yes. The inulin clearance of a healthy adult subject is around 120 ml per min.

16.31

(a)   Yes. There is approximate equality of osmolality comparing tubular fluid and peritubular fluid.

(b)   No. For the tubular fluid, the concentration of sodium chloride is about 1100 mosmol per litre (almost 4 times the plasma concentration) whereas in the peritubular fluid, it is around 600 mosmol per litre.

(c)   No. For the tubular fluid, the concentration of urea is around 80 mosmol per litre whereas in the peritubular fluid, it is around 600 mosmol per litre.

(d)   Yes.

(e)   No. In this region of the tubule, movements across the tubular epithelium are passive.

16.32

(a)   No. For a substance X that is only filtered, the concentration of X in the urine is greater than in the plasma because of tubular reabsorption of water.

(b)   Yes. Inulin is filtered but not secreted or reabsorbed. So if the concentration of X in the renal tubule increases to a greater extent than does the concentration of inulin, it must be being secreted.

(c)   Yes. Since X is not filtered at all at the glomerulus but is found in significant concentration in a midstream specimen of urine, it must have reached the urine by secretion.

(d)   Yes. If the value for the plasma clearance of X is sometimes found to exceed the glomerular filtration rate, then on those occasions X must be secreted.

(e)   No. If X is not reabsorbed, the reabsorption of water as the tubular fluid passes distally will cause a progressive increase in the concentration of X.

16.33

(a)   Yes. Excreted hydrogen ions are effectively exchanged for reabsorbed bicarbonate ions.

(b)   Yes. The increased excretion of ammonium ions is a homeostatic response to acidosis and contributes to the carriage of hydrogen ions.

(c)   Yes. Aciduria is a compensatory response to respiratory acidosis.

(d)   No. Inhibition of carbonic anhydrase in the kidneys reduces the tubular secretion of hydrogen ions.

(e)   No. The lower limit of urinary pH is about 4.5.

16.34

(a)   No. It is in the distal nephron that facultative (adjustable) reabsorption of water takes place.

(b)   No. A four-fold increase in the rate of excretion of water is accompanied by a profound fall in urine osmolarity.

(c)   Yes. Activation of the sympathetic nervous system reduces renal blood flow and hence reduces the diuresis.

(d)   Yes. Loss of 20% of the blood volume results in sympathetic outflow and hence reduces the diuresis.

(e)   Yes. Injection of hypertonic saline into the common carotid artery leads to the release of anti-diuretic hormone and so reduces the diuresis.

16.35

(a)   Yes. The proximal convoluted tubule cells are more metabolically active than the distal tubule cells and so contain more mitochondria.

(b)   Yes. The distal tubule cells are more metabolically active than the epithelial cells of the glomeruli and so contain more mitochondria.

(c)   Yes. The cells of Bowman's capsule have a purely filtering function and are thinner than those of the proximal tubule, which have a reabsorptive function.

(d)   No. Only filtration, not reabsorption, occurs at Bowman's capsule.

(e)   No. The Bowman's capsule consists of epithelial cells.

16.36

(a)   Yes. The proximal convoluted tubule and Bowman's capsule form a continuous epithelial lining.

(b)   Yes. The brush border of the proximal convoluted tubule is formed by numerous microvilli which enormously increase the surface available for absorption.

(c)   No. This is correlated with the fact that the descending limb of the loop of Henle has no active reabsorptive function.

(d)   Yes. Glomeruli that lie adjacent to the renal capsule have tubular loops that penetrate only a short way into the medulla and therefore contribute little to the establishment and maintenance of the medullary concentration gradient.

(e)   Yes. Juxtamedullary glomeruli have tubular loops that penetrate the medulla to near the tip of the renal papilla; these are the nephrons that are of prime importance in establishing and maintaining the medullary concentration gradient.

16.37

(a)   Yes. The anatomical arrangement is that the distal convoluted tubules of many nephrons join to form a single collecting duct.

(b)   Yes. All collecting ducts run through the medulla to the renal pelvis and drain into it.

(c)   Yes.

(d)   No. In the medulla, tubular loops do not become wider in their route from the cortex to near the tip of the renal papilla; the deepest part of the loop is thinnest.

(e)   Yes. As collecting ducts from different nephrons join, the ducts become wider in their route from the cortex to the tip of the renal papilla. Close to the cortex, the collecting ducts are narrower than the convoluted tubules but, as more and more nephrons drain into the ducts, they become progressively wider until, close to the papilla, they are many times wider than the convoluted tubules.

16.38

(a)   No. Renal tubular secretion is the term applied to movement across the tubular cells in the direction from interstitial fluid to tubular fluid.

(b)   No. Renal tubular secretion does not necessarily require metabolic energy. For chemicals moving down their electrochemical gradients, the movement may occur passively, e.g. secretion of potassium ions, which occurs mainly in the distal tubule, is probably passive and occurs down an electrochemical gradient, the distal tubular fluid being up to 100 mV negative to the interstitial fluid.

(c)   No. Only filtration occurs at the glomeruli.

(d)   No. The descending limb of the loop of Henle has no secretory function.
(e)   No. There is no secretion in the collecting ducts (although there is some active reabsorption of sodium chloride).

16.39
(a)   Yes. Due to filtration of glomerular fluid, the viscosity of blood is greater in the efferent than in the afferent arterioles.
(b)   Yes. Due to filtration of glomerular fluid, the haematocrit of blood is greater in the efferent than in the afferent arterioles.
(c)   No. Since the glomerular filtrate is isosmotic with plasma, the mean cell volume does not increase as the erythrocyte traverses the glomerulus. (In fact, because of the raised colloid osmotic pressure, the erythrocyte shrinks a little.).
(d)   No. Since the glomerular filtrate is an ultrafiltrate of plasma, the glucose concentration of the plasma is not altered as the plasma traverses the glomerular capillaries.
(e)   Yes. Since plasma proteins are retained by the glomerular filter, the plasma protein concentration is greater in the efferent than in the afferent arterioles.

16.40
(a)   Yes. The juxtaglomerular cells are modified vascular smooth muscle cells.
(b)   Yes.
(c)   Yes.
(d)   No. A rise in luminal pressure in the distal tubule causes the afferent arteriole to constrict, thus reducing the filtration pressure in the glomerulus and hence the glomerular filtration rate.
(e)   Yes.

16.41
(a)   No. The vasa recta of the kidney are wide capillaries; the wall consists only of endothelium and basement membrane.
(b)   Yes. The vasa recta are larger than the capillaries in muscle.
(c)   Yes.
(d)   No. The vasa recta travel parallel with the limbs of the loop of Henle.
(e)   Yes. The vasa recta altogether carry only about 10% of the renal blood flow. The remainder drains from the capillaries supplying distal convoluted tubules directly into the renal veins.

16.42

(a) No. The fenestrations occur in the endothelial cells of the glomerular capillaries. Podocytes are the epithelial cells of Bowman's capsule covering parts of the endothelial cells.

(b) No. Fluid passing through fenestrations is moving passively.

(c) Yes. Each fenestration houses many pores, which form a regular hexagonal array.

(d) Yes. The function of fenestrations is to allow the passage of more fluid (per square mm of capillary wall) than occurs in non-fenestrated capillaries.

(e) No. Fenestrations separate plasma and the fluid moving towards Bowman's capsule.

16.43

(a) No. The glomerular filtrate passes between, not through, the epithelial cells covering the glomerular capillaries.

(b) No. Glomerular filtration is a passive process, so the osmolarity of the glomerular fluid is unaffected if the kidneys are cooled.

(c) No. Erythrocytes are too large to be filtered at the glomerulus and so are not present in the glomerular filtrate.

(d) No. The obligatory loss of fluid in the urine of a 70 kg man is around 440 ml per 24 h.

(e) No. If the subject were to lose the ability to concentrate urine, the osmolarity of the urine would be close to that of the plasma, i.e. about 300 mosmol per litre.

16.44

(a) Yes. The ammonium ions in urine are carrying hydrogen ions without contributing to the fall in pH of the urine.

(b) No. The amount of titratable acid is determined by the amount of acid buffered by urinary buffers plus the amount carried as ammonium ions.

(c) No. By the Henderson–Hasselbalch equation, an acid urine implies a bicarbonate concentration below the plasma concentration.

(d) Yes. Transfer of hydrogen ions from tubular cell cytoplasm to tubular fluid is against a concentration gradient and so necessarily requires energy derived from metabolism.

(e) No. The concentration of urine, but not its acidification, depends on the countercurrent multiplier system.

16.45

(a) No. A meaty diet yields an excess of acid and the urine is consequently acid, not alkaline.

(b) Yes. By the Henderson–Hasselbalch equation, an alkaline urine implies a bicarbonate concentration above the plasma concentration of 24 mmol.

(c)   No. The maximum alkalinity that the kidney is capable of producing is around pH 8.

(d)   No. The fluid filtered in the renal glomeruli has the same pH as plasma.

(e)   No. Obstructive respiratory disorder results in acidaemia from CO_2 retention and production of an acid urine.

16.46

(a)   No. The kidney always extracts water from the renal plasma.

(b)   Yes. The kidney may generate bicarbonate from carbon dioxide and this bicarbonate is added to renal venous blood.

(c)   No. The kidney does not generate creatinine; creatinine is generated in muscle.

(d)   Yes. The kidney may generate ammonia, particularly in chronic acidosis and some of this ammonia overflows into the renal blood as ammonium ions.

(e)   No. Urine always contains sodium ions, so the total amount in renal venous blood must be less than in renal arterial blood.

16.47

(a)   No. X may not be filtered at all in the renal glomeruli; its transfer to tubular fluid could be entirely in the tubules.

(b)   Yes. Since 90% of renal blood flow does not traverse the renal medulla and yet the plasma is completely cleared of X, X must be actively secreted into the tubular fluid in the cortical region of the nephrons.

(c)   No. Even if the walls of the tubular loop of Henle were permeable to X, complete secretion could be occurring in the distal nephron.

(d)   No. The renal input of X equals its output, so there is no evidence that X is being generated in the kidney.

(e)   No. If X were firmly attached to the plasma proteins, it would not be available for secretion by the tubular cells.

16.48

(a)   Yes.

(b)   Yes.

(c)   Yes. Renal reabsorption of non-polar chemicals occurs primarily in the convoluted tubules and these lie in the cortex.

(d)   Yes. Renal reabsorption of inorganic electrolytes occurs both in the cortex (in the proximal and distal convoluted tubules) and in the medulla, notably in the thick part of the ascending limb of the loop of Henle.

(e)   Yes.

16.49

(a) No. Fenestrations are present in the glomerular capillaries, not in the vasa recta.

(b) No. Filtration of plasma occurs in the glomerular capillaries and the permeability of the walls of capillaries in the glomerulus is high, far greater than the permeability of capillaries in the convoluted tubules.

(c) No. The number of mitochondria reflects the metabolic activity of a cell. In the kidney, mitochondria are more numerous in the cells of the proximal than of the distal convoluted tubule because the cells of the proximal tubule are more metabolically active.

(d) No. The blood supply to the kidney comes via the renal artery, not via the sinusoids of the adrenal cortex.

(e) Yes. An erythrocyte traversing the kidney passes through two separate capillaries, the glomerular capillaries and then the capillaries around the renal tubules.

16.50

(a) Yes.

(b) No. As a result of the blockage, there is a rise in the pressure in the renal tract upstream of the obstruction. This impedes glomerular filtration.

(c) Yes. A drug inactivated by the liver readily leads to up or down regulation of hepatic mechanisms for inactivation of other drugs.

(d) No. Aldosterone controls sodium reabsorption in the distal nephron; about 70% of filtered sodium is reabsorbed in the proximal convoluted tubule and most of the remainder is reabsorbed in the loop of Henle. So only a small percentage reaches the region of the nephron in which aldosterone acts.

(e) No. Solute in the tubular fluid impedes the reabsorption of water.

16.51

(a) Yes. They contain smooth muscle that exhibits peristalsis.

(b) Yes. The epithelial lining is transitional epithelium and is several cells thick, so that as the diameter of the ureter changes, the cells can slide over each other and provide a continuous barrier between the urine and the tissues.

(c) Yes. The ureters contain nociceptive nerve endings that are stimulated when the ureter is distended, e.g. in passing a stone. This is the very painful condition of 'renal colic'.

(d)   Yes. Stimulation of ureteric nociceptors causes a reflex increase in sympathetic activity and hence a reduction in glomerular filtration.

(e)   No. The sphincter is at the uretero-vesical junction and consists of smooth muscle fibres.

16.52

(a)   Yes. The fluid injected via a catheter in the normal person initiates a transitory stretch reflex, so there is an initial sharp rise in pressure followed by a slower fall.

(b)   Yes. In spinal shock immediately after a spinal transection, the bladder responds purely passively to distension.

(c)   Yes. As the bladder volume rises, the pressure rises progressively more steeply. So doubling the volume from 200 ml to 400 ml will more than double the intravesicular pressure.

(d)   Yes. At a volume of 400 ml, in a normal person contraction waves occur and the intravesicular pressure exhibits transient rises.

(e)   Yes.

16.53

(a)   No. No concentration of the urine occurs in the bladder; the bladder has merely a storage function.

(b)   No. The lining epithelium is not keratinized. It consists of transitional epithelium.

(c)   No. The urine is frequently hypertonic and the lining epithelium is adapted to resist damage by hypertonic solutions.

(d)   No. The epithelium has no secretory nor reabsorptive function and so has no brush border.

(e)   No. The muscle in the bladder wall is smooth. Only the external urethral sphincter is striated.

16.54

(a)   No. The plasma has an osmolarity of around 300 mosmol/litre.

(b)   No. In diabetes insipidus the urine flow is always high and the urine osmolarity close to zero. This subject shows a progressive reduction in urine flow and rise in urine osmolarity with time.

(c)   No. The normal kidney can produce a urine four times as concentrated as plasma, i.e. around 1200 mosmol/litre.

(d)   Yes. This would account for the initially high urine flow and low urine osmolarity. It would also account for the progressive reduction in urine flow and increase in urine osmolarity as water was withheld.

(e)   No. In renal failure the kidney cannot produce a urine that is either more dilute or more concentrated than plasma. This subject produced urine with both these characteristics at different times.

16.55

(a)   Yes. The low pH with a low PCO_2 indicates a metabolic acidosis.

(b)   Yes. The PCO_2 is low, indicating hyperventilation.

(c)   Yes. The urine has a high titratable acidity, indicating that the subject is excreting an acid urine.

(d)   No. With a low plasma PCO_2 and a low pH, the bicarbonate concentration must be well below the normal value of 24 mmol.

(e)   No. If the subject were in renal failure, the kidney would not be able to produce significant titratable acidity or a significant concentration of ammonium ions.

16.56

(a)   Yes. The rate of renal hydrogen ion excretion is the sum of titratable acidity and concentration of ammonium ions.

(b)   Yes. Peripheral chemoreceptors are sensitive to a rise in plasma $[H^+]$.

(c)   No. In acidaemia the stimulus to ventilation is mainly via the peripheral chemoreceptors. Hydrogen ions in the blood do not readily cross the blood-brain-barrier.

(d)   Yes. A rate of ammonium ion excretion of 105 mmol/day is very high and only occurs in a person with chronic metabolic acidosis.

(e)   No. Ammonium chloride would dissociate to NH_4^+ and Cl^-. The ammonium is metabolized by the liver leaving HCl. This is equivalent to the administration of a strong acid and the metabolic acidosis would be exacerbated.

16.57

(a)   Yes. The osmolarity of glomerular filtrate is close to that of arterial plasma.

(b)   Yes. The junction between segments A and B corresponds to the end of the proximal convoluted tubule by which time about two-thirds of the filtered water has been reabsorbed. So the total flow of tubular fluid here is about one-third of the glomerular filtration rate.

(c)   No. The rise in osmolarity along segment B is due to passive movement of water out of the tubular fluid in the descending limb of the loop of Henle into the hypertonic interstitial fluid.

(d)   Yes. It is here, in the ascending limb of the loop of Henle, that active pumping occurs, electrolyte being pumped out of the tubular fluid.

(e)   Yes. For tubular fluid entering the distal convoluted tubule, the lowest osmolarity is about 100 mosmol per litre.

16.58

(a)   Yes.

(b)   No. The junction between B and C corresponds to the pelvic extremity of the renal medulla; the osmolarity of blood perfusing tissues here is the same as that of the concentrated interstital fluid, i.e. about four times as great as that of renal arterial plasma.

(c)   Yes.

(d)   No. The maximum degree of concentration of urine in the human is about four-fold.

(e)   Yes.

16.59

(a)   No. For inulin, the excretion rate is linearly related to the plasma concentration, as shown in Figure 16.59(b), and reflects the glomerular filtration rate.

(b)   No. At lower plasma concentrations, glucose is completely re-absorbed and the urine is glucose-free; glucose gives the relationship shown in Figure 16.59(a).

(c)   Yes. PAH is secreted into the tubular fluid and this process has a transfer maximum. This is why the slope is initially very steep, but, as the plasma concentration increases and the Tm (transport maximum) for secretion is exceeded, the slope is less steep and constant, this constancy reflecting the glomerular filtration rate.

(d)   Yes. Globulin is excluded from the urine.

(e)   Yes. For the lowest plasma concentrations of water shown, there is an obligatory water loss in the urine, essential for carrying away waste solutes. For higher water concentrations, there is a very steep rise, reflecting the homeostatic mechanisms concerned in maintaining a constant water concentration (and therefore osmolarity) of the plasma.

16.60

(a)   No. Inulin gives the relationship shown in Figure 16.60(b).

(b)   No. Glucose gives the relationship shown in Figure 16.60(a).

(c)   Yes. PAH is secreted into the tubular fluid and this process has a transfer maximum.

(d)   Yes.

(e)   No. At low plasma concentrations of sodium, the urine is almost sodium-free (the clearance is therefore very low) and as the plasma concentration rises, urinary sodium excretion rises very steeply, and the clearance reaches high levels.

16.61

(a)   No. Glomerular filtrate has a pH very close to that of plasma, i.e. pH = 7.4 (or slightly less in this acidotic subject).

(b)   Yes. This corresponds to the highest urinary concentration of hydrogen ions that the kidney can achieve.

(c)   Yes. Quantitatively, the amount of hydrogen ion secretion is greatest in the proximal convoluted tubule; these hydrogen ions comprise an essential step in the recapturing from the tubular fluid of filtered bicarbonate ions. Such hydrogen ions are not excreted.

(d)   Yes.

(e)   Yes.

16.62

(a)   No. In segment A (the proximal convoluted tubule), many hydrogen ions are pumped but against a trivial concentration gradient.

(b)   No. At the end of segment D, the pumping of hydrogen ions is from interstitial fluid (pH above 7) into the tubular fluid (pH around 4). So the hydrogen ions are pumped via the tubular cells against a concentration gradient in excess of 1000-fold.

(c)   No. Concentration of hydrogen ions depends on a very powerful pump, with no help from a countercurrent mechanism.

(d)   No. Hydrogen ions are being pumped into the tubular fluid and concurrently bicarbonate ions are transferred to the renal interstitial fluid. The latter is thus more alkaline than the pH of interstitial fluid elsewhere in the body.

(e)   No. An inhibitor of carbonic anhydrase greatly slows the tubular hydrogen secretion mechanism, so the urine is less acid and the body becomes more acid.

16.63

(a)   Yes. Inulin clearance $= UV/P = \dfrac{2 \times 0.4}{0.01} = 80\,\text{ml/min} = \text{GFR}$.

(b)   No. PAH clearance $= UV/P = \dfrac{2 \times 10}{0.05} = 400\,\text{ml/min} = $ plasma flow.

(c)   Yes. Clearance of X $= UV/P = \dfrac{2 \times 15}{1} = 30\,\text{ml/min}$.

(d)   Yes. Filtered load of X $=$ GFR $\times$ plasma concentration
$= 80 \times 1.0 = 80\,\text{mg/min}$.

(e)   No. Reabsorption rate $=$ filtration rate minus excretion rate $=$
$80 - (2 \times 15) = 50\,\text{mg/min}$.

16.64

(a)   No. The creatinine clearance gives the best estimate of the glomerular filtration rate.
Creatinine clearance $= UV/P = \dfrac{2 \times 1200}{30} = 80\,\text{ml/min}$.

(b)   No.
PAH clearance = UV/P = $\dfrac{2 \times 10\,000}{50}$ = 400 ml/min = plasma flow

(c)   Yes. Renal blood flow = $\dfrac{400 \times 1}{0.55}$ = 730 ml/min to 2 significant figs.

(d)   No. Filtered load of X = GFR × plasma concentration
= 80 × 4.0 = 320 mg/min.

(e)   Yes. The fractional reabsorption = amount reabsorbed/amount filtered.
Amount reabsorbed = amount filtered − amount excreted
= 320 − (2 × 40)
= 240 mg/min.
So fractional reabsorption = 240/320 = 0.75.

16.65

(a)   Yes. The glomerular filtration rate is equal to the inulin clearance. This is the filtered load divided by the plasma concentration:
$\dfrac{2.4}{20}$ = 0.12 litre per min.

(b)   No. The amount of glucose filtered per min is the same as the urinary excretion rate of inulin at the same plasma concentration, i.e. 2.4 mmol per min.

(c)   No. The glucose Tm (transfer maximum) is the filtered load minus the urinary excretion. Glucose Tm is thus (2.4 − 0.3) = 2.1 mmol per min.

(d)   Yes. PAH is freely filtered and also secreted into urine, so at any plasma concentration, more PAH than inulin appears in the urine, since inulin is only filtered, not secreted.

(e)   Yes. With complete blockade of glucose reabsorption, glucose and inulin are similarly handled by the kidney.

16.66

(a)   Yes. The nephrons with the lowest glucose Tm allow a little glucose to pass into the urine when the plasma concentration is such that nephrons with higher glucose Tm values reabsorb all filtered glucose.

(b)   No. When the GFR falls, the filtered load of glucose is reduced and, with normal tubular function, all glucose will be reabsorbed at a plasma glucose level above that at which glycosuria would occur if the GFR were normal.

(c)   No. In most normal people, ingestion of 100 g glucose results in a transient rise in the blood glucose concentration.

(d)   No. In a normal person, ingestion of 100 g glucose leads to secretion of insulin as the principal homeostatic mechanism for maintaining a near-constant plasma glucose concentration.

(e)   No. In a normal person, the movement of glucose into the cells that follows ingestion of 100 g glucose is accompanied by a movement of potassium ions in the same direction, so there is a tendency for the plasma potassium concentration to fall.

17 Acid-base physiology

QUESTIONS

17.1 Doubling of the partial pressure of CO_2 to which a sample of blood *in vitro* is exposed will result in:
(a) doubling of the concentration of CO_2 in physical solution.
(b) doubling of the concentration of H_2CO_3.
(c) doubling of the concentration of HCO_3^-.
(d) decrease in the concentration of H^+.
(e) decrease in the concentration of non-bicarbonate buffer base.

17.2 Suppose separated plasma and blood, both initially in equilibrium with the same PCO_2, were subjected to the same increase in PCO_2. By comparison with separated plasma, the plasma of the whole blood ('true plasma') would show a greater change in concentration of:
(a) CO_2 in physical solution.
(b) bicarbonate.
(c) hydrogen ions.
(d) carbonic acid.
(e) chloride concentration.

17.3 Concerning buffering:
(a) a solution of sodium bicarbonate buffers the pH changes due to increased concentration of carbon dioxide.
(b) a solution of sodium bicarbonate in equilibrium with CO_2 at a partial pressure of 50 mmHg buffers the pH changes due to addition of hydrochloric acid.
(c) the fact that blood pH is far removed from the pK of the CO_2–HCO_3^- buffer pair means that this system acts as an inefficient buffer in a closed system.
(d) physiologically, the efficacy of the CO_2–HCO_3^- buffer system is enhanced by the fact that the body can regulate the CO_2 concentration.
(e) physiologically, the efficacy of the CO_2–HCO_3^- buffer system is enhanced by the fact that the kidney can regulate the HCO_3^- concentration.

17.4 **In a patient suffering from chronic vomiting of gastric juice:**
(a)   the pH of the extracellular fluid is likely to be raised.
(b)   the plasma bicarbonate concentration is likely to be raised.
(c)   the plasma potassium concentration is likely to be raised.
(d)   the plasma chloride concentration is likely to be raised.
(e)   the urine may be acid.

17.5 **With reference to extracellular fluid (ECF) hydrogen ion concentration *in vivo*:**
(a)   a value of 10^{-4} mmol per litre indicates alkalosis.
(b)   to maintain normality on an average diet, the kidney must excrete 50–60 mmol of H^+ daily.
(c)   when ECF acidity increases, ventilation is stimulated.
(d)   when ECF acidity increases, arterial PCO_2 increases.
(e)   when ECF acidity increases, less bicarbonate is generated in renal tubular cells.

17.6 **Concerning acid-base physiology:**
(a)   plasma proteins are quantitatively more important than plasma phosphate in buffering.
(b)   the renal hydrogen ion secretion mechanism is transport maximum (Tm) limited.
(c)   when the arterial PCO_2 rises, the amount of bicarbonate reabsorbed by the tubules is increased.
(d)   bicarbonate reabsorption in the renal tubules is largely dependent on the tubular hydrogen ion pump mechanism.
(e)   as a result of the bicarbonate reabsorption mechanism, the body rids itself of excess acidity in the form of water.

17.7 **The Henderson–Hasselbalch equation applied to the CO_2 bicarbonate equilibrium at 37°C is: pH = 6.1 + log $([HCO_3^-])/(0.03\ PCO_2)$ where PCO_2 is measured in mmHg and $[HCO_3^-]$ is in mmol/litre. Take log 2 to be equal to 0.30:**
(a)   if $[HCO_3^-]$ = 24 mmol/l and PCO_2 = 40 mmHg, then the pH is 7.3.
(b)   if the pH falls by 0.3 of a unit with a constant PCO_2, the $[HCO_3^-]$ must fall by one-half.
(c)   in uncompensated respiratory acidosis, the plasma $[HCO_3^-]$ rises.
(d)   in uncompensated respiratory acidosis, it is the bicarbonate buffer system that limits the change in hydrogen ion concentration.
(e)   in metabolic acidosis the plasma bicarbonate concentration tends to be lowered.

17.8   Concerning acid-base physiology and body fluids:
(a)   the amount of undissociated carbonic acid in an aqueous solution is inversely proportional to the amount of dissolved carbon dioxide.
(b)   the amount of undissociated carbonic acid is approximately equal to the amount of dissolved carbon dioxide at a PCO_2 of 40 mmHg.
(c)   a rise in plasma carbon dioxide concentration associated with a proportional rise in bicarbonate ion concentration is accompanied by a fall in pH.
(d)   the renal compensation for a respiratory acidosis includes an increase in the rate of addition of bicarbonate to the blood by the renal tubules.
(e)   as a chemical buffer in a closed system, the bicarbonate buffer system is more efficient at a pH of 7.1 than at a pH of 7.4.

17.9   A patient with fully compensated respiratory acidosis has:
(a)   a normal arterial PCO_2.
(b)   a normal plasma pH.
(c)   a normal plasma bicarbonate concentration.
(d)   a normal bicarbonate: PCO_2 ratio in plasma.
(e)   a negative base excess.

17.10   With respect to acute respiratory disturbances of acid-base physiology:
(a)   retention of carbon dioxide due to respiratory depression increases the acidity in all body fluid compartments.
(b)   in either type of respiratory disturbance, cerebrospinal fluid pH will change in the same direction as blood pH.
(c)   in persistent hyperventilation, there will be a low rate of bicarbonate reabsorption in the kidneys.
(d)   in brief vigorous hyperventilation, cerebral blood vessels constrict.
(e)   if arterial PCO_2 rises, cerebral vasodilatation can help to protect against excessive tissue acidity in the brain.

17.11   The following tend to cause metabolic alkalosis:
(a)   ingested methionine.
(b)   sodium lactate in haemodialysis fluids.
(c)   a diet with a high content of meat.
(d)   strenuous exercise.
(e)   secretion of gastric acid.

17.12   Metabolic acidosis can be produced by:
(a)   persistent vomiting due to small bowel irritation.
(b)   severe hypoxia.
(c)   ingestion of sodium chloride.
(d)   a high protein diet.
(e)   a strict vegetarian diet.

17.13 Concerning lactic acid and lactate:
(a) the pK of this acid and conjugate base pair is 7.4.
(b) lactic acid release in the body leads to a metabolic acidosis.
(c) when lactic acid is released in the body, the main method available to the body for its removal is renal excretion of the lactic acid.
(d) in an isosmotic solution, sodium lactate is completely dissociated (into sodium ions and lactate ions).
(e) if an isosmotic solution of sodium lactate is infused, it causes a metabolic acidosis.

17.14 In metabolic alkalosis:
(a) there is net movement of potassium out of muscle cells.
(b) there is increased potassium excretion in the urine.
(c) the extracellular potassium concentration is above normal.
(d) renal excretion of ammonium ions is increased.
(e) the respiratory compensation consists of hyperventilation.

17.15 Are the circumstances below left appropriate causes for the type of primary acid-base disturbance below right:
(a) altitude hypoxia   respiratory alkalaemia.
    (at around 14 000 ft)
(b) persistent vomiting of
    gastric contents   metabolic acidaemia.
(c) renal failure   metabolic acidaemia.
(d) ventilatory failure   respiratory acidaemia.
(e) starvation   metabolic alkalaemia.

17.16 With reference to the acute disturbances listed below left, do the mechanisms below right play a part in compensatory mechanisms that would tend to restore pH towards normal?
(a) respiratory acidosis   generation of bicarbonate in renal tubule cells, in addition to that which is equivalent to the bicarbonate in the filtrate.
(b) metabolic acidosis   secretion of ammonia by the cells of the distal tubule.
(c) metabolic acidosis   stimulation of the carotid bodies.
(d) respiratory alkalosis   decrease in the rate of H^+ secretion by renal tubule cells.
(e) metabolic alkalosis   depression of respiratory centres by low arterial PCO_2.

17.17 **In a condition of long-term compensation in the chronic disturb-ances listed on the left, are the findings on the right appropriate?**

(a)   metabolic acidosis   low arterial PCO_2.
(b)   metabolic alkalosis   bicarbonate in the urine.
(c)   respiratory acidosis   low plasma bicarbonate.
(d)   respiratory alkalosis   low plasma bicarbonate.
(e)   metabolic acidosis   low plasma bicarbonate.

17.18 **Are the following likely to increase the acidity of the urine?**
(a)   a carbonic anhydrase inhibitor.
(b)   ingestion of sodium acetate.
(c)   ingestion of cystine.
(d)   ingestion of ammonium chloride.
(e)   hyperventilation syndrome.

17.19 **Concerning acid-base homeostasis and the kidney:**
(a)   the renal tubular reabsorption of bicarbonate involves the transfer of bicarbonate ions from the renal tubular fluid to the tubular cell cytoplasm.
(b)   the ingestion of sodium lactate will result in an increase in renal excretion of bicarbonate.
(c)   urinary ammonia is largely derived from urea.
(d)   the ammonium ions in the tubular fluid originate from molecular ammonia transferred across the tubular epithelial cell membrane.
(e)   acidosis is likely to be accompanied by an increased concentration of ammonium ions in the urine.

ANSWERS

17.1
(a)   Yes. One of the laws of physical chemistry states that the amount of gas in physical solution is directly proportional to the partial pressure of the gas with which the liquid is equilibrated.
(b)   Yes. $H_2O + CO_2 = H_2CO_3$. $[H_2O]$ is constant so, by the law of mass action, $[H_2CO_3]$ is directly proportional to $[CO_2]$.
(c)   No. This would only be the case if the hydrogen ion concentration were held constant, i.e. for a perfect buffer.
(d)   No. CO_2 reacting with water yields H_2CO_3 which dissociates to yield hydrogen ions, so there is an increase, not a decrease, in the concentration of H^+.
(e)   Yes. When the PCO_2 increases, most of the released hydrogen ions react with non-bicarbonate buffer base to yield non-bicarbonate buffer acid.

17.2

(a)   No. The amount of CO_2 in physical solution is directly proportional to the PCO_2 and would be the same in blood as in plasma.

(b)   Yes. Because the true plasma is in equilibrium with erythrocytes, which provide buffering capacity, true plasma is a better buffer than separated plasma, so true plasma will show the smaller change in $[H^+]$. By the Henderson–Hasselbalch equation, true plasma will show the larger change in bicarbonate concentration.

(c)   No. True plasma is a better buffer than separated plasma (see (b)), so true plasma will show the smaller change in $[H^+]$.

(d)   No. The concentration of carbonic acid is directly proportional to the concentration of CO_2. So the concentration of carbonic acid is the same in both fluids.

(e)   Yes. Separated plasma shows no change in chloride concentration with changes in PCO_2, whereas true plasma shows an increase with an increase in PCO_2 (the 'chloride shift').

17.3

(a)   No. A buffer cannot buffer itself; for the carbon dioxide–bicarbonate buffer pair, bicarbonate cannot buffer the pH changes due to increased concentration of carbon dioxide.

(b)   Yes. A solution of sodium bicarbonate in equilibrium with CO_2 at a partial pressure of 50 mmHg consists of the carbon dioxide–bicarbonate buffer pair, so it buffers the pH changes due to addition of hydrochloric acid.

(c)   Yes. In a closed system, a buffer pair operates efficiently only within about one pH unit on either side of the pK, so the fact that blood pH is far removed from the pK of the CO_2–HCO_3^- buffer pair means that this system acts as an inefficient buffer in a closed system.

(d)   Yes. The fact that the body can regulate the CO_2 concentration physiologically (by changing excretion rate from the lungs) means that the body can add or remove one member of the buffer pair and thus influence the pH in a way that it is not possible in a closed system (i.e. a system where members of the buffer pair cannot be added or withdrawn). So the efficacy of the CO_2–HCO_3^- buffer system is enhanced by the fact that the body can regulate the CO_2 concentration.

(e)   Yes. For reasons similar to those given in (d) but applied to bicarbonate, physiologically, the efficacy of the CO_2–HCO_3^- buffer system is enhanced by the fact that the kidney can regulate the HCO_3^- concentration.

17.4

(a)   Yes. Because of loss of hydrochloric acid.

(b)   Yes. Metabolic alkalosis is associated with a high plasma bicarbonate concentration.

(c)   No. Metabolic alkalosis is usually associated with a low potassium concentration.
(d)   No. Chloride is lost in the vomitus.
(e)   Yes. Despite the metabolic alkalosis, the loss of sodium from the body activates renal sodium retaining mechanisms. Preservation of electroneutrality involves increased excretion of hydrogen ions in the urine. Defence of body electrolytes takes precedence over the defence of pH.

17.5
(a)   No. 10^{-4} mmol per litre is 100 nmol per litre and this is indicative of a severe acidosis.
(b)   Yes. This is the approximate amount generated, and so this much must be excreted to remain in balance.
(c)   Yes. An increase in blood acidity stimulates ventilation, probably mainly via the arterial chemoreceptors (the blood–brain barrier is not freely permeable to H^+, so central chemoreceptors are not directly affected).
(d)   No. Ventilation is stimulated, which decreases the PCO_2, tending to correct acidity. (In a closed system, an increase in H^+ would increase the PCO_2 but in the body this is immediately lost in the lungs.)
(e)   No. When acidity decreases, less H^+ is excreted by the tubular cells into the tubular fluid, and less CO_2 moves into the cells to form bicarbonate. The effective result is less HCO_3^- 'reabsorption' in the kidney, which tends to correct the ECF change.

17.6
(a)   Yes. This is because the concentration of plasma proteins is higher than that of phosphates.
(b)   No. Renal hydrogen ion secretion is limited by the concentration gradient between tubular cell cytoplasm and tubular fluid.
(c)   Yes. This is partly by a mass action effect.
(d)   Yes.
(e)   No. Loss of a water molecule is equivalent to the loss of one hydrogen and one hydroxyl ion, so the net effect on acid-base balance is zero.

17.7
(a)   No. pH $= 6.1 + \log (24/(0.03 \times 40))$
        $= 6.1 + \log 20 = 7.4.$
(b)   Yes. If pH falls by 0.3, then $\log [HCO_3^-]/(0.03\ PCO_2)$ falls by the same amount. It is given that PCO_2 is unaltered. So $\log ([HCO_3^-])$ falls by 0.3. Now $\log 2 = 0.3$. So $[HCO_3^-]$ must fall by a factor of 2.
(c)   Yes.
(d)   No. The bicarbonate buffer system buffers acids and bases other than CO_2.

(e)   Yes. The type of reaction that takes place is: $H^+ + Cl^- + Na^+ + HCO_3^- = Na^+ + Cl^- + H_2O + CO_2$. Excess fixed acid plus plasma bicarbonate yields sodium and chloride ions, water and CO_2, the latter being blown off in the lungs.

17.8

(a)   No. There is a direct proportionality between these two variables.

(b)   No. $[HCO_3^-]/[CO_2]$ is approximately 1000.

(c)   No. From the Henderson–Hasselbalch equation, the pH is unaltered.

(d)   Yes. This is the principal way in which renal buffering of acidosis is effected.

(e)   Yes. Each buffer system is most effective at its pK (in this case 6.1) and progressively less effective as the pH moves away from the pK.

17.9

(a)   No. Respiratory acidosis, compensated or not, implies a raised arterial PCO_2.

(b)   Yes. 'Fully compensated' means that the pH has been restored to normal by the kidney.

(c)   No. The plasma bicarbonate concentration must be raised.

(d)   Yes. By the Henderson–Hasselbalch equation.

(e)   No. There will be a positive base excess due to addition to the blood of bicarbonate by the kidney.

17.10

(a)   Yes. CO_2 is readily diffusible across all membranes. pH change will be greater or less according to the amount of buffer present, but there is a decrease everywhere.

(b)   Yes. This is because CO_2 is freely transferable across the blood–brain barrier, not because H^+ is freely transferable.

(c)   Yes. The renal compensation for respiratory alkalosis is a diminished effective reabsorption of bicarbonate.

(d)   Yes. Cerebral vessels constrict when $PaCO_2$ is decreased; this leads to faintness/dizziness.

(e)   Yes. The greater the blood flow, the smaller will be the arterio-venous difference for CO_2, so that given a steady rate of tissue CO_2 production, the local rise in PCO_2 will be less. This applies in any tissue, but particularly in the brain where vessels are sensitively dilated by rises in PCO_2.

17.11

(a)   No. Methionine is a sulphur-containing amino acid and so ingested methionine, when metabolized, yields sulphuric acid, leading to metabolic acidosis.

(b) Yes. The lactate in sodium lactate in haemodialysis fluids is metabolized in the Krebs cycle, so effectively sodium hydroxide is being added to the body.

(c) No. A diet with a high content of meat tends to cause metabolic acidosis.

(d) No. Strenuous exercise results in the release of lactic acid and hence a transient metabolic acidosis.

(e) Yes. As a result of secretion of gastric acid into the gastro-intestinal tract, which is essentially outside the body, the body is left alkaline; this gives the so-called 'alkaline tide' after a meal.

17.12

(a) Yes. In persistent vomiting due to small bowel irritation, in some patients there is a net loss of alkaline juice and consequently a metabolic acidosis.

(b) Yes. With severe hypoxia, tissues such as muscle metabolize anaerobically with the release of acid metabolites, notably lactic acid.

(c) No. Ingestion of sodium chloride is without effect on acid-base status, because chloride is the base of hydrochloric acid, which is a very strong acid.

(d) Yes. A high protein diet yields acid when metabolized.

(e) No. A strict vegetarian diet, when metabolized, yields an excess of alkali, not acid.

17.13

(a) No. Lactic acid is a strong acid, so the pK of the lactic acid–lactate buffer pair is much lower than neutrality.

(b) Yes. Lactic acid is a strong acid and, when released in the body, leads to a metabolic acidosis.

(c) No. When lactic acid is released in the body, the main method of removal is uptake by the liver where most is converted to glucose.

(d) Yes. All salts completely dissociate in weak aqueous solutions.

(e) No. If sodium lactate solution is infused, the lactate is metabolized in the carboxylic acid cycle, leaving the sodium ions thus:
$$Na\ lactate + H_2O = Na^+ + OH^- + lactic\ acid$$
So the result is metabolic alkalosis.

17.14

(a) No. In metabolic alkalosis, the extracellular $[H^+]$ falls. This increases the concentration ratio across the membranes of cells and H^+ tend to move from intracellular to extracellular fluid. Electroneutrality is maintained partly by movement of potassium ions in the opposite direction, from extracellular to intracellular fluid.

(b)   Yes. By the mechanism of (a), potassium tends to move from the tubular cell cytoplasm into the tubular fluid. Consequently urinary potassium excretion is increased.

(c)   No. The extracellular potassium concentration is below normal.

(d)   No. In acidosis, renal excretion of ammonium ions contributes to excretion of the acid load, but in alkalosis, renal excretion of ammonium ions is not increased.

(e)   No. The respiratory compensation for metabolic alkalosis consists of hypoventilation.

17.15

(a)   Yes. At this altitude there is a significantly low but tolerable oxygen tension, to which the reflex response is hyperventilation, from stimulation of the arterial chemoreceptors. (The oxygen supply to the tissues can be maintained by means of this response and of increased cardiac output, so the metabolic acidosis of severe hypoxia does not arise.)

(b)   No. The loss of gastric acid causes metabolic alkalaemia (until or unless starvation supervenes, see part (e)).

(c)   Yes. Excretion of hydrogen ions by the kidneys is continuously essential to maintain balance.

(d)   Yes. Patients with chronic obstructive lung disease are liable to have a raised arterial PCO_2 and hence a respiratory acidosis which may ordinarily be compensated. When they develop an acute illness, ventilatory failure and acidaemia supervene.

(e)   No. Starvation results in production of ketone bodies which are acidic.

17.16

(a)   Yes. Increased extracellular fluid acidity ensures that all the bicarbonate in the filtrate is effectively reabsorbed by linkage to secreted H^+, and in addition the raised PCO_2 that characterizes respiratory acidosis promotes the formation of more H^+ (for secretion) and more HCO_3^- (for absorption) in the tubule cells.

(b)   Yes. The ammonia secreted into the filtrate buffers some of the excess H^+ that is secreted, thus assisting its loss from the body.

(c)   Yes. Blood acidity acts here to cause a reflex increase in ventilation, thus lowering the PCO_2 in body fluids, which tends towards alkalinity.

(d)   Yes. A decrease in hydrogen ion secretion follows simply from its lower concentration in body fluids, and from the decrease in PCO_2 which reduces its formation in renal tubule cells.

(e)   No. In metabolic alkalosis there is no decrease in PCO_2. The rise in blood pH itself has some inhibitory effect on the chemoreceptors, causing some depression of breathing and hence a rise in PCO_2 which tends to lower the pH. This respiratory mechanism is not so effective a compensation as the reverse effect for metabolic acidosis, because a rise in PCO_2 is such a strong central stimulus to breathing.

17.17

(a)   Yes.

(b)   Yes.

(c)   No. In respiratory acidosis, the plasma bicarbonate is high. This is due both to the raised PCO_2 and to renal retention of bicarbonate ions.

(d)   Yes.

(e)   Yes. Bicarbonate remains low in metabolic acidosis. All filtered bicarbonate is reabsorbed, but with low PCO_2, no additional bicarbonate is formed for absorption. Correction of pH is by increased H^+ secretion and lowering of PCO_2.

17.18

(a)   No. The secretion of acid urine is promoted by carbonic anhydrase in the renal tubular cells. The enzyme catalyses the release of hydrogen ions from carbonic acid derived from CO_2 and water. So an inhibitor of carbonic anhydrase will tend to result in a reduction of the acidity of the urine.

(b)   No. In the body, the acetate of sodium acetate is metabolized leaving, effectively, sodium hydroxide. So ingestion of sodium acetate results in a metabolic alkalosis and renal alkalinity.

(c)   Yes. Cystine is a sulphur-containing amino acid, the metabolism of which yields sulphuric acid. The renal compensation is to excrete acid.

(d)   Yes. The ammonium moiety is metabolized by the liver leaving hydrochloric acid, so ingestion of ammonium chloride results in aciduria.

(e)   No. Hyperventilation syndrome causes a respiratory alkalosis and the urine is alkaline.

17.19

(a)   No. In the renal tubular reabsorption of bicarbonate, hydrogen ions secreted into the tubular fluid combine with bicarbonate to yield carbon dioxide and water; it is the carbon dioxide that crosses into the renal tubular cell cytoplasm.

(b)   Yes. The lactate is metabolized so that effectively sodium hydroxide is released into the body. This metabolic alkalosis promotes renal excretion of bicarbonate.

(c)   No. Ammonia is formed from glutamine in the tubule cells.

(d)   Yes.

(e)   Yes. The major part of excess acid is excreted in the form of ammonium ions.

18 Endocrines

Endocrines in general	18.1–18.15
Hypothalamus and pituitary	18.16–18.26
Thyroid	18.27–18.32
Parathyroid, calcium and bone	18.33–18.40
Pancreatic endocrine function	18.41–18.48
Adrenal gland	18.49–18.53

QUESTIONS

Endocrines in general

18.1 With reference to endocrine function:
(a) growth hormone is involved in the control of growth of the long bones during adolescence.
(b) cortisol concentration in the plasma exerts a negative feedback effect on hypothalamic production of corticotrophin releasing factor.
(c) steroid hormones are normally bound to plasma proteins.
(d) adrenal androgens are normally secreted only in the male.
(c) release of anti-diuretic hormone (ADH) from the posterior pituitary is increased when osmolality of cerebral extracellular fluid increases.

18.2 Does the condition on the left lead to an increase in secretion of the hormone on the right?
(a) persistent exposure to cold   thyroxine.
(b) dietary deficiency of iodine   thyroid-stimulating hormone (TSH).
(c) increase in blood glucose   glucagon.
    concentration
(d) excessive water intake   aldosterone.
(e) dilatation of the cervix   oxytocin.
    uteri in labour

18.3 With reference to the features of endocrine function in general:
(a) all hormones reach their targets by means of dispersion throughout the whole circulation.
(b) the binding of a hormone to receptor sites on target cells increases in direct proportion to the plasma concentration of the hormone.
(c) hormones that are fat-soluble and of relatively low molecular weight may enter cells before acting in a specific manner.
(d) many hormones act by altering the rate at which some substance is transported across the cell membrane of the target cells.
(e) radioimmunoassay is a method of estimating the amount of antibody to a particular hormone.

18.4   **With reference to hormones:**
(a)   the concentration of a hormone bound to plasma protein is normally greater than the concentration of its free form.
(b)   plasma concentration of a hormone depends essentially on its secretion rate since inactivation and excretion rate vary relatively little.
(c)   the molecular weight of all hormones in the free form is such that they are too large to be lost in the glomerular filtrate.
(d)   thyroid-stimulating hormone (TSH) is secreted by an autotransplanted anterior pituitary gland.
(e)   prolactin is secreted by an autotransplanted anterior pituitary gland.

18.5   **In the 'stress syndrome' following injury, there is:**
(a)   release of corticotrophin-releasing hormone (CRH).
(b)   release of adrenocorticotrophic hormone (ACTH).
(c)   discharge of parasympathetic neurones.
(d)   release of adrenaline.
(e)   fall in blood glucose concentration.

18.6   **In the 'stress syndrome' following injury there is likely to be:**
(a)   retention of fluid.
(b)   increased metabolic rate.
(c)   retention of potassium.
(d)   negative nitrogen balance.
(e)   low heart rate.

18.7   **Concerning the structure of hormones:**
(a)   adrenaline is a catecholamine.
(b)   thyroxine is a steroid.
(c)   insulin is a protein.
(d)   aldosterone is a tyrosine derivative.
(e)   vasopressin is an oligopeptide.

18.8   **Concerning the actions of hormones on their targets:**
(a)   insulin acts on muscle by activation of tyrosine kinase.
(b)   anti-diuretic hormone (ADH) acts on the collecting duct cells of the renal tubules by causing an increase in the intracellular concentration of cAMP (cyclic adenosine monophosphate).
(c)   glucagon acts on liver cells by causing an increase in the intracellular concentration of cAMP (cyclic adenosine monophosphate).
(d)   the negative feedback loop that controls the tissue response to growth hormone (GH) is a simple one-stage loop.
(e)   the action of hormones that enter cells is more rapid than the action of those that act on the cell membrane.

18.9 **Are the following statements true?**

(a) the beta (insulin-secreting) cells of the islets of Langerhans are innervated.

(b) there are gastrin secreting cells in the pyloric antrum.

(c) somatostatin is produced in the anterior pituitary gland.

(d) growth hormone has the liver as one of its target organs.

(e) the myoepithelial cells of the mammary gland are concerned with lactogenesis (milk formation).

18.10 **Concerning the hormonal control of body fluid volume and osmolarity:**

(a) anti-diuretic hormone (ADH) secretion is reduced after drinking 2 litres of isotonic saline.

(b) ADH decreases the permeability of the collecting ducts of the kidney.

(c) aldosterone secretion is reduced after drinking 2 litres of isotonic saline.

(d) aldosterone acts on the distal convoluted tubule.

(e) aldosterone increases renal excretion of potassium.

18.11 **Concerning the renal handling of electrolytes:**

(a) the regulation of sodium excretion is primarily by changes in the glomerular filtration rate.

(b) distension of the right atrium results in release of atrial natriuretic factor.

(c) aldosterone operates by increasing renal tubular permeability.

(d) absence of aldosterone results in potassium retention.

(e) absence of aldosterone, if untreated, results in death.

18.12 **Concerning human sex hormones:**

(a) interstitial cells are prominent in the adult human ovary.

(b) interstitial cells are prominent in the adult testis.

(c) the pituitary of the adult male produces FSH (follicle-stimulating hormone).

(d) the pituitary of the adult male produces LH (luteinizing hormone).

(e) during pregnancy, ovulation is inhibited.

18.13 **Concerning hormone action:**

(a) LH (luteinizing hormone) is involved in a positive feedback loop.

(b) at six months, pregnancy would continue normally if the ovaries were removed.

(c) progesterone is without action on target organs unless they are primed by prior action of oestrogen.

(d) progesterone is secreted by the adrenal cortex.

(e) progesterone inhibits ovulation in women.

18.14   Concerning the cellular mechanism of actions of hormones:
(a)   thyroid hormones act via specific receptors on target cell membranes.
(b)   peptide hormones act after entering the cytoplasm of target cells.
(c)   steroid hormones act after entering the cytoplasm of target cells.
(d)   catecholamines act via specific receptors on target cell membranes.
(e)   hormones that enter their target cells operate via receptors within the nucleus.

18.15   With reference to endocrine systems:
(a)   secretion of hormones from the posterior pituitary is stimulated by releasing factors.
(b)   oestrogen in the normal woman causes development of secretory phase endometrium.
(c)   thyroglobulin is the bound form of thyroid hormone in the blood.
(d)   parathormone depletion leads to a high concentration of calcium in the renal tubular fluid.
(e)   aldosterone secretion is controlled primarily by the level of circulating adrenocorticotrophic hormone (ACTH).

Hypothalamus and pituitary

18.16   With reference to the secretions of the anterior pituitary:
(a)   the anterior pituitary contains much more growth hormone than any other hormone.
(b)   deficiencies produced by removal of the anterior pituitary could be corrected by reimplanting it at some other site in the body.
(c)   a fall in plasma glucose concentration leads to an increase in growth hormone (GH) secretion.
(d)   follicle-stimulating hormone (FSH) is secreted during pregnancy.
(e)   the period of peak prolactin secretion is around the time of parturition.

18.17   Concerning the anterior pituitary gland:
(a)   it arises embryologically as an outgrowth of the primitive brain.
(b)   it secretes growth hormone.
(c)   it secretes anti-diuretic hormone.
(d)   it is connected with the hypothalamus via a portal blood system.
(e)   the release of most of its hormones is controlled by releasing factors.

18.18 The hypothalamus:
(a) is situated in the medulla oblongata.
(b) secretes releasing factors for pituitary hormones.
(c) synthesizes hormones that are transported along axons to the pituitary gland.
(d) contains neurones that are specifically sensitive to temperature.
(e) contains neurones that are specifically sensitive to extracellular osmolarity.

18.19 Concerning anti-diuretic hormone (ADH):
(a) it is synthesized in neurones.
(b) it is carried to the pituitary gland via capillaries.
(c) its release into the blood is from the posterior pituitary.
(d) lack of ADH causes diabetes mellitus.
(e) in the kidney, ADH acts on the collecting ducts.

18.20 Concerning the pituitary gland:
(a) following hypophysectomy, there is an increase in the basal metabolic rate.
(b) the posterior pituitary controls the release of thyroxine from the thyroid gland.
(c) following hypophysectomy in the adult, there is regression of the mature testis.
(d) in the absence of pituitary function, testosterone secretion ceases.
(e) vasopressin is released by the posterior pituitary gland.

18.21 Concerning the anterior pituitary:
(a) its hormones are synthesized in the hypothalamus.
(b) some of the chromophobe cells are reserve cells that can differentiate into chromophils.
(c) acidophils and basophils secrete the same hormones.
(d) the pars intermedia secretes MSH (melanocyte-stimulating hormone).
(e) it secretes parathormone.

18.22 Concerning the anterior pituitary gland:
(a) its blood supply is sparse.
(b) the secretions are elaborated by the Golgi complex within the cells.
(c) the secretion diffuses through the cytoplasm to the cell surface.
(d) lysosomes degrade some of the secretion.
(e) the secretory cells all stain similarly with standard stains.

18.23 Concerning the posterior pituitary gland:
(a) it contains many neuronal cell bodies.
(b) it contains many non-medullated nerve fibres.
(c) it contains secretory cells.
(d) the capillaries are fenestrated.
(e) it releases hormones whose function is to influence the activity of other endocrine glands.

18.24 Concerning the anterior pituitary gland:
(a) its hormones are all proteins.
(b) it synthesizes the hormones that are released by the posterior pituitary gland.
(c) its secretory cells are innervated.
(d) the capillaries are fenestrated.
(e) it releases hormones whose function is to influence the activity of other endocrine glands.

18.25 With reference to pituitary function:
(a) adrenocorticotrophic hormone secretion is inhibited by a rise in blood cortisol.
(b) growth hormone is secreted only before adulthood.
(c) the hypothalamus secretes both growth hormone-releasing factor and growth hormone-inhibiting factor.
(d) oxytocin migrates in neurones from hypothalamus to posterior pituitary.
(e) storage of anti-diuretic hormone is in the posterior pituitary.

18.26 Deficiency of the anterior pituitary gland results in:
(a) reduced ability to respond to stress.
(b) gigantism.
(c) infertility.
(d) the person appearing older than his years.
(e) excessive libido.

Thyroid

18.27 Concerning thyroid hormones:
(a) they increase whole body oxygen consumption.
(b) their secretion depends on the integrity of the pituitary gland.
(c) they potentiate the action of catecholamines on the heart.
(d) hormones from the thyroid gland enter the blood as thyroglobulin.
(e) thyroid hormones are secreted in excess when iodine is deficient in the diet.

18.28 The follicular cells of the thyroid:
(a) collect iodine from the blood.
(b) synthesize thyroglobulin.
(c) secrete thyroglobulin into the blood.
(d) remove thyroglobulin from the colloid.
(e) remove thyroid hormones from thyroglobulin.

18.29 Calcitonin:
(a) is produced by cells concentrated mainly in the parathyroid gland.
(b) causes a fall in blood calcium concentration.
(c) promotes bone reabsorption.
(d) influences calcium retention in the kidney.
(e) influences calcium absorption from the gut.

18.30 Concerning the thyroid gland:
(a) it is the only endocrine gland that stores its secretions in follicles.
(b) its large storage capacity is connected with the fact that dietary intake of iodine fluctuates around the deficiency level in many parts of the world.
(c) the store of iodine is mainly extracellular.
(d) 95% of the body store of iodine is in the thyroid gland.
(e) dietary deficiency of iodine causes hypertrophy of the gland.

18.31 Concerning the thyroid:
(a) the side of the follicular cell facing the colloid has a brush border.
(b) the follicular cells secrete thyroxine into the blood.
(c) the follicular cells secrete thyroxine into the colloid.
(d) secretion passing from the follicular cells to the blood must cross two basement membranes.
(e) each molecule of thyroglobulin has many molecules of hormone attached to it.

18.32 Concerning the thyroid gland and its secretions:
(a) thyroid hormones are coupled and iodinated globulins.
(b) the thyroid hormones are synthesised on the surface of the thyroglobulin molecule.
(c) deficiency of thyroid hormones in children causes rickets.
(d) deficiency of thyroid hormones in children causes premature maturation.
(e) deficiency of thyroid hormones from birth causes low mental ability.

Parathyroid, calcium and bone

18.33 Injection of parathyroid hormone leads to:
(a)   an increase in urinary phosphate.
(b)   increased production of dihydroxycholecalciferol in the kidney.
(c)   an increase in the number of osteoblasts.
(d)   a rise in plasma calcium.
(e)   increased reabsorption of calcium in the kidney.

18.34 A low serum calcium may be associated with:
(a)   hyperexcitability of peripheral nerves.
(b)   increased calcitonin release.
(c)   an increased serum phosphate concentration.
(d)   vitamin D deficiency.
(e)   reduced parathormone release.

18.35 With reference to calcium:
(a)   calcitonin can start to correct a rise in plasma calcium level within
       a few minutes.
(b)   calcium is released from smooth muscle cells when they contract.
(c)   calcium is necessary for blood clotting.
(d)   parathormone decreases calcium absorption from the gut.
(e)   calcium ion concentration in interstitial fluid is about 1.2 mmol per
       litre.

18.36 With respect to calcium in humans:
(a)   there is a higher concentration of free calcium ions inside cells than
       outside.
(b)   bound calcium in the plasma dissociates more when pH decreases.
(c)   low plasma calcium concentration leads to the release of more
       1,25-dihydroxycholecalciferol.
(d)   phytic acid in the diet diminishes absorption of calcium from the
       gut.
(e)   a minimum daily dietary requirement in an adult is about 100 mg.

18.37 In bone in the mature person:
(a)   three-quarters of the substance is mineral, one-quarter organic.
(b)   bed-rest can deplete the mineral content.
(c)   osteoblasts are associated with areas where reabsorption is taking
       place.
(d)   alkaline phosphatase is associated with the laying down of mineral.
(e)   calcium is transferred to the extracellular fluid in response to an
       increase in calcitonin.

18.38 Concerning parathyroid hormone (parathormone):
(a) it is produced by parafollicular cells of the thyroid.
(b) its secretion is controlled by the pituitary gland.
(c) it increases bone reabsorption.
(d) it increases phosphate reabsorption by the kidney.
(e) it stimulates the production of vitamin D in the skin.

18.39 Concerning blood calcium concentration:
(a) parathormone is the most important hormone involved in calcium homeostasis.
(b) administration of vitamin D to a D-deficient person increases the level of parathormone (PTH) in the peripheral blood.
(c) parathormone has a life in the circulation of around 6 hr.
(d) a rise in plasma calcium concentration causes a rise in parathormone release.
(e) calcitonin is produced in the thyroid glands.

18.40 Concerning calcium regulation:
(a) the plasma calcium concentration is lowered in a subject as a result of his receiving a blood transfusion.
(b) calcium influx into the axoplasm is essential for the release of transmitter from the terminal of a motor nerve.
(c) calcium release into muscle cell cytoplasm is essential in excitation-contraction coupling.
(d) the vitamin D group of substances promotes the uptake of calcium from the gut.
(e) calcitonin stimulates the action of osteoclasts.

Pancreatic endocrine function

18.41 In uncontrolled diabetes mellitus:
(a) the large volume of urine excreted is principally due to a lack of secretion of anti-diuretic hormone.
(b) the specific gravity of the urine is typically 1000 units.
(c) the renal tubular reabsorption mechanism for glucose is working at its maximum rate.
(d) the concentration of glucose in the intracellular fluid of skeletal muscles is high.
(e) energy requirements of the body are largely met by metabolism of fats.

18.42 In an uncontrolled diabetic:
(a)   there is likely to be a metabolic alkalosis.
(b)   there is likely to be hyperventilation.
(c)   the blood is hypo-osmotic.
(d)   the thirst that is a feature of the condition is due to the polyuria.
(e)   administration of insulin causes a fall in extracellular concentration of potassium.

18.43 Concerning the endocrine secretions of the pancreas:
(a)   the blood supply of the islets of Langerhans is denser than that of the exocrine part of the gland.
(b)   the half-life of insulin is about 20 min.
(c)   the insulin secreting cells outnumber the glucagon secreting cells by about 3 to 1.
(d)   insulin secreted into the bloodstream goes straight to the liver.
(e)   the pancreas contains gastrin-secreting cells.

18.44 In a normal person, insulin secretion:
(a)   is depressed by a high blood glucose level.
(b)   is unaffected by an infusion of mannose.
(c)   is increased by vagal nerve stimulation.
(d)   is primarily controlled by the anterior pituitary gland.
(e)   results in increased transfer of glucose into muscle cells.

18.45 Concerning glucagon:
(a)   it is secreted by the islets of Langerhans.
(b)   it is secreted by cells in the gastric mucosa.
(c)   hypoglycaemia promotes glucagon secretion.
(d)   glucagon promotes hepatic gluconeogenesis.
(e)   glucagon promotes hepatic glycogenesis.

18.46 Concerning blood glucose:
(a)   after a heavy carbohydrate meal, the plasma concentration of glucagon falls.
(b)   glucagon stimulates the pancreatic secretion of insulin.
(c)   insulin secretion is promoted by sympathetic nerve activity.
(d)   glucagon secretion is promoted by sympathetic nerve activity.
(e)   sympathetic stimulation promotes hepatic glycogenolysis.

18.47 Concerning insulin and its actions:
(a) insulin binds to the outer surface of its target cells.
(b) glycogen synthesis in the liver is enhanced by insulin.
(c) in the liver, the intracellular concentration of glucose is raised by insulin.
(d) glucose movement across the hepatocyte cell membrane is directly enhanced by insulin.
(e) glucose movement across the cell membrane in a skeletal muscle cell is directly enhanced by insulin.

18.48 Concerning the metabolic disturbances in diabetes mellitus:
(a) oxidation of free fatty acids in the liver is impeded at the acetyl co-enzyme A (CoA) stage.
(b) the formation of ketone bodies (acetone and aceto-acetic acid) is from acetyl CoA.
(c) ketone bodies are formed in skeletal muscle.
(d) ketoacids are excreted in the urine.
(e) a high concentration of ketoacids in the blood leads to delirium.

Adrenal gland

18.49 Aldosterone:
(a) is secreted by the zona glomerulosa of the adrenal cortex.
(b) output is principally dependent on adrenocorticotrophic hormone secretion.
(c) greatly stimulates hepatic gluconeogenesis.
(d) assists in compensation for depletion of blood volume by haemorrhage.
(e) promotes renal loss of potassium.

18.50 Concerning aldosterone:
(a) in the kidney, it acts mainly on the proximal convoluted tubule.
(b) it promotes renal excretion of sodium ions.
(c) angiotensin promotes its secretion.
(d) over-secretion results in a rise in the extracellular potassium concentration.
(e) over-secretion results in a rise in the extracellular hydrogen ion concentration.

18.51 Concerning the adrenal gland:
(a) it contains much more medullary than cortical tissue.
(b) the blood supply of tissues is via sinusoids.
(c) the flow of blood is from cortex to medulla.
(d) glucocorticoids are released by the zona fasciculata of the cortex.
(e) glucocorticoids inhibit the medullary release of catecholamines.

18.52   Concerning the adrenal cortex:
(a)   the zona glomerulosa lies just beneath the capsule.
(b)   the secretory cells contain much smooth endoplasmic reticulum.
(c)   progesterone is formed as an intermediary in the synthesis of glucocorticoids and mineralocorticoids.
(d)   adrenal cortical androgens have a stronger masculinizing effect than testosterone.
(e)   the adrenal cortex is the only site in the body where steroid hormones are produced.

18.53   Concerning cortisol:
(a)   it is a protein.
(b)   it is the main glucocorticoid in humans.
(c)   it is under the control of the posterior pituitary gland.
(d)   it causes a reduction in blood glucose concentration.
(e)   it is broken down in the tissues on which it exerts its physiological actions.

ANSWERS

18.1
(a)   Yes.
(b)   Yes.
(c)   Yes.
(d)   No. They are secreted in the female also.
(e)   Yes. Cerebral extracellular fluid includes that to which hypothalamic osmoreceptors are exposed; increase in osmolality stimulates neuro-endocrine secretion of ADH so that more water is retained in the kidney, and the extracellular compartment is 'diluted' back to normal.

18.2
(a)   Yes. This tends to raise temperature by increasing metabolic rate at rest.
(b)   Yes. Low iodine leads to low production of thyroid hormone, which stimulates secretion of TSH.
(c)   No. Insulin is secreted.
(d)   No. Aldosterone increases sodium and water retention.
(e)   Yes. This is a neuro-endocrine positive feedback mechanism.

18.3
(a)   No. The hypothalamic releasing hormones, for example, are distributed through a special portal system.
(b)   No. A limit is reached when receptor sites are fully occupied.

(c)   Yes. Although the protein hormones and the thyroid hormones act at a membrane, the fat-soluble hormones of low molecular weight (steroid hormones and catecholamines) enter first and act within.

(d)   Yes. Insulin, for example.

(e)   No. Radioimmunoassay measures the amount of hormone in a sample after that sample has been treated with a serum containing antibody to the hormone.

18.4

(a)   Yes. For example, over 99% of T4 and T3 in the blood is bound.

(b)   Yes.

(c)   No. Many hormones in the free form have a small enough molecular weight to be filtered.

(d)   No. Because TSH secretion depends on TSH releasing factor from the hypothalamus.

(e)   Yes. Because prolactin secretion is ordinarily suppressed by prolactin inhibiting hormone.

18.5

(a)   Yes. In the 'stress syndrome' the adrenal cortex and medulla are both major participants. Release of CRH from the hypothalamus is the first step in the sequence of activation of the adrenal cortex.

(b)   Yes. Release of ACTH from the anterior pituitary is the second step in the sequence of activation from the hypothalamus to the adrenal cortex.

(c)   No. In the stress syndrome, on the whole there is a reduction in discharge of parasympathetic neurones and an increase in discharge of sympathetic neurones.

(d)   Yes.

(e)   No. In the stress syndrome, there is a rise in blood glucose concentration due to adrenaline and cortisol release. This is part of the mobilization of resources to provide substrates to tissues important in the repair of the organism.

18.6

(a)   Yes. Retention of fluid is caused by cortisol secretion.

(b)   Yes. Increased metabolic rate is caused by adrenaline secretion.

(c)   No. Cortisol secretion causes sodium retention and potassium excretion; these actions of cortisol are much weaker than the actions of aldosterone.

(d)   Yes. Breakdown of protein is a feature of the stress syndrome and is evidenced by negative nitrogen balance.

(e)   No. The secretion of adrenaline causes a rise in heart rate.

18.7

(a)   Yes.

(b)   No. Thyroxine is an amine hormone, derived from the amino acid tyrosine.

(c)   Yes.
(d)   No. Aldosterone is a steroid hormone, as its name suggests.
(e)   Yes. It is a small peptide nine amino acids in length.

18.8
(a)   Yes. The receptors for insulin are proteins with a glycosylated extracellular domain, a single transmembranal sequence and an intracellular domain with protein tyrosine kinase activity.
(b)   Yes. ADH binds to a receptor on the basolateral aspects of the collecting duct cells. This receptor is coupled to adrenyl cyclase and increases the intracellular concentration of cAMP. This in turn activates protein kinases.
(c)   Yes.
(d)   No. It is a two-stage loop. GH stimulates synthesis of somatostatin which in turn dampens the tissue response to GH.
(e)   No. The action of hormones which enter cells is much less rapid than the action of those which act on the cell membrane because those acting intracellularly do so via intracellular messenger systems which are relatively slow.

18.9
(a)   Yes. The beta (insulin-secreting) cells of the islets of Langerhans receive a parasympathetic secretogogue innervation from the vagus nerve.
(b)   Yes.
(c)   No. Somatostatin is produced in the hypothalamus.
(d)   Yes. Growth hormone acting on the liver promotes RNA synthesis, protein synthesis and gluconeogenesis.
(e)   No. The myoepithelial cells of the mammary gland are concerned with expulsion of milk, not with lactogenesis.

18.10
(a)   No. ADH secretion depends primarily on the osmolarity of the blood and so is not reduced after drinking 2 litres of isotonic saline.
(b)   No. ADH increases the permeability of the collecting ducts of the kidney, thereby allowing water to move from duct fluid to the renal interstitium and promoting water reabsorption.
(c)   Yes. Aldosterone promotes sodium reabsorption; its secretion is reduced after drinking 2 litres of isotonic saline.
(d)   Yes.
(e)   Yes.

18.11

(a)   No. Changes in the glomerular filtration rate are not employed by the organism in the regulation of sodium excretion.

(b)   Yes. The release of atrial natriuretic factor as a result of distension of the right atrium is the most important factor in the control of fluid volume initiated by the right atrium.

(c)   No. Aldosterone operates by stimulating active reabsorption of sodium in the distal convoluted tubule.

(d)   Yes.

(e)   Yes.

18.12

(a)   No. They are prominent in other species and they are present in the ovaries of girls, but they virtually disappear in women.

(b)   Yes. They produce testosterone.

(c)   Yes. It stimulates Sertoli cells of the testis.

(d)   Yes. It stimulates the interstitial cells of the testis to secrete testosterone.

(e)   Yes. During pregnancy, ovulation is inhibited by progesterone, first from the corpus luteum and then from the placenta.

18.13

(a)   Yes. As a component of the hormonal changes during the menstrual cycle.

(b)   Yes. By six months, the placenta has taken over the hormonal functions earlier subserved by ovarian hormones.

(c)   Yes.

(d)   No. Progesterone is secreted by the corpus luteum and the placenta.

(e)   Yes. Progesterone inhibits ovulation in women, probably by inhibiting release of LH-releasing factor from the hypothalamus.

18.14

(a)   No. Thyroid hormones act after entering the cytoplasm of target cells.

(b)   No. Peptide hormones act via specific receptors on target cell membranes.

(c)   Yes.

(d)   Yes.

(e)   Yes. Hormones that enter their target cells operate via receptors within the nucleus. These are specific intranuclear receptors and, when the hormone binds, it produces a configurational change in a nearby DNA-binding site to influence gene transcription and synthesis of proteins.

18.15

(a)   No. Releasing factors act on the anterior pituitary. Posterior pituitary hormones are released from the nerve endings as a result of action potentials originating in their cell bodies in the hypothalamus.

(b)   No. Oestrogen is responsible for the proliferation phase, and progesterone for the secretory phase.

(c)   No. Thyroglobulin is the form in which the hormone is stored in the thyroid gland.

(d)   Yes. Parathormone's action on the kidney is to promote phosphate excretion and calcium retention.

(e)   No. ACTH has some action, but the main control is by the renin–angiotensin system.

18.16

(a)   Yes.

(b)   No. The secretions are controlled by releasing factors from the hypothalamus which reach the anterior pituitary via the local portal blood system.

(c)   Yes. Via the hypothalamus and the secretion of GH-releasing hormone; GH decreases peripheral glucose utilization and promotes lipid utilization; hence the brain is protected from shortage.

(d)   No. Secretion is inhibited during pregnancy.

(e)   Yes. Secretion rises during pregnancy.

18.17

(a)   No. The anterior pituitary arises embryologically as an outgrowth of the primitive mouth.

(b)   Yes.

(c)   No. Anti-diuretic hormone is secreted by the posterior pituitary.

(d)   Yes. The anterior pituitary is connected with the hypothalamus via a portal blood system and it is via this that control from the hypothalamus is exerted.

(e)   Yes. The release of most anterior pituitary hormones is controlled by releasing factors from the hypothalamus.

18.18

(a)   No. The hypothalamus is situated in the diencephalon.

(b)   Yes.

(c)   Yes.

(d)   Yes. The hypothalamus contains neurones that are specifically sensitive to temperature and is the regulating centre for temperature control.

(e)   Yes. The hypothalamus contains neurones that are specifically sensitive to extracellular osmolarity; this is associated with its role in regulating osmolarity via anti-diuretic hormone.

18.19

(a)   Yes. Anti-diuretic hormone is synthesized in the neurones whose axons form the supraoptico-hypophyseal tract.

(b) No. ADH is transported along the axons of the neurones of the supraoptico-hypophyseal tract to the posterior pituitary gland.

(c) Yes. From nerve terminals in the posterior pituitary gland ADH is released into the blood.

(d) No. Lack of ADH causes diabetes insipidus ('tasteless' diabetes, so-called because the urine is not sugary).

(e) Yes. It increases the permeability of the cells of the collecting ducts to water, thus allowing water to move from the tubular fluid to the interstitium by osmosis; this is an essential part of the mechanism of producing a concentrated urine.

18.20

(a) No. Following hypophysectomy, there is a decrease in the basal metabolic rate.

(b) No. It is the anterior pituitary that controls the release of thyroxine from the thyroid gland.

(c) No. In the absence of pituitary function, there is sufficient production of testosterone by the testis to maintain normal function.

(d) No. Testosterone secretion continues even after hypophysectomy.

(e) Yes.

18.21

(a) No. This would be true of the posterior pituitary.

(b) Yes.

(c) No. Acidophils secrete growth hormone and prolactin; basophils secrete thyroid-stimulating hormone, follicle-stimulating hormone and luteinizing hormone.

(d) Yes.

(e) No. Parathormone is secreted by the parathyroid glands.

18.22

(a) No. The blood supply is rich.

(b) Yes.

(c) No. It is transported as secretory vesicles.

(d) Yes.

(e) No. Cells stain in three different ways: this allows the cells to be classified into chromophobe, acidophil and basophil.

18.23

(a) No. The posterior pituitary gland is the site of termination of axons; it does not contain neuronal cell bodies.

(b) Yes. The posterior pituitary gland contains many non-medullated nerve fibres, these being the termination of nerve fibres from the hypothalamus.

(c)   No. The posterior pituitary does not contain secretory cells; it contains the terminals of axons from the hypothalamus.

(d)   Yes. In the posterior pituitary gland, the capillaries are fenestrated. This allows the hormones, which are relatively large molecules, to pass into the blood when released from the nerve.

(e)   No. The actions of posterior pituitary hormones are directly on target tissues.

18.24

(a)   Yes.

(b)   No. The hormones that are released by the posterior pituitary gland are synthesized in the hypothalamus, not in the anterior pituitary gland.

(c)   No. The secretory cells of the anterior pituitary are not innervated; secretion is controlled by releasing factors.

(d)   Yes. The capillaries are fenestrated. This allows the hormones, which are relatively large molecules, to pass into the blood when released.

(e)   Yes. One function of the anterior pituitary gland is to release hormones whose function is to influence the activity of other endocrine glands.

18.25

(a)   Yes.

(b)   No. Secretion of growth hormone continues into adulthood.

(c)   Yes.

(d)   Yes.

(e)   Yes.

18.26

(a)   Yes. The ability to respond to stress depends on adrenocorticotrophic hormone acting on the adrenal cortex.

(b)   No. The anterior pituitary secretes growth hormone; deficiency results in pituitary dwarfism.

(c)   Yes. Fertility depends on follicle-stimulating hormone and luteinizing hormone stimulating the generative cells.

(d)   No. There is retardation of maturation and the subject typically appears juvenile.

(e)   No. There is loss of libido due to lack of follicle-stimulating hormone and luteinizing hormone.

18.27

(a)   Yes. Thyroid hormones increase the basal metabolic rate.

(b)   Yes. Thyroid hormone secretion depends on adrenocorticotrophic hormone from the anterior pituitary gland.

(c)   Yes.

(d)   No. Thyroid hormones from the thyroid gland enter the blood as iodothyronine hormones.

(e)   No. Deficiency of thyroid hormone secretion results when iodine is deficient in the diet.

18.28
(a)   Yes.
(b)   Yes.
(c)   No. The follicular cells of the thyroid secrete thyroglobulin into the colloid of the follicle.
(d)   Yes.
(e)   Yes.

18.29
(a)   No. Calcitonin is produced by parafollicular cells distributed in the thyroid tissue.
(b)   Yes.
(c)   No. Calcitonin inhibits bone reabsorption.
(d)   No. Unlike parathormone, calcitonin acts only on bone.
(e)   No. Unlike parathormone, calcitonin acts only on bone.

18.30
(a)   Yes.
(b)   Yes.
(c)   Yes.
(d)   Yes.
(e)   Yes.

18.31
(a)   Yes.
(b)   Yes.
(c)   No. Thyroglobulin is secreted into the follicle.
(d)   Yes. Secretion passing from the follicular cells to the blood must cross two basement membranes, that of the epithelium and that of the endothelium.
(e)   Yes.

18.32
(a)   No. Thyroid hormones are coupled and iodinated amino acids. The globuloin from thyroglobulin is retained for recycling.
(b)   Yes.
(c)   No. Rickets occurs as a result of Vitamin D deficiency.
(d)   No. Deficiency of thyroid hormones leads to delayed occurrence of the normal stages of development, with holding up the head, sitting, walking and speech occurring later than normal.
(e)   Yes. Deficiency of thyroid hormones from birth leads to 'cretinism'.

18.33

(a) Yes. Reabsorption of phosphate by the proximal tubule is depressed.
(b) Yes. This metabolite of vitamin D promotes calcium reabsorption from the gut.
(c) No. Parathormone stimulates osteoclast activity.
(d) Yes.
(e) Yes.

18.34

(a) Yes. This is the cause of tetany, e.g. in excessive hyperventilation.
(b) Yes. Low calcium can result from an increase in the release of calcitonin.
(c) Yes. The combination of low calcium and high phosphate concentration is found in hypoparathyroidism.
(d) Yes. This interferes with absorption.
(e) Yes. A primary defect of parathormone output allows calcium to decrease.

18.35

(a) Yes.
(b) No. Calcium enters smooth muscle cells when they contract.
(c) Yes.
(d) No. It increases calcium absorption.
(e) Yes. This is the value of ionized calcium concentration in plasma with which interstitial fluid is in equilibrium.

18.36

(a) No. $[Ca^{2+}]$ outside is many orders of magnitude greater than inside.
(b) Yes.
(c) Yes. This assists restoration of the calcium level by aiding absorption.
(d) Yes.
(e) No. The requirement is twice as much, and the usual intake is nearer 1000 mg/day. 100 mg is the normal average value for net absorption.

18.37

(a) Yes.
(b) Yes.
(c) No. -Blasts are for 'building' -clasts are for breaking down.
(d) Yes.
(e) No. Calcitonin decreases the removal of calcium from bone.

18.38

(a) No. Parathormone is produced by the parathyroid glands, which lie in the thyroid gland.

(b)   No. Parathormone is not under the control of the pituitary gland; its release is promoted by a fall in calcium concentration in the secretory cells of the parathyroid gland.

(c)   Yes.

(d)   No. Parathormone increases renal excretion of phosphate.

(e)   No.

18.39

(a)   Yes. Parathormone is the most important hormone involved in calcium homeostasis, although calcitonin has a possible role in reducing hypercalcaemia.

(b)   No. Administration of vitamin D to a D-deficient person reduces the level of PTH in the peripheral blood, although the blood calcium concentration remains unaltered.

(c)   No. Parathormone has a life in the circulation of around 20 min.

(d)   No. A rise in plasma calcium concentration causes a fall in parathormone release. This is the negative feedback loop controlling plasma calcium concentration.

(e)   Yes. Calcitonin is produced in the parafollicular cells of the thyroid gland.

18.40

(a)   Yes. The plasma calcium concentration is lowered in a subject as a result of his receiving a blood transfusion because the stored blood contains citrate which binds calcium.

(b)   Yes.

(c)   Yes.

(d)   Yes.

(e)   No. Calcitonin inhibits the action of osteoclasts.

18.41

(a)   No. The large volume of urine excreted is principally due to the osmotic diuretic action of urinary glucose.

(b)   No. 1000 is the specific gravity of water. The specific gravity of the urine is high due to its glucose content.

(c)   Yes. Despite the fact that the renal tubular reabsorption mechanism for glucose is working at its maximum rate, an excess of glucose is filtered and this is why there is overspill into the urine.

(d)   No. Insulin is required for the transport of glucose across the skeletal muscle membrane; in uncontrolled diabetes mellitus, the concentration of glucose in the intracellular fluid of skeletal muscles is low.

(e)   Yes. As a result of the derangement of metabolism resulting from insulin lack, energy requirements of the body are largely met by metabolism of fats.

18.42

(a)   No. Because of the production of ketone bodies, which are fixed acids, there is a metabolic acidosis.

(b)   Yes. Because of the metabolic acidosis, there is likely to be hyperventilation.

(c)   No. Due to excess glucose, the blood is hyperosmotic.

(d)   Yes.

(e)   Yes. Insulin causes potassium uptake in association with glucose uptake by cells and hence a fall in extracellular concentration of potassium.

18.43

(a)   Yes. All endocrine secretory tissue has a high blood flow.

(b)   Yes.

(c)   Yes.

(d)   Yes. The pancreatic venous drainage is into the portal venous system.

(e)   Yes. In the islets of Langerhans, the alpha cells which secrete glucagon comprise 15–25% of the cells and the beta cells, which secrete insulin, comprise 70–80%. There are also a few delta cells, which secrete gastrin.

18.44

(a)   No. A high blood glucose level stimulates insulin secretion.

(b)   No. Mannose is also a stimulant for insulin secretion.

(c)   Yes. Vagal stimulation increases insulin secretion by release of acetylcholine; this effect is blocked by atropine.

(d)   No.

(e)   Yes.

18.45

(a)   Yes. It is secreted by the alpha cells.

(b)   Yes. It is secreted by the mucosa of the stomach and the duodenum.

(c)   Yes.

(d)   Yes. This contributes to its function of raising the blood glucose concentration.

(e)   No. Glucagon promotes hepatic glycogenolysis.

18.46

(a)   Yes. This fall is in response to the rise in blood glucose concentration.

(b)   Yes. This is partly a direct effect and partly secondary to the rise in blood glucose concentration that it causes.

(c)   No. Insulin secretion is inhibited by sympathetic nerve activity.

(d) Yes. The increase in glucagon secretion by sympathetic nerve activity contributes to the increase in blood glucose concentration caused by sympathetic activity.

(e) Yes. Sympathetic stimulation promotes glycogenolysis and this contributes to the rise in blood glucose as a component of the 'fight-or-flight' reaction. It similarly contributes to maintaining blood glucose when utilization increases in exercise.

18.47

(a) Yes.

(b) Yes. Glycogen synthesis in the liver is enhanced by insulin, thus laying down energy stores.

(c) No. By promoting glycogen synthesis, insulin lowers the intracellular concentration of glucose.

(d) No. Insulin has no direct effect on glucose movement across the hepatocyte cell membrane; the effect of insulin is to promote glycogen synthesis, lower the intracellular concentration of glucose and then, because of the inwardly-directed concentration gradient for glucose, glucose entry is increased.

(e) Yes. Glucose movement across the cell membrane in a skeletal muscle cell is directly enhanced by insulin; in this respect hepatocytes and skeletal muscle cells differ.

18.48

(a) Yes.

(b) Yes.

(c) No. Ketone bodies are formed only in the liver.

(d) Yes. The renal excretion of ketoacids is accompanied by ammonium excretion (as buffer) and, later in the disease, by sodium excretion (to balance the electrical charge on the acids). This leads to severe dehydration.

(e) No. A high concentration of ketoacids in the blood leads to 'ketoacidaemic coma'.

18.49

(a) Yes.

(b) No. Aldosterone secretion is mainly controlled by angiotensin.

(c) No. The main action of aldosterone is in the control of electrolyte balance.

(d) Yes. By promoting retention of sodium and water in the kidney.

(e) Yes. Aldosterone promotes renal reabsorption of sodium and, as part of the movement of other ions to maintain electroneutrality, potassium ions are excreted. So aldosterone promotes renal loss of potassium.

18.50

(a)   No. Aldosterone acts mainly on the distal convoluted tubule.

(b)   No. Aldosterone promotes renal retention of sodium ions.

(c)   Yes. The principal stimulus for secretion of aldosterone is angiotensin.

(d)   No. Over-secretion of aldosterone, by promoting urinary excretion of potassium in exchange for sodium reabsorption, results in a fall in the extracellular potassium concentration.

(e)   No. Over-secretion of aldosterone, by reducing the extracellular potassium concentration, results in an exit of potassium from cells; to maintain electrical neutrality, positively-charged ions including hydrogen ions enter cells and this leads to a fall in the extracellular hydrogen ion concentration.

18.51

(a)   No. The adrenal gland contains much more cortical than medullary tissue.

(b)   Yes. Sinusoids are wide capillaries; these are needed to carry away the viscous secretions of the glandular cells.

(c)   Yes. This has functional significance in carrying glucocorticoids to the medulla.

(d)   Yes.

(e)   No. Glucocorticoids promote the medullary release of catechol-amines.

18.52

(a)   Yes.

(b)   Yes. Steroid-secreting cells possess much smooth endoplasmic reticulum, because it is on this that steroids are synthesized.

(c)   Yes.

(d)   No. Adrenal cortical androgens have a much weaker masculinizing effect than testosterone.

(e)   No. Steroid hormones are produced in the adrenal cortex, the gonads and the placenta.

18.53

(a)   No. Cortisol is a steroid.

(b)   Yes. Cortisol is the main glucocorticoid in humans, corticosterone being present in much smaller amounts.

(c)   No. Cortisol is under the control of the anterior pituitary gland.

(d)   No. It is a glucocorticoid; these hormones are so-named because they enhance glucose formation and cause a rise in blood glucose concentration.

(e)   No. Cortisol is not broken down in the tissues on which it exerts its physiological actions. It is broken down in the liver.

19 Temperature regulation

19.1 When a healthy individual is exposed to cold:
(a) metabolic heat production is increased by catecholamine secretion.
(b) the total peripheral vascular resistance decreases.
(c) surface temperature decreases more than core temperature.
(d) adjustments are controlled from centres in the medulla.
(e) shivering further decreases the body temperature.

19.2 A survivor of a shipwreck with a core temperature of 30°C:
(a) has a higher metabolic rate than a normal subject at rest.
(b) shivers violently.
(c) is unconscious.
(d) has a decreased blood pressure.
(e) has a raised peripheral resistance.

19.3 If a normal individual is exposed to a hot environment:
(a) the additional heat loss through sweating depends on evaporation of the sweat.
(b) a reflex increase in ventilation is a major way of increasing heat loss.
(c) if sweating is excessive, salt intake should be cut down.
(d) in the process of maintaining water balance, urine output can decrease to about 200 ml per day.
(e) resting cardiac output will be higher than in his usual environment.

19.4 With reference to the maintenance of body temperature in the human:
(a) during prolonged exposure to hot environments, the metabolic rate increases.
(b) all mechanisms controlling heat loss from the skin surface are served by noradrenergic sympathetic nerves.
(c) changes in temperature of the skin are more potent than changes in temperature of the hypothalamus in evoking homeostatic responses.
(d) when the environmental temperature is high, a high relative humidity facilitates the loss of heat by the subject.
(e) in a fever of rapid onset when the core temperature is rising, the subject is likely to feel cold.

19.5   Concerning body temperature and its control in the human:
(a)   evaporation of water from the body surface occurs only when the sweat glands secrete.
(b)   if the core temperature rises, the subject will sweat even if the fluid loss results in circulatory collapse.
(c)   in a trained athlete, the sodium concentration is the same in plasma and sweat.
(d)   the loss by a healthy adult of 4 litres of sweat during a working shift in a hot environment endangers life.
(e)   a core temperature of 43°C signifies a danger to life.

19.6   With reference to maintenance of a normal body temperature:
(a)   during prolonged exposure to hot environments, secretion of thyroid hormones increases.
(b)   heat can be lost from the skin by convection at an environmental temperature of 40°C.
(c)   the loss of heat in expired air constitutes more than half the unavoidable heat loss in average environmental and physiological conditions.
(d)   the hypothalamus contains neurones specifically responsive to temperature.
(e)   shivering may treble the resting metabolic rate.

19.7   When the core temperature of a subject is rising because of a bacterial infection:
(a)   there is an excess of heat loss over heat production by the body.
(b)   the subject feels hot.
(c)   the subject shivers.
(d)   the cause of the condition is an increase in the set point of the central temperature regulator.
(e)   respiration is depressed.

19.8   The core temperature is above normal in a subject:
(a)   with a deficiency of thyroid function.
(b)   exercising strenuously.
(c)   as a result of administration of pyrogens.
(d)   as a result of administration of progesterone.
(e)   as a result of administration of adrenaline.

19.9   When a normal adult human from a temperate climate adapts to a tropical climate, there is a decrease in:
(a)   the overall rate of heat loss from the body.
(b)   the basal metabolic rate.
(c)   thyroxine production.
(d)   the vascular peripheral resistance.
(e)   the salt concentration of sweat.

19.10 **With reference to maintenance of a normal body temperature:**
(a) exposure of part of the body surface to an external heat source results in increased skin blood flow in that part.
(b) the thermoregulatory centre lies in the cerebral cortex.
(c) the thermoregulatory centre receives information from temperature receptors in the skin.
(d) the hypothalamus contains neurones that increase their firing rate specifically in response to an increase in their temperature.
(e) the hypothalamus contains neurones that increase their firing rate specifically in response to a decrease in their temperature.

19.11 **With reference to maintenance of a normal body temperature:**
(a) shivering is due to contraction of smooth muscle fibres.
(b) the efferent nerve fibres causing shivering are sympathetic nerve fibres.
(c) shivering is a spinal reflex.
(d) in excessive sweating, the inorganic ion whose loss is the main cause of collapse is potassium.
(e) in an individual undertaking strenuous muscular exercise in a hot environment, the main vehicle for heat loss is the evaporation of sweat.

19.12 **Concerning environmental factors:**
(a) when the environmental temperature is 38°C and the air is dry, a person can lose heat by conduction.
(b) when the environmental temperature is 38°C and the air is dry, a person can lose heat by evaporation.
(c) it is sufficient for sweat to be produced for it to be a mechanism for heat loss from the body.
(d) it is possible for a person to survive for prolonged periods at an environmental temperature of 38°C if the air is saturated with water vapour.
(e) a black-skinned person loses more than twice the amount of heat by radiation than is lost by a white-skinned person.

ANSWERS

19.1
(a) Yes.
(b) No. It rises due to increased sympathetic activity.
(c) Yes. Peripheral vasoconstriction reduces heat loss through the skin and contributes to conserving the core temperature.
(d) No. Centres are in the hypothalamus.
(e) No. Shivering produces heat, which helps to raise temperature.

19.2

(a)   No. His metabolic rate is depressed.

(b)   No. The shivering reflex is paralysed at this temperature.

(c)   Yes.

(d)   Yes.

(e)   No. Vasomotor tone is absent.

19.3

(a)   Yes. Sweating is ineffective if you rub the sweat off with a towel.

(b)   No. Not in humans, only in panting animals, which are furry and cannot use sweating.

(c)   No. Sweat contains NaCl; sodium loss can be a problem, and intake should be increased.

(d)   No. The minimum volume of maximally concentrated urine is 400–500 ml/day; 200 ml per day would indicate failure of excretory function.

(e)   Yes. Increased blood flow through the skin requires this.

19.4

(a)   No. It decreases; thyroid activity decreases.

(b)   No. The sweat glands are cholinergically innervated.

(c)   No. In order to elicit similar reflex responses, the fall in temperature of peripheral receptors must be 50 times as great as the fall in temperature of hypothalmic receptors.

(d)   No. A high relative humidity decreases evaporation from the body surface.

(e)   Yes. The set point of the hypothalamic integrating centre has risen to a high level, so the subject feels cold until his core temperature is raised to match the new set point.

19.5

(a)   No. Insensible perspiration also provides fluid for evaporation.

(b)   Yes. A rise in core temperture is so life-threatening that, if the body is both overheated and fluid-depleted, homeostatic mechanisms for heat loss, including sweating, take precedence over those for fluid conservation.

(c)   No. There is normally some reabsorption of sodium in the ducts of the sweat glands; this increases with habituation to high levels of physical activity.

(d)   No. In a healthy adult, the loss of 4 litres of fluid is not sufficiently great to result in severe side-effects.

(e)   Yes. At this temperature heat stroke develops, there is circulatory collapse and the outcome is commonly fatal.

19.6

(a) No. During prolonged exposure to hot environments, secretion of thyroid hormones decreases.

(b) No. Heat can be lost from the skin by convection only at environmental temperatures below body temperature.

(c) No. The loss of heat in expired air constitutes a tiny proportion of the unavoidable heat loss in average environmental and physiological conditions.

(d) Yes.

(e) Yes. Shivering may increase the resting metabolic rate by as much as five-fold.

19.7

(a) No. If the temperature of the body is rising, there must be more heat production than heat loss.

(b) No. The subject feels cold because his core temperature is below the set point of his central regulator.

(c) Yes. He shivers as one of the heat production mechanisms.

(d) Yes.

(e) No. Hyperthermia stimulates respiration.

19.8

(a) No. Thyroxine stimulates metabolism, so thyroid deficiency leads to a depression of core temperature.

(b) Yes. The body cannot immediately rid itself of all the heat generated by the exercise.

(c) Yes. Pyrogens reset the central temperature reference to a higher value than normal.

(d) Yes. Progesterone raises the body temperature slightly; progesterone secretion during the luteal phase of the ovarian (and menstrual) cycle accounts for the rise in body temperature occurring at the time of ovulation.

(e) Yes. Adrenaline stimulates heat production.

19.9

(a) Yes.

(b) Yes.

(c) Yes. This is the origin of the fall in basal metabolic rate.

(d) Yes. Due to vasodilatation.

(e) Yes.

19.10

(a) Yes.

(b) No. The thermoregulatory centre lies in the hypothalamus.

(c)   Yes.
(d)   Yes.
(e)   Yes.

19.11
(a)   No. Shivering is due to contraction of skeletal muscle fibres.
(b)   No. The efferent nerve fibres causing shivering are somatic nerve fibres.
(c)   No. Shivering depends on impulses from the hypothalamus descending to the motoneurones in the spinal cord. After a spinal transection, shivering never reappears; shivering is not a spinal reflex.
(d)   No. In excessive sweating, the inorganic ion whose loss is the main cause of collapse is sodium.
(e)   Yes. In a hot environment, conduction and convection are ineffectual because the temperature of the air is close to that of the skin, and so the main vehicle for heat loss is the evaporation of sweat.

19.12
(a)   No. When the environmental temperature is 38°C, a person cannot lose heat by conduction because the environmental temperature exceeds the body temperature.
(b)   Yes.
(c)   No. For sweating to be a mechanism for heat loss from the body, the sweat must evaporate.
(d)   No. It is impossible for a person to survive for prolonged periods at an environmental temperature of 38°C if the air is saturated with water vapour because there is no vehicle for loss of heat from the body. The body is always producing heat at a basal rate and if this cannot be lost, the body temperature rises and death ensues.
(e)   No. For the wavelengths at which radiation occurs at 37°C, there is almost no difference between a black and a white skin. The difference in skin colour is only apparent in the visible part of the electromagnetic spectrum.

20 The life cycle: reproductive function

Female reproductive system	20.1–20.6
Male reproductive system	20.7–20.9
Fertilization and implantation	20.10–20.11
Pregnancy	20.12–20.13
Fetal physiology	20.14–20.16
Neonate and lactation	20.17–20.18

QUESTIONS

Female reproductive system

20.1 During the normal ovarian cycle:
(a) ova multiply during the first half of the cycle.
(b) a single mature Graafian follicle discharges its oocyte about the middle of the cycle.
(c) oestradiol secretion increases during the first half of the cycle.
(d) progesterone secretion inhibits follicle-stimulating hormone (FSH) secretion.
(e) a corpus luteum develops only if the ovum is fertilized.

20.2 During the normal uterine cycle:
(a) the endometrium proliferates in the first half of the cycle.
(b) the endometrium secretes gonadotrophins in the second half of the cycle.
(c) a decrease in secretion of both oestrogen and progesterone at the end of the cycle brings about the breakdown of the endometrium.
(d) the mucus secretion of the cervix becomes thicker at mid-cycle.
(e) a typical menstrual blood loss is about 200 ml.

20.3 With reference to the menstrual cycle:
(a) a surge of luteinizing hormone (LH) secretion is associated with ovulation.
(b) oestrogens tend to inhibit the production of follicle-stimulating hormone (FSH) by the anterior pituitary gland.
(c) ovulation occurs about 14 days after the end of menstrual flow.
(d) progesterone production during the menstrual cycle is largely under the control of luteinizing hormone (LH).
(e) throughout the part of the menstrual cycle that follows ovulation, there is a rise in body temperature.

20.4 Concerning reproduction:
(a) each Graffian follicle contains an oocyte that has been present, undivided, since before the woman's birth.
(b) the cells of the theca interna produce oestrogen.
(c) the zona pellucida surrounding the oocyte is a barrier to movement of antibodies.
(d) the cells of the theca externa produce progesterone.
(e) the follicle is filled with clotted blood.

20.5 Concerning the human corpus luteum:
(a) the granulosa luteal cells produce progesterone.
(b) the thecal luteal cells produce oestrogen.
(c) in an ovary with a corpus luteum, there will also be Graafian follicles.
(d) the corpus luteum arises from a Graafian follicle.
(e) the corpus haemorrhagica is a degenerating corpus luteum.

20.6 Oestrogen in the normal human female causes:
(a) development of secondary sex characteristics.
(b) development of secretory phase endometrium.
(c) thickening of the cervical secretions at the time of ovulation.
(d) decrease of sebaceous gland activity.
(e) the alveolar growth that may cause breast enlargement during the menstrual cycle.

Male reproductive system

20.7 The secretion of testosterone from the testis:
(a) starts during fetal life.
(b) causes the development of the external genitalia.
(c) stimulates androgen secretion from the adrenal cortex.
(d) is controlled by the male equivalent of luteinizing hormone.
(e) is without influence on spermatogenesis.

20.8 Concerning the testis:
(a) the interstitial cells are found among the germinal cells of the seminiferous tubules.
(b) the interstitial cells secrete testosterone.
(c) the interstitial cells secrete a fluid to nourish spermatozoa.
(d) the Sertoli cells secrete the hormone inhibin.
(e) testosterone secretion is controlled by FSH (from the anterior pituitary).

20.9 **Concerning sperm production and storage:**
(a) the germ cells are protected from changes in blood chemistry by the barrier function of Sertoli cells.
(b) Sertoli cells secrete androgen binding protein.
(c) when they have separated from Sertoli cells and are free in the tubular fluid, spermatozoa are fully mature and fertile.
(d) most of the seminal fluid comes from the seminiferous tubules.
(e) spermatozoa are stored pending ejaculation in the rete testis.

Fertilization and implantation

20.10 **Fertilization of an ovum:**
(a) usually occurs (if at all) within an hour of coitus.
(b) usually occurs in one of the fallopian tubes.
(c) results in a cell with the haploid number of chromosomes.
(d) may sometimes involve two spermatozoa, resulting in twin pregnancy.
(e) is followed by implantation in the uterus within 24 hours.

20.11 **Concerning implantation of the embryo:**
(a) by the time of implantation, the embryo has become a multicellular blastocyst.
(b) the embryo develops microvilli before implantation.
(c) implantation is normally in the fundus of the uterus.
(d) by the time of implantation trophoblast cells are secreting human chorionic gonadotrophin.
(e) progestin used alone as a birth control pill acts by rendering the endometrium unsuitable for implantation.

Pregnancy

20.12 **During the first three months of pregnancy:**
(a) chorionic gonadotrophin acts to maintain the corpus luteum.
(b) prolactin is secreted in increasing amounts by the maternal anterior pituitary gland.
(c) the smooth muscle of the uterus is relatively inexcitable because of the action of progesterone.
(d) pregnancy can be diagnosed by means of tests based on the presence in the maternal urine of pituitary gonadotrophins.
(e) there is a progressive reduction in the mother's total vascular peripheral resistance.

20.13   Concerning a mother at the 36th week of pregnancy:
(a)   plasma osmolarity is less than in the non-pregnant state.
(b)   red cell mass has increased by the same proportion as plasma volume.
(c)   cardiac output is higher than at the fourth week of pregnancy.
(d)   the corpus luteum is synthesizing significant quantities of progesterone.
(e)   arterial PCO_2 is lower than in early pregnancy.

Fetal physiology

20.14   During intrauterine life:
(a)   all the fetal blood returning from the placenta flows directly into the inferior vena cava.
(b)   haemoglobin in fetal blood is more saturated with oxygen than haemoglobin in maternal blood at the same PO_2 of 60 mmHg.
(c)   many antibodies are transferred freely between maternal and fetal circulations.
(d)   blood in the right side of the fetal heart is slightly better oxygenated than blood in the left side.
(e)   pulmonary vascular resistance is higher than after birth.

20.15   Concerning the fetus and newborn:
(a)   erythropoiesis in the fetus occurs in the spleen and the liver.
(b)   fetal blood can carry more oxygen per litre at any given PO_2 than can maternal blood.
(c)   fetal oxygen tension in the umbilical vein is similar to that in the maternal uterine artery.
(d)   surfactant production is stimulated by the release of cortisol from the fetal adrenal cortex.
(e)   changes in the circulation at birth result in an increase in the pulmonary vascular resistance.

20.16   Concerning the human fetus:
(a)   intrauterine weight gain is greatest in the middle trimester of gestation.
(b)   the testes of the male fetus usually descend before birth.
(c)   regular breathing movements are present towards the end of gestation.
(d)   a decrease in fetal heart rate during labour is a sign of hypoxia.
(e)   pulmonary surfactant production is established by the 30th week of gestation.

Neonate and lactation

20.17 The newborn infant:
(a)   is able to sweat.
(b)   is able to shiver.
(c)   has an increasing haemoglobin concentration.
(d)   has 10–15% of its body weight as fat.
(e)   after the first few days, requires about four times the calorie intake per kg of an adult.

20.18 Concerning lactation:
(a)   milk production is only fully developed three to four days after delivery.
(b)   the hypertrophy of the mammary glands early in pregnancy is caused by both progesterone and oestrogens.
(c)   suckling acts as a stimulus for the release of oxytocin.
(d)   conception can occur during lactation.
(e)   the secretion of milk only occurs if the infant is suckled.

ANSWERS

20.1
(a)   No. All multiplication (mitosis) of ova is complete at birth: meiotic division occurs just before ovulation.
(b)   Yes. Many Graafian follicles contain oocytes that develop during the first half of the cycle, reaching different stages; only one usually discharges at ovulation.
(c)   Yes. The developing follicles secrete oestradiol under the influence of follicle-stimulating hormone.
(d)   No. The progesterone that is secreted during the second half of the cycle has a negative feedback effect on luteinizing hormone (which maintains the corpus luteum and its secretions); it is oestrogens that have a negative feedback effect on FSH.
(e)   No. The Graafian follicle which has discharged its egg cell becomes a corpus luteum in the second half of the cycle; this is maintained into pregnancy if fertilization occurs.

20.2
(a)   Yes. The endometrium and its blood vessels proliferate under the influence of the increasing oestrogen secretion from the developing follicles in the ovary.
(b)   No. The second half of the cycle is the secretory phase, but it is mucus that is secreted; gonadotrophins start to be secreted by fetal tissue before the end of a cycle in which fertilization and implantation has occurred.

(c)   Yes. As the second half of the cycle progresses, the secretion of both the hormones by the corpus luteum rises, and then falls; the fall is followed by disintegration and shedding of the endometrium.

(d)   No. It becomes thinner at mid-cycle, facilitating the passage of sperm.

(e)   No. Typical menstrual blood loss is only about 50 ml.

20.3

(a)   Yes.

(b)   Yes.

(c)   No. Ovulation occurs typically 14 days after the start of menstrual flow.

(d)   Yes. LH promotes progesterone secretion by the granulosa cells of the corpus luteum, after ovulation.

(e)   Yes. Temperature rises by 0.5–1 °C at the time of ovulation and remains higher until menstruation.

20.4

(a)   Yes. All potential ova are present in the ovary from birth – unlike the male, whose germ cells continually divide and replenish the supply.

(b)   Yes.

(c)   Yes.

(d)   No. Only very small amounts of progesterone are produced by the Graafian follicle and by granulosa cells.

(e)   No. This occurs after ovulation.

20.5

(a)   Yes.

(b)   Yes.

(c)   Yes. Usually only one Graafian follicle releases its ovum.

(d)   Yes. Regeneration and luteinization follow ovulation.

(e)   No. The corpus haemorrhagica arises from the Graafian follicle after release of the ovum, and rapidly develops into the corpus luteum. Corpus albicans is the name for a degenerating follicle.

20.6

(a)   Yes.

(b)   No. Oestrogens are predominant in the postmenstrual, proliferative phase of the endometrial cycle.

(c)   No. Oestrogens are responsible for a major increase in cervical secretion around the time of ovulation, but it becomes more watery, and adapted to facilitate movement of sperm.

(d)   No. This activity is stimulated, e.g. causing acne problems at puberty.

(e)   No. This occurs in the premenstrual phase of the cycle, and is attributable to progesterone.

20.7

(a)   Yes. The development of a testis rather than an ovary is genetically determined, and the secretion of testosterone by that testis governs the further development of male characteristics.

(b)   Yes. Testosterone secretion influences both the fetal and the pubertal development.

(c)   No. Androgen secretion is controlled by adrenocorticotrophic hormone.

(d)   Yes. Luteinizing hormone controls testosterone secretion, otherwise known in the male as interstitial cell stimulating hormone.

(e)   No. Testosterone, as well as pituitary gonadotrophins, are necessary for spermatogenesis.

20.8

(a)   No. The interstitial cells lie between the tubules, as their name suggests.

(b)   Yes.

(c)   No. This is a function of the Sertoli cells, in the wall of the tubules.

(d)   Yes. Inhibin is a component of negative feedback regulation of pituitary follicle-stimulating hormone secretion.

(e)   No. Testosterone secretion is regulated by luteinizing hormone. Follicle-stimulating hormone has its major effect on Sertoli cell function, and hence on the control of spermatogenesis.

20.9

(a)   Yes.

(b)   Yes. Testosterone binds to the androgen binding sites of the Sertoli cells: a necessary step in spermatogenesis; androgen binding protein is secreted with testosterone into the tubular fluid.

(c)   No. Further development takes place during their one to two week journey through the rete testis and epididymis.

(d)   No. Testicular fluid provides only about a fifth of the volume of the semen, and of this, most comes from the rete testis. The major component is from the seminal vesicles, and somewhat less from the prostate gland.

(e)   No. Storage is at the far end (cauda) of the long coiled tube of the epididymis.

20.10

(a)   No. The transit time of the sperm to the fallopian tube is usually a few hours.

(b)   Yes.

(c)   No. Haploid is the number in each of the germ cells, resulting from meiosis; the zygote – the cell after fertilization – has the diploid number.

(d)   No. Only one sperm can fertilize an ovum. The zona pellucida instantaneously becomes impenetrable to any other. Twin pregnancy results either from two ova being released and fertilized (non-identical) or by later division from one fertilized ovum (identical).

(e)   No. The dividing zygote takes nearly a week to reach the uterine cavity.

20.11

(a)   Yes.

(b)   Yes.

(c)   Yes.

(d)   Yes.

(e)   Yes.

20.12

(a)   Yes. Secretion of gonadotrophins starts as soon as implantation has occurred and they take over from maternal hormones in maintaining the corpus luteum.

(b)   Yes. This causes enlargement and proliferation of the alveoli of mammary glands.

(c)   Yes.

(d)   No. Chorionic gonadotrophin, which is fetal, is the relevant hormone.

(e)   Yes. The cardiac output increases; the blood pressure does not increase; total peripheral resistance is therefore lower.

20.13

(a)   Yes. There is relative retention of water.

(b)   No. The red cell mass does increase but not to the same extent as the plasma volume. There is therefore a decrease in Hb and red blood cell count. The decrease in viscosity is advantageous.

(c)   Yes. The increasing uterine blood flow is associated with a progressively increasing cardiac output.

(d)   No. The corpus luteum is not functional after the third month. Progesterone is secreted by the fetoplacental unit.

(e)   Yes. Ventilation increases disproportionately to the increase in metabolic rate: there is hyperventilation, reducing PCO_2.

20.14

(a) No. Some of the blood flows through the portal vein to the liver; the rest passes via the ductus venosus to the inferior vena cava.

(b) Yes. This is another way of saying that the oxyhaemoglobin dissociation curve is further to the left for haemoglobin in fetal than in adult blood.

(c) Yes.

(d) Yes. The fetal lungs take up some oxygen from the relatively small pulmonary blood flow. The rest of the blood goes directly from right to left.

(e) Yes. The uninflated lungs present a greater vascular resistance; only a small fraction of blood returning to the right heart passes through the pulmonary circulation: most flows through the pathways of lower resistance – the foramen ovale and ductus arteriosus.

20.15

(a) Yes.

(b) Yes. Fetal blood carries more oxygen per litre for two reasons: the oxygen dissociation curve for fetal blood lies to the left of that for adult blood (greater 'affinity' for oxygen), associated with the absence from fetal haemoglobin of binding sites for 2, 3–DPG; also the fetal Hb concentration is higher than in the adult. The PO_2 is always relatively low, but these properties allow adequate amounts to be carried.

(c) No. Because the barrier for gas exchange in the placenta is thick compared to that in adult lungs, and the maternal arterial blood flow is sluggish, equilibration is far from complete; fetal blood returns from the placenta at a PO_2 of only about 30 mmHg, but at this, the Hb is 60% saturated (see b).

(d) Yes.

(e) No. There is a dramatic decrease in pulmonary vascular resistance, with expansion of the lungs at the first breath.

20.16

(a) No. Weight gain is greatest from the 28th week until full-term.

(b) Yes.

(c) Yes. The fetus 'breathes' progressively more regularly during gestation, and for most of the time in the final weeks.

(d) Yes.

(e) No. Pulmonary surfactant does not appear until the final weeks; its absence presents a problem in premature infants.

20.17

(a) No.

(b) No.

(c)   No. The haemoglobin concentration decreases; the haemolysis that occurs in the first week causes a high serum bilirubin concentration and frequently a noticeable jaundice.

(d)   Yes. Fat stores start to be laid down at about five months' gestation and reach this level by full-term.

(e)   Yes. As well as provision for growth, the high surface to volume ratio of the newborn relative to the adult is linked to the relatively high metabolic rate and hence energy intake requirement.

20.18

(a)   Yes. Only colostrum is secreted in the first days.

(b)   Yes.

(c)   Yes. This is a reflex with a neural afferent and neuro-endocrine efferent pathway.

(d)   Yes. The likelihood of conception is reduced during lactation, but it is not uncommon.

(e)   No. Secretion of milk occurs even without suckling, but soon dries up unless the milk is artificially expressed.

21 Integrative questions

Control systems	21.1–21.3
Cell structure and function	21.4–21.16
General questions	21.17–21.44

QUESTIONS

Control systems

21.1 With reference to control systems:
(a) a gland secretes substance A into the blood; when the plasma concentration of A rises, secretion is inhibited. Is this a positive feedback mechanism?
(b) a feedback system with a low gain will permit only changes in the controlled variable that are so small as to be virtually undetectable.
(c) the only sensors involved in the control of body temperature are in the skin.
(d) arterial blood pressure is regulated only by neural mechanisms.
(e) reflex adjustments to a fall in blood pressure include effects depending on noradrenaline as the transmitter at neuro-effector junctions.

21.2 In the following situations, each involving feedback, decide whether the described effect is part of a NEGATIVE feedback system:
(a) the secretion of secretin into the blood in response to acidity of the duodenal contents.
(b) the opening of sodium channels in the nerve membrane in response to depolarization of the membrane.
(c) the secretion of bile salts by the liver into the hepatic bile in response to bile salts in the plasma.
(d) the release of TSH (thyroid-stimulating hormone) in response to a low plasma concentration of thyroxine.
(e) the secretion of LH (luteinizing hormone) just before ovulation in response to a rise in circulating oestrogen levels.

21.3 **With reference to sensors for homeostatic regulatory mechanisms:**
(a) hypothalamic receptors sense alterations in extracellular osmolality.
(b) the carotid sinus receptors sense alterations in arterial PO_2.
(c) atrial wall receptors sense changes in central venous pressure.
(d) receptors in the liver account for the response that corrects alterations in blood glucose.
(e) the need for adjustment of sodium reabsorption is sensed in the kidneys.

Cell structure and function

21.4 **With reference to microscopic structure:**
(a) the blood/air barrier in lung alveoli is typically less than 1 μm thick.
(b) the trachea is lined by ciliated epithelium.
(c) there are mucus-secreting cells along the whole length of the alimentary tract.
(d) cytoplasmic bridges connect the cells of single-unit smooth muscle.
(e) neutrophil polymorphs are normally the commonest of the white cells in circulating blood.

21.5 **With reference to microscopic structure and function:**
(a) the T-tubes of skeletal muscle release Ca^{2+} into the muscle fibre.
(b) the oxyntic cells of the gastric mucosa secrete pepsinogen.
(c) the type II alveolar cells of the lung secrete surfactant.
(d) the interstitial cells of the testis have an endocrine function.
(e) a renal tubule starts as an open-ended duct in direct continuity with the interstitial fluid.

21.6 **With reference to the functional significance of microscopic structure:**
(a) the function of microvilli of small intestinal mucosal cells is entirely to provide a large surface for absorption of the products of digestion.
(b) the microvilli (brush border) of the proximal convoluted tubule in the kidney are associated with passive movement of Na^+ into the cells down a diffusion gradient.
(c) cells of the juxtaglomerular apparatus secrete renin.
(d) microvilli on the surface of thyroid follicular cells aid in the re-absorption of colloid from the store.
(e) in the stomach, intrinsic factor is secreted by cells in the mucosa of the antrum (the distal fifth).

21.7   With reference to mitochondria:
(a)   they are more numerous in cardiac than in any other kind of muscle.
(b)   they are one type of intracellular vesicle.
(c)   they are most numerous in cells whose primary source of energy is anaerobic glycolysis.
(d)   they are numerous in red blood cells.
(e)   they contain chromosomes.

21.8   Active transport across cell membranes:
(a)   is increased by hypothermia.
(b)   transfers hydrogen ions into gastric juice against a concentration gradient.
(c)   requires energy production by the cell.
(d)   aids hydrogen ion secretion by kidney tubule cells.
(e)   prevents an excess of water from entering the cell.

21.9   Concerning the skin:
(a)   collagen fibres are present in the epidermis.
(b)   free nerve endings are present in the epidermis.
(c)   capillaries are present in the epidermis.
(d)   Meissner's corpuscles are sited in dermal papillae.
(e)   sweat glands are supplied by myelinated nerve fibres.

21.10   Concerning structure and function:
(a)   valves are present in the larger lymphatic vessels.
(b)   all erythrocytes entering the kidney pass via glomerular capillaries.
(c)   all erythrocytes entering the kidney pass via the vasa recta.
(d)   vesicles in the surface cells of transitional epithelium are thought to provide reserves of cell membrane.
(e)   in the male, the urethra within the penis is lined with transitional epithelium.

21.11   Are the following all different types of direct cytosolic communication between cells through ultramicroscopic channels?
(a)   nexuses in cardiac muscle.
(b)   gap junctions between secretory cells.
(c)   neuromuscular junctions.
(d)   electrical synapses in the central nervous system.
(e)   nerve terminals subserving presynaptic inhibition.

21.12 **Do the cells listed below left secrete a substance that binds to receptors in the membrane of other cells (on the right) and thereby modify their function?**

(a)	aldosterone-secreting cells in the adrenal cortex	distal convoluted tubule cells in the nephron.
(b)	sympathetic preganglionic neurones	secretory cells of the adrenal medulla.
(c)	type II cells in the lung alveoli	alveolar epithelial lining cells.
(d)	G cells in the gastric antrum	parietal cells in the gastric mucosa.
(e)	neurones in the hypothalamus	secretory cells in the anterior pituitary.

21.13 **Epithelial cells in many sites perform an important part of their function by actively extruding sodium ions across only the baso-lateral parts of the cell membranes. Does this occur in the lining of:**

(a) the colon
(b) sweat gland ducts
(c) the urinary bladder
(d) the gall bladder
(e) the proximal convoluted tubules of the kidney

21.14 **With respect to the ways in which substances enter and leave cells:**

(a) potassium ions move in and out through water-filled 'pores'.
(b) glucose enters by dissolving in the cell membrane.
(c) amino acids enter by a carrier-mediated transport mechanism.
(d) all healthy cells have sodium pumps that extrude sodium ions against a concentration gradient.
(e) only water-soluble substances can cross cell walls.

21.15 **Concerning the contents of cells:**

(a) the cytosol is the term for the intracellular fluid.
(b) microtubules provide routes for internal transport.
(c) microfilaments can change a cell's shape.
(d) messenger RNA (mRNA) is made in the endoplasmic reticu-lum.
(e) lysosomes contain enzymes in a package of internal membrane.

21.16 The cell membrane:
(a)   has hydrophilic heads of lipid molecules pointing only to the outer side.
(b)   allows movement of water across it over the whole of its surface.
(c)   allows movement of oxygen and carbon dioxide across it over the whole of its surface.
(d)   has protein molecules embedded in it.
(e)   has glycogen granules embedded in it.

General questions

21.17 Are these associations appropriate between receptor and stimulus?
(a)   muscle spindles   tapping the patellar tendon.
(b)   receptor cells in the   linear acceleration of the
       utricle   head.
(c)   receptor cells in the   movement of the basilar
       auditory system   membrane of the cochlea.
(d)   rod photoreceptor   red light.
(e)   Pacinian corpuscle   heat receptor.

21.18 Are these associations appropriate between receptor and stimulus?
(a)   receptor cells in the   rotation of the head.
       semicircular canals
(b)   receptor cells in the cochlear   sound reception.
       basilar membrane
(c)   cone photoreceptors   sensitive to colour of light.
(d)   carotid sinus receptors   fall in arterial oxygen tension.
(e)   Golgi tendon organs in   contraction of quadriceps
       patellar tendon   muscle.

21.19 With reference to variations in plasma constituents:
(a)   plasma sodium concentration rises when aldosterone secretion is deficient.
(b)   the concentration of calcium ions in the plasma is decreased by vigorous hyperventilation.
(c)   arterial carbon dioxide tension is normal in compensated respiratory alkalosis.
(d)   arterial oxygen tension is below normal in anaemia.
(e)   plasma pH is low during exhausting muscular work.

21.20 With reference to the mechanisms of regulation of concentrations in the plasma of several substances:

(a) a fall in blood glucose is corrected mainly by replacement from muscle glycogen.

(b) a rise in blood urea is corrected by a rise in the filtered load of urea in the glomeruli.

(c) a rise in blood glucose is partly corrected by lowering the renal transport maximum (Tm) for reabsorption.

(d) a rise in plasma Ca^{2+} leads to greater deposition of calcium salts in bone.

(e) plasma albumin is replenished by the liver.

21.21 In each case, can the item or method on the left be used to estimate the variable on the right?

(a) haemocytometer — haemoglobin concentration.

(b) blood smear stained with Leishman's stain — differential white cell count.

(c) blood diluted with Hayem's fluid — reticulocyte count.

(d) intravenous injection of tritated water — volume of the extra-cellular space.

(e) intravenous injection of radioactively labelled albumin — plasma volume.

21.22 There is a continuous net movement of the following into active muscle cells of:

(a) oxygen.

(b) carbon dioxide.

(c) glucose.

(d) water.

(e) lactate.

21.23 Concerning the circulation:

(a) autoregulation of blood flow during elevation of renal arterial blood pressure involves vasodilatation of renal afferent arterioles.

(b) after drinking 1 litre of an isotonic solution of sodium chloride, the osmolarity of the blood falls.

(c) after an acute haemorrhage, the right atrial pressure is increased.

(d) after an acute haemorrhage, there is an increase in plasma protein concentration.

(e) after prolonged dietary sodium deprivation, plasma aldosterone levels are increased.

21.24 **Below is a set of values representing measurements made on a male subject at rest breathing air. You must select the descriptions that fit his condition:**

Weight	**70 kg**
Arterial blood pressure	**100/60 mmHg**
Blood volume	**5.5 litres**
Arterial blood pH	**7.30**
Arterial PCO$_2$	**60 mmHg**
Right atrial pressure	**20 mmHg**

In this person:
(a) there must be a degree of arterial hypoxaemia.
(b) bicarbonate reabsorption in the kidneys is likely to be proceeding at a lower rate than normal.
This picture is consistent with:
(c) hypovolaemic shock.
(d) failure of the heart as a pump.
(e) heavy exercise in a healthy subject.

21.25 **With further reference to the subject of the previous question, the picture is consistent with:**
(a) hypoventilation.
(b) exposure of a healthy subject to low ambient pressure.
(c) persistent vomiting of gastric contents.
(d) diabetes mellitus.
(e) pulmonary hypertension.

21.26 **Are the values given appropriate for a healthy 70 kg man?**
(a) the pulmonary blood flow is approximately 500 ml per min at rest.
(b) the minimal daily water intake to maintain fluid balance in temperate conditions is approximately 250 ml.
(c) a suitable daily energy intake for moderate physical activity would be 1500 kcal.
(d) the glomerular filtration rate (both kidneys) is approximately 1200 ml per min.
(e) plasma osmolarity is about 300 mosmol per litre.

21.27 In relation to oxygen consumption and its estimation in a normal adult man:

(a) during muscular exercise, the energy expenditure can be estimated by measuring only the oxygen percentage in expired gas.

(b) if the subject is at rest and hyperventilates, the percentage of O_2 in expired air will decrease.

(c) the oxygen consumption can be measured from the rate of emptying of a spirometer bell, when the subject breathes in and out of it without a CO_2 absorber in the circuit.

(d) the average resting oxygen consumption is about 0.25 litres per minute.

(e) with increasing work rates, the heart rate increases in direct proportion to the work rate.

21.28 The force favouring the movement of fluid out of the capillary lumen is:

(a) greater in pulmonary than in bronchial vessels.

(b) greater in glomerular capillaries than in those of resting skeletal muscle.

(c) decreased by an increase in the colloid osmotic pressure of the plasma.

(d) decreased by an increase in the colloid osmotic pressure of the interstitial fluid.

(e) decreased by an increase in the hydrostatic pressure of the extra-cellular fluid.

21.29 Concerning the body:

(a) cells are continually making water.

(b) infusion of 0.9% sodium chloride solution decreases the colloid osmotic pressure of the plasma.

(c) the renal blood flow (both kidneys) is about one-20th of the cardiac output.

(d) about one-tenth of the renal blood flow is filtered in the renal glomeruli.

(e) when a person drinks an alcoholic beverage, alcohol is absorbed through the wall of the stomach.

21.30 Is it possible for a person to survive indefinitely if the following are reduced to half their normal value?

(a) arterial PO_2.

(b) arterial PCO_2.

(c) acid in gastric juice.

(d) body temperature (from 37°C to 18°C).

(e) concentration of water in the extracellular fluid.

21.31 With reference to body fluid and electrolytes:
(a)   the body's total potassium is greater than the total sodium.
(b)   insulin takes part in regulation of plasma potassium ion concentration.
(c)   the resting membrane potential of excitable tissue is close to the potassium equilibrium potential.
(d)   an average adult body contains about 40 kg of water.
(e)   total body potassium is closely linked to the control of extracellular fluid volume.

21.32 Are these associations appropriate?
(a)   sympathetic activity in the male   penile erection.
(b)   parasympathetic activity in the male   ejaculation of semen.
(c)   parasympathetic activity   lachrymation.
(d)   myogenic contraction of arteriolar smooth muscle in response to stretching   autoregulation of blood supply.
(e)   excessive activity of the parasympathetic nervous system   cold clammy skin.

21.33 Concerning the nervous system and nervous mechanisms:
(a)   all efferent nerve fibres leaving the spinal chord are cholinergic.
(b)   the postjunctional receptors for acetylcholine at the parasympathetic ganglionic relay have the same properties as those at the parasympathetic neuro-effector junction.
(c)   the neurotransmitter chemical at the junction between a primary afferent nerve fibre and a motoneurone is glutamate.
(d)   the neurotransmitter chemical in presynaptic inhibition in the cord is GABA (gamma-aminobutyric acid).
(e)   the neurotransmitter chemical in postsynaptic inhibition in the cord is glycine.

21.34 When skeletal muscles become vigorously active:
(a)   there is a continuous net movement of heat into the muscle cells.
(b)   the oxyhaemoglobin dissociation curve of blood traversing the muscle is shifted to the left.
(c)   there is a fall in the plasma concentration of potassium ions.
(d)   the oxygen content of arterial blood to the muscle is greater than when the muscle is at rest.
(e)   the oxygen content of venous blood from the muscle is greater than when the muscle is at rest.

21.35 The following are examples of active transport:
(a)   chloride shift between red blood cells and the plasma.
(b)   sodium reabsorption in the distal tubules of the kidney.
(c)   movement of oxygen from pulmonary alveoli into the blood.
(d)   uptake of calcium by the sarcoplasmic reticulum of muscle.
(e)   oxygen movement within a muscle fibre.

21.36 Three patches of a red colour, A, B, and C, have the same spectral components. Patches A and B are indistinguishable to one observer; to this same observer, B also appears to be identical with patch C.
(a)   it follows that A and C will appear to this same observer to be identical.
(b)   it follows that A and B will appear to be identical to a different observer.
(c)   a subject with red–green colour-blindness is likely to find it harder to distinguish such patches than a subject with normal colour vision.
(d)   in a dim light, distinguishing differences in red patches is harder than distinguishing differences in green patches.
(e)   any estimation that depends on visual matching of intensity involves matching both when the intensity is just less than and when it is just greater than the standard.

21.37 Concerning lactate:
(a)   it is the end-product of aerobic respiration.
(b)   it is released in strenuously contracting skeletal muscle.
(c)   its release into the extracellular tissue is usually accompanied by an increase in extracellular pH.
(d)   most of the lactate that reaches the blood is excreted in the urine.
(e)   it can be taken up from the blood by the liver.

21.38 By comparison with someone whose respiratory quotient (RQ) is 1, for a subject with RQ 0.7:
(a)   his ratio of expiratory volume to minute volume is greater.
(b)   he is metabolizing a greater proportion of carbohydrates.
(c)   he gets more energy for every gram of foodstuff that he metabolizes.
(d)   assuming that both subjects have the same basal metabolic rate and the same cardiac output, for the subject with an RQ of 0.7, the change in hydrogen ion concentration of the blood, as it passes through the lungs, is less.
(e)   if both subjects have the same alveolar PCO_2, the subject with RQ 0.7 has a lower alveolar PO_2.

21.39 **With reference to movement of substances in the body:**
(a)   all living cells take up amino acids.
(b)   most of the water filtered in the renal glomeruli is excreted in the urine.
(c)   in the small intestine, iron is absorbed more easily in the Fe^{2+} (ferrous) than the Fe^{3+} (ferric) form.
(d)   antibodies against AB red cell antigens normally cross the placenta.
(e)   oxygen traverses lipid membranes.

21.40 **Are the following statements true?**
(a)   plasma $[K^+]$ can rise by 25% during muscular work.
(b) Ca^{2+} concentration in the plasma is decreased by vigorous hyperventilation.
(c)   arterial partial pressure of carbon dioxide is normal in compensated respiratory acidosis.
(d)   arterial partial pressure of oxygen can be normal in severe anaemia.
(e)   plasma pH is high during exhausting muscular work.

21.41 **By comparison with normal, there is likely to be an elevation of:**
(a)   plasma potassium concentration in metabolic alkalosis.
(b)   plasma calcium concentration when the parathyroid glands have been removed.
(c)   arterial tension of CO_2 at high altitude, where atmospheric pressure is halved.
(d)   arterial tension of O_2 during a dive (breathing air) to 30 feet.
(e)   plasma bicarbonate concentration in compensated respiratory acidosis.

21.42 **With reference to microscopic structure and function:**
(a)   the presence of smooth endoplasmic reticulum is characteristic of cells synthesizing polypeptide hormones.
(b)   the presence of rough endoplasmic reticulum is characteristic of cells synthesizing steroid hormones.
(c)   the terminals of the nerves supplying the smooth muscle of muscular arteries lie next to the endothelium.
(d)   elastic fibres in the lung are confined to the pleura.
(e)   the lamellated bodies in type II alveolar cells are phagocytosed foreign particles.

21.43 **Concerning the endothelial cells lining blood vessels:**
(a)   they can secrete vasodilator substances.
(b)   they can secrete vasoconstrictor substances.
(c)   they synthesize enzymes that catalyse the conversion of substances in the bloodstream.
(d)   endothelial cells bordering on injury site release prostacyclin.
(e)   on their luminal surface, endothelial cells have molecules that inhibit blood clotting.

21.44 **Concerning structure:**
(a)   there is a higher proportion of elastic tissue in the wall of an arteriole than in the wall of the aorta.
(b)   for blood vessels of similar diameter, the muscle layer is thicker in an artery than in a vein.
(c)   the diameter of a capillary is usually about twice the diameter of a red blood cell.
(d)   capillaries actively constrict in response to sympathetic stimulation.
(e)   fenestrated capillaries are characteristic of brain tissue.

ANSWERS

21.1
(a)   No. The situation described is a negative feedback mechanism.
(b)   No. This statement is nonsense. A feedback system permitting only small changes in the controlled variable to be compensated needs higher gain than one compensating for larger changes.
(c)   No. There are sensors involved in the control of body temperature in the hypothalamus as well as in the skin.
(d)   No. Arterial blood pressure is regulated by neural and humoral mechanisms; for instance, aldosterone, by retaining sodium and fluid, is a mechanism for restoring blood pressure depressed due to hypovolaemia.
(e)   Yes. An example of reflex adjustments to a fall in blood pressure is arteriolar constriction, mediated by sympathetic nerves influencing vascular smooth muscle using adrenaline as neurotransmitter.

21.2
(a)   Yes. Secretin acts to reduce duodenal acidity by stimulation of pancreatic (alkaline) secretion.
(b)   No. Opening of sodium channels assists the progress of depolarization. This is positive feedback.

(c)   No. Secretion of bile salts by the liver into the bile does not reduce the plasma concentration, so this is not negative feedback.

(d)   Yes. TSH, by stimulating release of thyroid hormone, tends to correct the low plasma level.

(e)   No. Just before ovulation, the secretion of LH is stimulated by circulating oestrogen; this is positive feedback.

21.3

(a)   Yes. There are osmoreceptors in the hypothalamus.

(b)   No. These are stretch receptors in the arterial wall, sensing changes in arterial blood pressure.

(c)   Yes. Reflex responses are both neural and endocrine, altering venous capacity and blood volume.

(d)   Yes. The main control is the negative feedback effect of glucose concentration on insulin secretion.

(e)   Yes. Renin-secreting cells of the juxtaglomerular apparatus are activated as a result of decreased blood volume or increased sodium load, probably via sensors in the macula densa or in the walls of the glomerular arterioles.

21.4

(a)   Yes.

(b)   Yes. This is associated with protective function: foreign particles and mucus are continually carried upwards.

(c)   Yes. There is no exception to this, from mouth to anus.

(d)   Yes. These allow transmission of excitation through a sheet of muscle fibres.

(e)   Yes. They normally constitute 60–70% of all white cells.

21.5

(a)   No. Calcium is released from the endoplasmic reticulum.

(b)   No. Oxyntic cells secrete acid.

(c)   Yes.

(d)   Yes. They secrete testosterone.

(e)   No. A renal tubule starts with a blind end called the 'Bowman's capsule'.

21.6

(a)   No. They harbour enzymes and these take part in the final processes of digestion itself.

(b)   Yes. Active transport of Na^+ out of the cell occurs on other surfaces, thus maintaining low intracellular Na^+ and causing passive movement into the cell from the tubular fluid.

(c)   Yes.
(d)   Yes. They are concerned both with synthesis and with reabsorption of colloid.
(e)   No. The antrum is the part of the stomach where there are not any parietal (oxyntic) cells: no acid, and no intrinsic factor originates here.

21.7
(a)   Yes.
(b)   No. They are lamellar structures, not vesicles.
(c)   No. They are associated essentially with aerobic metabolism.
(d)   No. There are none in red blood cells, which metabolize anaerobically.
(e)   No. Chromosomes are nuclear material.

21.8
(a)   No. Hypothermia slows down energy-dependent processes.
(b)   Yes.
(c)   Yes.
(d)   Yes.
(e)   Yes. When cells stop actively adjusting the distribution of ions across the membrane, they swell.

21.9
(a)   Yes.
(b)   Yes. Nociceptive endings are free nerve endings and they penetrate into the epidermis.
(c)   No. The capillaries permeate the dermis but not the epidermis.
(d)   Yes.
(e)   No. Sweat glands are supplied by postganglionic sympathetic nerve fibres, which are unmyelinated.

21.10
(a)   Yes. The valves present in the larger lymphatic vessels ensure flow of lymph back to the thoracic duct.
(b)   Yes.
(c)   No. Erythrocytes in blood supplying the juxtamedullary glomeruli pass via the vasa recta but those in blood supplying the glomeruli just beneath the capsule do not.
(d)   Yes.
(e)   Yes.

21.11

(a)   Yes. These allow direct transmission of the cardiac action potential from cell to cell.

(b)   Yes. Gap junctions allow spread of excitation among adjacent secretory cells.

(c)   No. Neuromuscular junctions involve secretion of a transmitter substance which crosses an extracellular cleft from nerve terminal to muscle fibre receptor.

(d)   Yes. Electrical synapses in the central nervous system provide direct electrical linkage, via cytosol, between neurones.

(e)   No. Nerve terminals subserving presynaptic inhibition form chemical synapses on presynaptic terminals; there is no continuity of cytoplasm between these nerve terminals and the presynaptic terminals they innervate.

21.12

(a)   No. The target is correct, but the mechanism of action is not. Steroid hormones do not bind to membrane receptors, but enter cells and act within them.

(b)   Yes. Acetylcholine released at the nerve terminals binds to receptors in the membrane of the catecholamine secreting cells.

(c)   No. Type II cells secrete surfactant, which has a physicochemical action by spreading over the alveolar lining.

(d)   Yes. G cells secrete gastrin, a peptide hormone which targets parietal cells. Peptide hormones all act by binding to membrane receptors.

(e)   Yes. There are neurones in the hypothalamus which synthesize releasing factors (hormones) for the several anterior pituitary secretions. These are extruded at the nerve terminals into blood capillaries in the hypothalamus, and thence reach the anterior pituitary directly via the portal vessels. Being peptide hormones, they act on the secretory cells by binding to membrane receptors.

21.13

(a)   Yes. Sodium continues to be absorbed in the colon, as in the small intestine. Absorption entails active extrusion of sodium ions across surfaces other than the luminal one, thus facilitating its movement into the cell from the lumen.

(b)   Yes. The fluid entering the sweat gland ducts has the same ionic concentrations as plasma. Reabsorption of sodium occurs along the length of the duct.

(c)   No. The transitional epithelium of the bladder wall does not have an absorptive function.

(d)   Yes. The gall bladder epithelium reabsorbs sodium ions as an essential part of the concentrating function.

(e)   Yes. The proximal convoluted tubule cells reabsorb sodium ions; this function is crucial to the reabsorption also of water and other solutes.

21.14

(a)   Yes.
(b)   No. Glucose is not lipid-soluble.
(c)   Yes.
(d)   Yes.
(e)   No. Lipid-soluble substances enter by dissolving in the membrane.

21.15

(a)   Yes.
(b)   Yes.
(c)   Yes.
(d)   No. mRNA is made in the nucleus, then moves out.
(e)   Yes.

21.16

(a)   No. There are two rows of molecules, with heads on the inner and outer sides of the membrane.
(b)   No. The lipid itself is waterproof; water enters and leaves through submicroscopic pores in the membrane.
(c)   Yes. The respiratory gases are lipid-soluble.
(d)   Yes. There may be thousands in the membrane of a single cell. They include enzyme molecules, which act as 'pumps', and receptor molecules, which provide binding sites for hormones or transmitters.
(e)   No. Glycogen stores are intracellular.

21.17

(a)   Yes. Tapping the patellar tendon stretches the quadriceps muscle and therefore the spindles within it.
(b)   Yes.
(c)   Yes.
(d)   No. Rods are sensitive to the green part of the spectrum. If one wears red spectacles in bright light, rods are not bleached; this is a means of dark-adapting the eyes in a bright environment.
(e)   No. Pacinian corpuscles are sensitive to pressure.

21.18

(a)   Yes.
(b)   Yes.

(c)   Yes.

(d)   No. The carotid sinus receptors are sensitive to stretch; the carotid body receptors are the ones sensitive to a fall in arterial oxygen tension.

(e)   Yes. The contracting quadriceps exerts tension on the patellar tendon and stimulates its Golgi tendon organs.

21.19

(a)   No. Aldosterone promotes sodium reabsorption.

(b)   Yes. The respiratory alkalaemia due to lowered blood PCO_2 causes a reduction in the concentration of ionized calcium.

(c)   No. By definition, respiratory alkalosis implies a low $PaCO_2$, even though pH may have been corrected back to normal.

(d)   No. Not unless the lungs are abnormal. The oxygen content is low.

(e)   Yes. Lactic acidosis causes a fall in pH.

21.20

(a)   No. Liver glycogen is the source.

(b)   Yes. Plasma urea concentration depends on metabolic production; concentration in glomerular filtrate follows plasma concentration; increased filtered load leads to increased excretion.

(c)   No. The renal transport maximum for reabsorption of glucose does not change with a change in concentration of glucose in the blood. The spill-over of glucose into the urine when the glucose Tm is exceeded does contribute to limiting the rise in blood glucose concentration.

(d)   Yes. A rise in plasma $[Ca^{2+}]$ inhibits parathormone release; parathormone causes reabsorption of calcium salts in bone and inhibits their deposition in bone. So a rise in plasma $[Ca^{2+}]$ has an overall effect of increasing the deposition of calcium salts in bone.

(e)   Yes. The liver is the source of plasma albumin.

21.21

(a)   No. The haemocytometer is the engraved slide used for estimating the red or white cell count.

(b)   Yes.

(c)   No. In blood diluted with Hayem's fluid, it is not possible to discriminate between reticulocytes and mature red cells.

(d)   No. Tritiated water mixes with the whole of the body water, not just water in the extracellular space.

(e)   Yes.

21.22

(a)   Yes.

(b)   No. The net movement of carbon dioxide produced by metabolic reactions is out of the cells.

(c)   Yes.

(d)   No. Like CO_2, water is an end product of metabolism. So there is a net outward movement of water.

(e)   No. Lactate is a metabolite released from active muscle.

21.23

(a)   No. Pressure autoregulation tends to keep blood flow constant, so when the renal arterial blood pressure rises, the afferent arterioles constrict.

(b)   No. Drinking isotonic sodium chloride solution is without effect on the osmolarity of the blood.

(c)   No. After an acute haemorrhage, there is hypovolaemia, with a decrease in the right atrial pressure.

(d)   No. After an acute haemorrhage, there is a net reabsorption of interstitial fluid into the plasma, with a consequent decrease in plasma protein concentration.

(e)   Yes. A component of the response to sodium deprivation is an increase in aldosterone secretion.

21.24

(a)   Yes. If the arterial PCO_2 is high, there must be a degree of arterial hypoxaemia.

(b)   No. There is an acidosis, so bicarbonate reabsorption in the kidneys is likely to be proceeding at a higher rate than normal.

(c)   No. In hypovolaemic shock the blood volume would be low and the right atrial pressure would not be high.

(d)   Yes. The low arterial blood pressure and the high right atrial pressure are consistent with failure of the heart as a pump.

(e)   No. In the healthy subject, exercise does not result in a high arterial PCO_2.

21.25

(a)   Yes. The definition of hypoventilation is an arterial PCO_2 above normal.

(b)   No. With exposure of a healthy subject exposed to low ambient pressure, the arterial PCO_2 is low, not high.

(c)   No. With persistent vomiting of gastric contents, there is alkalaemia, not acidaemia as in this subject.

(d)   No. In diabetes mellitus, the acidaemia results in hyperventilation with a low, not a high, arterial PCO_2.

(e)   Yes. Raised pulmonary arterial pressure, associated with obstructive lung disease, can result in right heart failure and would be consistent with the hypoventilation.

21.26

(a)   No. The pulmonary blood flow is equal to the cardiac output, typically 5 litres per min at rest.

(b)   No. The minimal daily water intake to maintain fluid balance in temperate conditions is approximately 450 ml.

(c)   Yes. A suitable daily calorie intake for moderate physical activity would be 1500 kcal.

(d)   No. The glomerular filtration rate (both kidneys) is approximately 120 ml per min.

(e)   Yes.

21.27

(a)   No. To estimate the energy expenditure, one must measure both the oxygen percentage in expired gas and the expiratory minute volume.

(b)   No. If the subject is at rest and hyperventilates, the expiratory minute volume increases with negligible increase in oxygen usage by the body. So the difference between the percentage of O_2 in expired gas compared with atmospheric air decreases, i.e. the percentage of O_2 in expired air will increase.

(c)   No. In order to measure the oxygen consumption from the rate of emptying of a spirometer bell, when the subject breathes in and out of it, a CO_2 absorber is needed in the circuit, otherwise CO_2 accumulates as oxygen is removed.

(d)   Yes.

(e)   No. Initially with increasing work rates the heart rate increases as the level of oxygen consumption increases, but at very high work rates the rise in heart rate reaches a plateau. If the heart rate were to increase above this plateau there would be insufficient time for ventricular filling during diastole.

21.28

(a)   No. The reverse is the case because the hydrostatic pressure is greater in the bronchial capillaries (systemic capillaries) than in the pulmonary capillaries.

(b)   Yes. The mean capillary pressures are around 50 mmHg and 25 mmHg respectively.

(c)   Yes. An increase in the colloid osmotic pressure of plasma tends to retain water in the blood.

(d)   No. An increase in the colloid osmotic pressure of the interstitial fluid tends to retain water in the interstitial fluid.

(e)   Yes.

21.29

(a)   Yes. Normal metabolic processes yield water, so cells are continually making water.

(b)   Yes. Infusion of 0.9% sodium chloride solution dilutes the plasma proteins and so decreases the colloid osmotic pressure of the plasma.

(c)   No. The renal blood flow is about one-fifth of the cardiac output.

(d)   Yes. About one-fifth of the renal plasma flow is filtered in the renal glomeruli; this is approximately one-tenth of the renal blood flow.

(e)   Yes. Alcohol is the only commonly-ingested chemical that is absorbed in significant amounts through the wall of the stomach.

21.30

(a)   Yes. Halving of the arterial PO_2 to 50 mmHg reduces the oxygen saturation of the blood to around 82% and this is sufficient to provide normal tissue requirements. Oxygen delivery is maintained partly by an increase in cardiac output.

(b)   Yes. Hyperventilation may halve the arterial PCO_2 to 20 mmHg; there will be various symptoms but the low PCO_2 can be survived.

(c)   Yes. People can survive with achlorhydria.

(d)   No. If the body temperature is reduced to half of 37°C, the subject becomes comatose and dies.

(e)   No. Reduction of the concentration of water in the extracellular fluid will be fatal long before it is as low as half normal.

21.31

(a)   No. Intracellular $[K^+]$ is similar to extracellular $[Na^+]$, and there is twice as much intracellular fluid as extracellular; this might suggest a preponderance of potassium in the body. However, there is a large quantity of sodium in bone so that its whole body total exceeds that of potassium.

(b)   Yes. The 'extrarenal' regulation of $[K^+]$ includes the action of insulin, which assists transfer from extracellular to intracellular fluid.

(c)   Yes.

(d)   Yes.

(e)   No. Total body sodium is closely linked to the extracellular fluid volume control because it is the main extracellular cation; NaCl accounts for most of the extracellular osmolarity.

21.32

(a) No. Penile erection is primarily a function of the parasympathetic system, with parasympathetic discharge causing dilatation of the penile arterioles.

(b) No. Ejaculation of semen, the movement of semen from seminal vesicles to the urethra and thence to the exterior is due to contraction of smooth muscle, under the influence of sympathetic innervation.

(c) Yes. The parasympathetic nervous system provides the motor innervation of the lachrymal glands.

(d) Yes.

(e) No. Over-activity of the sympathetic, not the parasympathetic, nervous system gives cold clammy skin. The coldness is due to intense cutaneous vasoconstriction and the clamminess is due to sweating induced by the impulses in the sympathetic sudomotor supply to the skin.

21.33

(a) Yes. The efferent nerve fibres leaving the spinal chord are somatic, sympathetic preganglionic fibres and parasympathetic preganglionic fibres; these are all cholinergic.

(b) No. The postjunctional receptors for acetylcholine at the para-sympathetic ganglionic relay are nicotinic whereas those at the parasympathetic neuro-effector junction are muscarinic.

(c) Yes.

(d) Yes.

(e) Yes.

21.34

(a) No. There is a continuous net movement of heat out of the muscle cells.

(b) No. Increase in temperature together with increase in content of CO_2 cause the oxyhaemoglobin of blood traversing the muscle to shift to the right; this assists off-loading of oxygen.

(c) No. In muscular exercise there is a rise in the plasma concentration of potassium ions.

(d) No. In the subject at rest, the arterial blood is normally virtually saturated with oxygen, so there is no possibility of increase as a mechanism of providing more oxygen when muscle becomes active.

(e) No. The extraction of oxygen from the blood increases in exercise, so the oxygen content of venous blood from the muscles is less than when the muscle is at rest.

21.35

(a) No. The chloride shift between red blood cells and the plasma is a passive exchange mechanism, chloride exchanging with bicarbonate.

(b)   Yes. In the distal tubules of the kidney, sodium is reabsorbed against a concentration gradient; this is an active process.

(c)   No. All movement of oxygen, including that from pulmonary alveoli into the blood, is passive in the higher mammals including humans.

(d)   Yes.

(e)   No. Oxygen movement within a muscle fibre is by passive diffusion.

21.36

(a)   No. A may, for instance, be indistinguishably paler than B, and B indistinguishably paler than C. The difference between A and C may, however, be distinguishable.

(b)   No. Since a different observer may have more sensitive vision, A and B may be distinguishable to him or her.

(c)   No. Since A, B and C have the same spectral components, a subject with red-green colour-blindness is at no disadvantage. Indeed colour-blind subjects are frequently more sensitive to small differences in intensity than are people with normal colour vision.

(d)   Yes. In a dim light, vision depends on rods and they are less sensitive to red light than to green light. So distinguishing differences in red patches is harder than distinguishing differences in green patches.

(e)   Yes. The mean of the two measurements is the best estimate of the match.

21.37

(a)   No. Lactate is the endproduct of anaerobic respiration.

(b)   Yes. Strenuously contracting skeletal muscle metabolizes anaerobically, with the production of lactate.

(c)   No. Lactate is the conjugate base of a relatively strong acid. So its release into the extracellular tissue is usually accompanied by a decrease, not an increase, in extracellular pH.

(d)   No. Most of the lactate that reaches the blood is taken up by the liver and the major part of this is converted back to glucose.

(e)   Yes. Lactate is taken up from the blood by the liver.

21.38

(a)   No. He is expiring less carbon dioxide than he is absorbing, so his ratio of expiratory to inspiratory minute volume is less.

(b)   No. He must be metabolizing almost entirely fat, since fat has an RQ of 0.7, protein of 0.85 and carbohydrate of 1.0.

(c)   Yes. Gram for gram, fat yields more than twice as much energy as carbohydrate. So this subject gets more energy for every gram of foodstuff that he metabolizes.

(d)   Yes. Since less carbon dioxide is being excreted for the same oxygen usage, the change in hydrogen ion concentration of his blood, as it passes through the lungs, is less.

(e)   Yes. The fall in PO_2 from atmosphere to alveolar gas multiplied by the RQ is equal to the alveolar PCO_2. Thus if the RQ is 1.0, the fall from atmosphere to alveolar gas is equal to the alveolar PCO_2; if the RQ is 0.7, this fall is 1/0.7 times as great. So if both subjects have the same alveolar PCO_2, the subject with RQ 0.7 has a lower alveolar PO_2.

21.39

(a)   Yes.

(b)   No. Almost all the water filtered in the renal glomeruli is reabsorbed in the tubules; typically only 1% but 10% at most, is excreted in the urine.

(c)   Yes. One of the functions of stomach acid is to keep iron in the Fe^{2+} form because, in the small intestine, iron is absorbed more easily in the Fe^{2+} (ferrous) than the Fe^{3+} (ferric) form.

(d)   No. Antibodies against AB red cell antigens do not normally cross the placenta; there are very rare instances where this does occur and the fetus dies.

(e)   Yes. Oxygen is lipid-soluble and traverses lipid membranes.

21.40

(a)   Yes.

(b)   Yes. Due to the lowering of the hydrogen ion concentration, the Ca^{2+} concentration in the plasma is decreased by vigorous hyperventilation. This may lead to hypocalcaemic tetany.

(c)   No. In compensated respiratory acidosis, there is a persistently high PCO_2, compensation is for the increased hydrogen ion concentration and involves bicarbonate retention, restoring pH towards normal.

(d)   Yes. It is the oxygen carrying capacity of the blood, not the arterial partial pressure of oxygen, that is depressed in anaemia.

(e)   No. The plasma pH is low during exhausting muscular work, due to anaerobic metabolism and the release of lactic acid.

21.41

(a)   No. In the extracellular fluid, the concentration of potassium and hydrogen ions tend to move together in the same direction.

(b)   No. Parathormone elevates plasma calcium concentration.

(c)   No. The low PO_2 in inspired air results in hyperventilation.

(d)   Yes. The gas in the lungs is compressed about two-fold, with a concomitant increase in alveolar PO_2.

(e)   Yes. The plasma bicarbonate concentration is increased both by the increase in PCO_2 and by renal retention of bicarbonate.

21.42

(a)   No. The presence of smooth endoplasmic reticulum is characteristic of cells synthesizing steroid, not polypeptide hormones.

(b)   No. The presence of rough endoplasmic reticulum is characteristic of cells synthesizing polypeptide, not steroid hormones.

(c)   No. The terminals of the nerves supplying the smooth muscle of muscular arteries lie in the smooth muscle coat, not next to the endothelium.

(d)   No. Elastic fibres in the lung are found throughout the lung tissue; they are not confined to the pleura.

(e)   No. The lamellated bodies in type II alveolar cells are stores of surfactant, ready to be liberated into the fluid lining the alveoli; they are not phagocytosed foreign particles.

21.43

(a)   Yes. Nitric oxide (endothelium-derived relaxing factor) and prostacyclin.

(b)   Yes. Endothelin and thromboxane.

(c)   Yes. Among others, converting enzymes catalyse the formation of angiotensin II, and the breakdown of bradykinin.

(d)   Yes. Endothelial cells bordering an injury site release prostacyclin, a prostaglandin that impedes platelet aggregation.

(e)   Yes. Endothelial cells have heparin-like molecules on the luminal surface of the membrane.

21.44

(a)   No. The wall of the aorta contains much elastic tissue, connected with its function of passive stretching during ventricular systole, partially storing the stroke volume, and its passive recoil during diastole which provides a continuous flow of blood to the tissues throughout the cardiac cycle. The walls of arterioles are rich in smooth muscle connected with the function of being a resistance vessel whose diameter can be controlled for appropriate regional distribution of blood. So there is a lower, not a higher, proportion of elastic tissue in the wall of an arteriole than in the wall of the aorta.

(b)   Yes. It is typical of blood vessels that the muscle layer is thicker in an artery than in a vein.

(c)   No. The diameter of a capillary is about the same as, or even slightly less than, the diameter of a red blood cell.

(d)   No. Capillaries possess no smooth muscle coat; changes in diameter are dependent, for instance, on changes in tone in the smooth muscle of the precapillary sphincter.

(e)   No. Capillaries in brain tissue impede the transfer of fluid and solutes; fenestrations are found in capillaries where there is a large flow of fluid, e.g. glomerular capillaries.

22 Sample MCQ papers

Paper 1	22.1–22.20
Paper 2	22.21–22.40
Paper 3	22.41–22.60

QUESTIONS

Paper 1

22.1 Concerning epithelia:
(a)   secretory epithelial cells are rich in mitochondria.
(b)   secretory epithelial cells form a thin pavement membrane.
(c)   capillaries supplying skeletal muscle have an epithelial covering.
(d)   epithelial cells covering a membrane involved in ultrafiltration form a continuous lining of the membrane.
(e)   the existence of a brush border is associated with absorptive function.

22.2 The packed cell volume (PCV, haemotocrit) is likely to be increased:
(a)   by a widespread increase in capillary blood pressure.
(b)   following haemorrhage.
(c)   following widespread hypoxic damage to capillary walls.
(d)   by a reduction in the concentration of albumin in the plasma.
(e)   by an increase in the concentration of urea in the plasma.

22.3 By comparison with someone depleted of water, a person depleted of an equal amount of isotonic fluid is likely to show a greater degree of:
(a)   intracellular dehydration.
(b)   circulatory collapse.
(c)   increase in haematocrit (packed cell volume).
(d)   thirst.
(e)   clouding of consciousness.

22.4   If the left optic nerve is damaged:
(a)   light shone in the right eye will cause pupillary constriction of the left eye.
(b)   light shone in the left eye will cause pupillary constriction of the right eye.
(c)   convergence will be accompanied by constriction of both pupils.
(d)   the subject will be able to see objects to the left of the mid-line.
(e)   as the right eye moves in scanning the visual field, the left eye will move too.

22.5   With reference to breathing and gas exchange:
(a)   if a little air were introduced between the two layers of pleura and the resulting space connected to a pressure transducer, the measured pressure would be below atmospheric throughout both inspiration and expiration during normal quiet breathing.
(b)   increased resistance to airflow in the bronchioles can best be detected by measurements made during forced rapid inspiration rather than expiration.
(c)   in normal circumstances the ventilation is regulated so as to maintain a constant arterial PCO_2.
(d)   in an area of the lungs where the ventilation/perfusion ratio is low, the pulmonary venous blood leaving that area will have a lower PO_2 than the average for the whole lung.
(e)   during voluntary hyperventilation, the arterial PO_2 will stay the same.

22.6   Hyperventilation at rest could cause:
(a)   uptake of about 1.5 times as much oxygen into the blood in the lungs compared with normal quiet breathing.
(b)   an increase in loss of carbon dioxide from the body to 1.5 times the normal rate.
(c)   a reduction in the plasma concentration of ionized calcium.
(d)   more negative intrathoracic pressure during inspiration than in quiet breathing.
(e)   vasodilatation in the cerebral circulation.

22.7   Accompanying moderately severe haemorrhagic shock, there is likely to be:
(a)   thirst.
(b)   decreased urinary output.
(c)   sweating.
(d)   cutaneous flushing.
(e)   hypercapnia (raised arterial PCO_2).

22.8 **Concerning gastro-intestinal function:**
(a) neutralization of acid from the stomach occurs mainly in the pancreatic duct.
(b) the pancreatic and biliary secretions enter the gastro-intestinal tract via a common duct.
(c) gastrin is a digestive enzyme.
(d) alcohol is absorbed through the wall of the stomach.
(e) the absorption of Fe^{2+} ions occurs in the stomach.

22.9 **Concerning renal function:**
(a) Bowman's capsule allows all particles below a certain size to pass.
(b) in the glomerulus, almost all the plasma is filtered.
(c) the glomerular filtration path is through the cytoplasm of the endothelial cells of the glomerular capillaries.
(d) the net filtration pressure increases along the glomerular capillary.
(e) about half the tubular reabsorption of glucose is by passive diffusion across the tubular wall.

22.10 **A previously well-controlled subject with insulin-dependent diabetes mellitus ceases to take insulin. This will result in:**
(a) an increase in urine osmolarity.
(b) an increase in ventilation.
(c) an increase in urinary excretion of acid.
(d) an increase in the renal plasma clearance of glucose.
(e) an increase in the plasma bicarbonate concentration.

22.11 **Concerning the adrenal gland:**
(a) the only site of action of aldosterone is in the kidney.
(b) the secretions of the adrenal cortex cease if the gland is denervated.
(c) the secretions of the adrenal medulla cease if the gland is denervated.
(d) the nerve fibres innervating the adrenal medullary secretory cells are unmyelinated.
(e) the nerve endings in the renal medulla are analogous to those on postganglionic nerve cells in sympathetic ganglia.

22.12 **Concerning environmental factors:**
(a) shivering requires a functioning hypothalamus.
(b) sweating requires a functioning hypothalamus.
(c) in a dehydrated subject the urine osmolarity may rise to 1200 mosmol per litre.
In a 70 kg man:
(d) in a temperate climate fluid loss from the lungs and insensible perspiration amounts to about 500 ml in 24 hrs.
(e) dehydration by 6 litres is liable to be fatal.

22.13 Cerebrospinal fluid:
(a)   is formed by the arachnoid villi.
(b)   normally has a pH lower than that of plasma.
(c)   has a greater buffering capacity than blood.
(d)   contains sodium in a concentration similar to that of plasma.
(e)   drains into the lymphatic system.

22.14 The endplate potential in mammalian skeletal muscle:
(a)   is a hyperpolarization.
(b)   is produced by noradrenaline released from the nerve endings.
(c)   is due to a specific increase in the permeability of the muscle membrane at the endplate to sodium.
(d)   lasts typically for 1 sec.
(e)   is propagated without decrement along the muscle fibre membrane.

22.15 The equilibrium potential of a given ion across a membrane is:
(a)   the membrane potential that would be required to balance the concentration gradient for that ion.
(b)   a function of the concentrations of that ion on the two sides of the membrane.
(c)   a function of the membrane potential.
(d)   the potential at which there is no net movement of that ion across the membrane due to electrical and concentration forces.
(e)   the potential that would exist across the membrane if the membrane were permeable only to that ion.

22.16 Concerning the nervous system and nervous mechanisms:
(a)   there are efferent nerve fibres leaving the spinal cord that are adrenergic.
(b)   an inhibitory postsynaptic potential (IPSP) in a mammalian motoneurone may prevent an excitatory postsynaptic potential (EPSP) from initiating an action potential.
(c)   an inhibitory postsynaptic potential in a mammalian motoneurone is enhanced by strychnine.
(d)   an excitatory postsynaptic potential in a mammalian motoneurone is due to the opening of channels specific for chloride ions.
(e)   the neurotransmitter for excitatory postsynaptic potentials in mammalian motoneurones is glycine.

22.17 **An individual has 1 dioptre of hypermetropia (hyperopia) and his range of accommodation is 2 dioptres:**

(a)   his near point is 1 m in front of his cornea.

(b)   his far point is 1 m behind his cornea.

(c)   he can clearly see distant objects.

(d)   if his accommodation is paralysed by atropine applied to the eye, he can clearly see objects 10 m in front of him.

(e)   if his accommodation is paralysed, a +2D spectacle lens will allow him to see clearly an object 25 cm in front of him.

22.18 **The sympathetic division of the autonomic nervous system is responsible for producing:**

(a)   a constriction of the pupil.

(b)   constriction of the internal sphincter of the urinary bladder.

(c)   acceleration of the heart.

(d)   dilatation of skin blood vessels.

(e)   relaxation of bronchial smooth muscle.

22.19 **With regard to acid base physiology:**

(a)   human urine is always acid.

(b)   in disorders of acid base status, the concentrations of potassium and hydrogen ions in the extracellular fluid tend to move in opposite directions.

(c)   respiratory compensation in metabolic acidosis involves a fall in arterial PCO_2.

(d)   compensation of respiratory alkalosis involves increased renal excretion of bicarbonate ions.

(e)   if in the compensated phase of respiratory acidosis a sample of arterial blood is equilibrated with a gas mixture containing CO_2 at a partial pressure of 40 mmHg, the pH of the sample is above normal.

22.20 **Concerning the anterior pituitary gland:**

(a)   the main control of release of its secretions is by direct innervation of its secretory cells.

(b)   its secretions are transported back via a local portal system to the hypothalamus.

(c)   it contains secretory cells.

(d)   the capillaries are fenestrated.

(e)   it releases hormones whose function is to influence the activity of other endocrine glands.

Paper 2

22.21   The circulating erythrocytes in a normal person:
(a)   are spherical in shape.
(b)   contain nuclei.
(c)   respire aerobically.
(d)   have a life-span of around 12 days.
(e)   have a specific gravity lower than that of plasma.

22.22   Compared with intracellular fluid, extracellular fluid:
(a)   has a lower pH.
(b)   constitutes a greater proportion of the total body water.
(c)   has a lower protein concentration.
(d)   has a higher chloride ion concentration.
(e)   has a lower potassium ion concentration.

22.23   A person loses a solution similar in composition to extracellular fluid, as in watery diarrhoea. This will result in:
(a)   a reduction in the volume of extracellular fluid.
(b)   a reduction in the volume of intracellular fluid.
(c)   an increase in the osmolarity of the extracellular fluid.
(d)   an increase in the osmolarity of the intracellular fluid.
(e)   a reduction in the total quantity of osmotically active material in the body.

22.24   Concerning the alimentary tract:
(a)   loss of the terminal 2 ft of the ileum is far more debilitating than the loss of an equal length of jejunum.
(b)   the parasympathetic nerve supply is excitatory to colonic motility.
(c)   the sympathetic nerve supply is excitatory to the internal (involuntary) anal sphincter.
(d)   constipation results in the absorption of toxic substances from the bowel.
(e)   persistent diarrhoea leads to metabolic acidosis.

22.25   Are the following associations appropriate?
(a)   lack of pulmonary surfactant leads to increased work of breathing.
(b)   multiple blockage of pulmonary capillaries leads to an abnormally large difference between end-expired and arterial PCO_2.
(c)   collapse of some alveoli leads to an increase in the alveolar-arterial difference for oxygen partial pressure (PO_2).
(d)   increased resistance to airflow causes an increase in functional residual capacity.
(e)   increased resistance to airflow causes a proportionate decrease in both vital capacity and FEV_1 (forced expiratory volume in one second).

22.26 **If a diver is at a depth of about 60 ft of water (i.e. about 3 atmospheres) and is breathing air:**
(a) PO_2 of arterial blood will be about six times the normal value.
(b) the arterial PCO_2 is likely to be near normal.
(c) there will be more N_2 than usual dissolved in the tissues.
(d) the alveolar partial pressure of H_2O will be about three times the normal value.
(e) ill effects are unlikely if he comes rapidly to the surface from a depth as moderate as this.

22.27 **The renal mechanisms involved in acid-base homeostasis include:**
(a) varying the urinary excretion of carbon dioxide.
(b) varying the urinary excretion of bicarbonate ions.
(c) the synthesis of ammonia.
(d) the synthesis of organic acids to buffer alkalosis.
(e) the metabolism of organic acids to buffer acidosis.

22.28 **Concerning the heart and great vessels in a healthy adult:**
(a) the systolic-diastolic pressure in the left ventricle is typically 120/5 mmHg.
(b) the systolic/diastolic pressure in the aorta is typically 120/70 mmHg.
(c) the systolic/diastolic pressure in the right ventricle is typically 25/5 mmHg.
(d) the systolic/diastolic pressure in the pulmonary artery is typically 25/8 mmHg.
(e) the maximum pressure drop across the mitral valve is typically 25 mmHg.

22.29 **Concerning glucose:**
(a) at blood glucose concentrations below the renal transport maximum (Tm) for glucose reabsorption, the amount of glucose reabsorbed is independent of the blood glucose concentration.
(b) at blood glucose concentrations above the renal Tm for glucose reabsorption, the amount of glucose excreted in the urine is independent of the blood glucose concentration.
(c) in a subject with a high blood glucose concentration and glycosuria, lowering of the glomerular filtration rate results in an increase in the amount of glucose in the urine.
(d) when the blood glucose concentration rises, the spill-over of glucose into the urine when the glucose Tm is exceeded contributes to limiting the rise in blood glucose concentration.
(e) with damage to the renal tubules, the glucose Tm is typically higher than normal.

22.30 Are these associations appropriate?

(a)	improved physical fitness	decreased cardiac stroke volume at rest.
(b)	improved physical fitness	decreased heart rate at rest.
(c)	excessive sweating	haemoconcentration.
(d)	haemorrhage	haemoconcentration.
(e)	reduced conduction velocity through the ventricles	reduced amplitude or inversion of the T wave of the ECG.

22.31 In a healthy human in anti-diuresis:

(a) the wall of the descending limb of the loop of Henle is readily permeable to water.

(b) the wall of the ascending limb of the loop of Henle, as it joins the distal convoluted tubule, is permeable to water.

(c) as an erythrocyte travels along the descending limb of one of the vasa recta to the top of the renal papilla, it loses at least a half of its intracellular water.

(d) as tubular fluid flows along the several components of the nephron, there is at least one segment where the volume of the tubular fluid increases.

(e) as tubular fluid flows along the several components of the nephron, there is at least one segment where the osmolarity of the tubular fluid decreases.

22.32 Consider an individual who is an emmetrope and whose near point is 100 cm:

(a) his eye has to accommodate for him to see distant objects clearly.

(b) his power of accommodation is 1 dioptre.

(c) with a spectacle lens of +3 dioptres, he will clearly read print held at 25 cm in front of him.

(d) if his accommodation is paralysed pharmacologically, he will be able to see clearly objects 100 cm ahead of him.

(e) if his lens were to be removed, his near point would recede.

22.33 Concerning sensory receptors:

(a) in the skin there are separate receptors for hot and for cold.

(b) a receptor sensitive to cold and a receptor sensitive to touch may connect to a common sensory nerve fibre.

(c) several receptors of the same type may be innervated by one sensory nerve fibre.

(d) a rapidly adapting receptor signals the rate of change of strength of a signal rather than its absolute intensity.

(e) for somaesthetic receptors (receptors subserving general body senses), there is a chemical junction between the receptor and the ending of the sensory nerve fibre.

22.34 **The result of severe damage to the visual system in the region of:**

(a) the left optic tract is blindness in the right half of the visual fields of both eyes (right homonymous hemianopia).

(b) the optic chiasma (e.g. by a pituitary tumour) is blindness in the nasal half of each visual field (binasal hemianopia).

(c) the occipital cortex of one hemisphere is loss of foveal vision with preservation of peripheral vision.

(d) the left optic nerve is loss of reflex constriction of the left pupil when light is shone in the right eye.

(e) the occipital cortex of both cerebral hemispheres is a loss of the direct light reflex.

22.35 **Concerning the posterior pituitary gland:**

(a) its hormones are all proteins.

(b) it synthesizes the hormones that are released by the anterior pituitary gland.

(c) its secretions are synthesized in the gland itself.

(d) the capillaries are fenestrated.

(e) it releases hormones whose function is to influence the activity of other endocrine glands.

22.36 **In a patient with metabolic alkalosis:**

(a) the condition may be caused by vomiting of gastric contents.

(b) the $[HCO_3^-]$ of arterial blood is raised.

(c) the urine is alkaline.

(d) the kidney retains bicarbonate.

(e) there is likely to be hyperventilation.

22.37 **In a person excreting acid urine, as the tubular fluid passes along the nephron:**

(a) there are regions of the nephron in which the hydrogen ion concentration is less than in the plasma.

(b) the reabsorption of water assists in the excretion of hydrogen ions.

(c) the reabsorption of water contributes to the rise in hydrogen ion concentration.

(d) the lower limit of urinary acidity is a pH of around 6.0.

(e) in the distal convoluted tubule, hydrogen ions flowing from within the tubular cell cytoplasm to the tubular fluid are moving down their electrochemical gradient.

22.38 Concerning the effects of a complete transection of the spinal cord:

(a) an hour after a complete transection in the lower cervical region, an electrical stimulus applied percutaneously to a nerve in a limb will cause a contraction of the muscles that it innervates.

(b) spinal shock is due to release of toxins from the cord at the site of injury.

(c) in spinal shock the muscle spindle stretch receptors generate action potentials in the afferent nerve fibres when the muscle is stretched.

(d) the lack of muscle tone in spinal shock is due to interruption of proprioceptive input to the cord.

(e) recovery of spinal reflex activity after the phase of shock is due to regeneration of peripheral nerve fibres.

22.39 Concerning the function of the cerebral hemispheres:

(a) it is mainly the association areas that show asymmetry of function.

(b) mathematical ability and logic are attributes of the right hemisphere in most subjects.

(c) creative and artistic ability are attributes of the right hemisphere in most subjects.

(d) a subject with a split brain (section of the corpus callosum) can name an object presented in the right visual field.

(e) it takes longer for a split-brain subject to identify, by pointing, a face presented in the left visual field than if the face is presented in the right visual field.

22.40 Concerning glutamate:

(a) it is the principal inhibitory transmitter in higher centres of the brain.

(b) it is involved in the general amino acid metabolism of the body.

(c) the increase in the intracellular calcium concentration induced by glutamate is due partly to calcium influx from the extracellular fluid.

(d) the increase in the intracellular calcium concentration induced by glutamate is due partly to calcium release from intracellular stores.

(e) in hypoxic brain, there is a decrease in release of glutamate.

Paper 3

22.41   With reference to water in the body:
(a)   the total body water accounts for approximately 60% of body weight in an adult man who has about 15% of his body weight as fat.
(b)   approximately two-thirds of the total volume of water in the body is intracellular.
(c)   in a patient with severe diarrhoea, the intracellular/extracellular volume ratio would increase.
(d)   the total body water volume is controlled from centres in the thalamus.
(e)   the total volume of the body water may be estimated using labelled albumin injected intravenously.

22.42   Simple diffusion of molecules across a cell membrane:
(a)   will occur even if there is no concentration difference between the two solutions on either side of the membrane.
(b)   approximately halves in rate if the temperature of the system drops from 37°C to 25°C.
(c)   involves the formation of chemical bonds with structures in the cell membrane.
(d)   occurs at a rate determined by the permeability constant of the membrane.
(e)   occurs at a rate that is independent of the size of the molecule.

22.43   In relation to the formation and absorption of interstitial (tissue) fluid:
(a)   local arteriolar constriction results in less tissue fluid formation.
(b)   reduction of plasma globulin level by a half would halve the plasma colloid osmotic pressure.
(c)   the fluid drained away in lymphatic channels is protein-free.
(d)   the fluid that is formed when the capillary permeability is increased by histamine will contain a higher concentration of protein than normal.
(e)   the rate of formation of tissue fluid at the ankle will be greater when standing still than when lying down.

22.44   In acute respiratory obstruction, there is:
(a)   a rise in arterial PCO_2.
(b)   a rise in arterial concentration of CO_2.
(c)   a rise in arterial bicarbonate concentration.
(d)   a rise in arterial pH.
(e)   a rise in the pK in the Henderson–Hasselbalch equation for the reaction $H_2O + CO_2 = H^+ + HCO_3^-$.

22.45   With reference to renal mechanisms:
(a)   glucose molecules entering renal venous blood as a result of re-absorption in the proximal convoluted tubule are the same molecules that were in the tubular fluid.
(b)   bicarbonate ions entering renal venous blood as a result of reabsorption in the proximal convoluted tubule are the same ions that were in the tubular fluid.
(c)   the proximal tubule reabsorbs more hydrogen ions than does the distal tubule.
(d)   the transport of hydrogen ions is against a greater gradient in the proximal tubule than in the distal tubule.
(e)   the change in hydrogen ion concentration as tubular fluid passes through the proximal convoluted tubule is greater than the change as the fluid passes through the distal convoluted tubule.

22.46   In uncontrolled diabetes mellitus:
(a)   diabetic coma is due to a direct effect of the high blood glucose concentration on brain cells.
(b)   the concentration of glucose in brain cells is above normal.
(c)   the concentration of glucose in liver cells is above normal.
(d)   the concentration of free fatty acids in the blood is below normal.
(e)   there is haemodilution.

22.47   Concerning the posterior pituitary gland:
(a)   it arises embryologically as an outgrowth of the primitive brain.
(b)   it secretes growth hormone.
(c)   it secretes anti-diuretic hormone.
(d)   it is connected with the hypothalamus via a portal blood system.
(e)   its hormones are released as a result of action potentials in hypothalamic neurones.

22.48   Lowered plasma potassium:
(a)   tends to decrease renal H^+ secretion.
(b)   is commonly associated with an extracellular alkalosis.
(c)   is commonly associated with an intracellular acidosis.
(d)   is a consequence of aldosteronism.
(e)   may occur as a consequence of administration of insulin.

22.49   With regard to buffering:
(a)   in plasma, phosphate is quantitatively more important than other non-bicarbonate buffers.
(b)   interstitial fluid in an inflamed area is better buffered than that in non-inflamed tissue.
(c)   the CO_2 bicarbonate buffer system is an efficient buffer system in a closed system at body pH.
(d)   the CO_2 bicarbonate buffer system is an efficient physiological buffer system.

(e)   a buffer pair is most effective as a buffer at pH values far from their pK value.

22.50   Concerning skeletal muscle in a healthy human adult:

(a)   when the endplate of an extrafusal muscle fibre is depolarized to threshold, the contraction that is initiated occurs along the whole length of the muscle fibre.

(b)   the endplates of intrafusal muscle fibres are usually in the equatorial region.

(c)   the initiation of impulses in afferent nerve fibres by spindle receptors is via the intermediary of a chemical synapse.

(d)   when extrafusal muscle fibres shorten, the equatorial region of the intrafusal muscle fibres are stretched.

(e)   contraction of all the intrafusal fibres in a muscle results in the development of a smaller tension than if all the extrafusal fibres contract.

22.51   Concerning the human eye:

(a)   the fovea contains more cones than rods.

(b)   there is a greater density of rods around the optic disc than at its centre.

(c)   close to the optic disc, the density of cones exceeds the density of rods.

(d)   the photosensitive receptors are expansions of the terminals of optic nerve fibres.

(e)   rhodopsin, the visual pigment in rods, is broken down by smaller amounts of blue light than is photopsin, the pigment in cones.

22.52   Concerning the speech areas in the cerebral cortex:

(a)   these areas all lie together in the same lobe of the cerebral hemisphere.

(b)   disordered function of the speech areas results in difficulty with articulation.

(c)   the motor speech area (Broca's area) lies just posterior to the primary motor area.

(d)   disordered function of the auditory speech area (Wernicke's area) results in reduction in the amount of speaking.

(e)   if in an adult the hemisphere housing the speech areas is destroyed, the remaining hemisphere is able to take over the speech functions.

22.53   Concerning renal function:

(a)   the kidney contributes to acid-base homeostasis by regulating the urinary excretion of carbon dioxide.

(b)   in alkalosis, the kidney excretes alkali as ammonium salts.

(c)   the titratable acid in the urine measures the total urinary output of acid.

(d)   in a healthy person excreting a concentrated urine, at least 90% of the osmolarity of the urine is due to sodium chloride.

(e)   in a patient with renal failure, the urine osmolarity is less than one-tenth of the osmolarity of plasma.

22.54 In a patient with no brain-stem function, it may be possible to elicit:

(a)   reflex withdrawal of the foot when a toe is pinched.

(b)   spontaneous respiratory movements when the arterial PCO_2 is raised to 50 mmHg.

(c)   grimacing on pressing over the supraorbital notch.

(d)   ocular deviation in response to infusing cold water into the external auditory meatus.

(e)   intelligible speech.

22.55 Concerning the cerebral cortex:

(a)   a greater proportion is devoted to primary sensory and motor functions in human than in non-human mammals.

(b)   during development, myelination of the association areas occurs before that of the primary sensory areas.

(c)   at birth, myelination of the central nervous system is complete in humans.

(d)   the primary motor area of cortex lies behind most of the primary sensory areas.

(e)   first order sensory neurones project to the primary somatosensory area of the cortex without a synaptic relay.

22.56 With reference to cardiovascular responses in healthy human subjects:

(a)   when tilted from the horizontal to the vertical position, the arterial blood pressure decreases and remains at a lower level.

(b)   the mean arterial blood pressure increases more during sustained muscular contraction ('static exercise') than during rhythmic muscular contraction ('dynamic exercise').

(c)   digital pressure on the carotid sinus may stimulate the baroreceptors and cause a fall in blood pressure.

(d)   excessive overbreathing leads to cerebral vasoconstriction.

(e)   the duration of ventricular diastole increases during inspiration.

22.57 With reference to the spinal cord and spinal reflexes in a normal person:

(a)   in the spinal cord, the cell bodies of autonomic preganglionic fibres lie in the lateral horn.

(b)   in the spinal cord, the cell bodies of autonomic preganglionic fibres aggregate in segments innervating the limbs.

(c)   a motoneurone in the cord supplies muscle fibres on the opposite side of the body.

(d)   a reflex contraction of one muscle is accompanied by reflex inhibition of its antagonist.

(e)   a reflex response may involve the discharge of all the neurones in a motoneurone pool.

22.58 Concerning the liver:
(a)   portal venous blood has a lower oxygen saturation than hepatic venous blood.
(b)   the portal vein provides the liver with more oxygen per min than the hepatic artery.
(c)   during digestion, the portal blood flow decreases.
(d)   during digestion, the oxygen saturation of the portal blood decreases.
(e)   in portal hypertension, ascites is a common feature.

22.59 Active transport:
(a)   across the cell membrane is essential to prevent cells from swelling and bursting.
(b)   depends on energy from metabolism.
(c)   is required for net movement of a chemical down its electrochemical gradient.
(d)   is required for the production of urine with a concentration higher than that of blood plasma.
(e)   is required for the production of urine with a concentration lower than that of blood plasma.

22.60 Concerning saliva:
(a)   in the primary acinar secretion, the concentration of potassium is less than in plasma.
(b)   as saliva passes along the ducts of the salivary glands, sodium ions are reabsorbed.
(c)   as saliva passes along the ducts of the salivary glands, its osmolarity falls.
(d)   as saliva passes along the ducts of the salivary glands, potassium ions are secreted into it.
(e)   at low salivary flow rates, the salivary concentration of potassium is greater than at high flow rates.

ANSWERS

22.1
(a)   Yes. Secretory epithelial cells are metabolically very active and so are rich in mitochondria.
(b)   No. Associated with their high metabolic activity, secretory epithelial cells are thick.
(c)   No. Capillaries supplying skeletal muscle are surrounded by a basement membrane, but they have no epithelial covering.
(d)   No. Epithelial cells covering a membrane involved in ultrafiltration have gaps between to allow the ultrafiltrate to pass.
(e)   Yes. The brush border provides a large surface area for reabsorption.

22.2

(a)   Yes. A widespread increase in capillary blood pressure will result in net movement of fluid from the plasma to the interstitial fluid, resulting in an increase in PCV.

(b)   No. Following haemorrhage, there is widespread arteriolar constriction; this results in a lowering of the capillary pressure, a net transfer of fluid from interstitial fluid to the plasma and hence a decrease in PCV.

(c)   Yes. Hypoxic damage to capillary walls allows plasma proteins to leak into the interstitial fluid; this results in an increase in PCV.

(d)   Yes. Reduced concentration of albumin in the plasma results in a reduction in the colloid osmotic pressure sucking fluid from interstitial fluid to the plasma; fluid leaves the plasma leading to a rise in PCV.

(e)   No. Urea permeates capillary walls, so its concentration in the plasma is without influence on fluid transfer across capillary walls.

22.3

(a)   No. Depletion of isotonic fluid results in a reduction mainly of the volume of the extracellular compartment.

(b)   Yes. Depletion of isotonic fluid results in a depletion mainly of the extracellular compartment including the plasma, while water depletion is at the expense of both extra and intracellular fluid. Circulatory collapse is therefore more likely to occur with depletion of isotonic fluid than with depletion of water.

(c)   Yes. By the same logic as (b), the haematocrit is increased more by depletion of isotonic fluid than by depletion of water.

(d)   No. Depletion of water results in hypertonicity of the body fluids, and hypertonicity is a strong stimulus for thirst; depletion of isotonic fluid has little effect on the tonicity of the body fluids.

(e)   No. Clouding of consciousness is a feature of intracellular dehydration and this occurs to a greater extent with deprivation of water than with deprivation of isosmotic solution.

22.4

(a)   Yes. The input pathway is the right optic nerve and the output pathway is the parasympathetic nerve supply to the left eye; both these pathways are intact.

(b)   No. The left optic nerve is damaged so the input pathway for the reflex is interrupted.

(c)   Yes. This reflex does not depend on visual input.

(d)   Yes. The seeing eye has a visual field to both sides.

(e)   Yes. The nerve supply to the extrinsic ocular muscles is intact and both eyes move.

22.5

(a)   Yes. Intrapleural pressure is below atmospheric ('negative') throughout the whole respiratory cycle in quiet breathing; it is most negative at the end of inspiration, because when the lungs are stretched they pull away more (by 'elastic recoil') from the chest wall.

(b) No. During forced expiration, the bronchioles tend to shut down because positive pressure is exerted on the lungs; any tendency to obstruction is therefore enhanced.

(c) Yes.

(d) Yes. Where blood flow is excessive relative to ventilation, the gas concentrations in the alveoli and in the blood leaving them become closer to those in mixed venous blood.

(e) No. During hyperventilation, as carbon dioxide tension decreases, oxygen tension rises. It is the haemoglobin oxygen saturation and arterial oxygen content that are virtually unchanged by the increase in PO_2.

22.6

(a) No. The additional oxygen would reflect only a tiny extra amount dissolved because of the increase in alveolar PO_2, from 100 mmHg to not more than 130 mmHg (say, 1 ml per litre, an increase of 0.5%). The increased work of breathing would require some extra oxygen uptake, but not 1.5 times.

(b) Yes. Normal alveolar ventilation might be losing, say, 5% of 4 litres per min = 200 ml per min. Hyperventilation, although it progressively reduces the carbon dioxide percentage, could lose 3% of 10 litres per min = 300 ml per min. (If hyperventilation were maintained at a tolerable steady rate, the CO_2 output would return to the original volume per min at a stable low alveolar CO_2 percentage.)

(c) Yes. The respiratory alkalaemia increases binding of calcium to plasma proteins. The resulting hypocalcaemia can cause tetany.

(d) Yes. The more the lungs are inflated, the greater is their elastic recoil, and the lower the intrathoracic pressure.

(e) No. Low PCO_2 causes cerebral vasoconstriction, reduction in cerebral blood flow and hence faintness/dizziness if severe enough.

22.7

(a) Yes. As a result of the reduced blood volume, after haemorrhage there is thirst.

(b) Yes. The response to haemorrhage includes vasoconstriction of afferent renal arterioles, a reduction in glomerular filtration rate and a decreased urinary output.

(c) Yes. The intense sympathetic outflow leads to sweating.

(d) No. There is cutaneous vasoconstriction.

(e) No. Ventilation is stimulated and this leads to a reduction, not an increase, in arterial PCO_2.

22.8

(a) No. The pancreas secretes much of the alkali that neutralizes gastric acid but the mixture of the juices from stomach and pancreas occurs in the duodenum, not in the pancreatic duct.

(b) Yes. The pancreatic duct terminates by joining the bile duct to form a short dilated duct, the 'ampulla of Vater', which drains into the second part of the duodenum; entry of secretions is controlled here by the 'sphincter of Oddi'.

(c) No. Gastrin is a hormone.

(d) Yes. Alcohol and water are the only substances absorbed through the wall of the stomach to any significant extent.

(e) No. The absorption of Fe^{2+} ions occurs in the small intestine; stomach acidity is important in maintaining iron in the Fe^{2+} form.

22.9

(a) Yes. Bowman's capsule behaves rather like a physical filter.

(b) No. In the glomerulus, about 20% of the plasma is filtered.

(c) No. The glomerular filtration path is between the endothelial cells and through fenestrations.

(d) No. The net filtration pressure decreases along the glomerular capillary due to the rise in colloid osmotic pressure as the concentration of plasma proteins rises.

(e) No. The tubular reabsorption of glucose is active.

22.10

(a) Yes. Glucose in the urine causes an increase in urine osmolarity.

(b) Yes. Acidaemia due to ketosis stimulates ventilation.

(c) Yes. In the metabolic acidosis accompanying diabetes mellitus, the renal compensation is the production of an acid urine.

(d) Yes. In normal subjects, there is no glucose in the urine so the renal clearance of glucose is zero. In an uncontrolled diabetic, there is glucose in the urine and hence an increase in the renal clearance of glucose.

(e) No. Metabolic acidosis is accompanied by a decrease in the plasma bicarbonate concentration.

22.11

(a) No. Aldosterone also acts on sweat glands, regulating sodium reabsorption in the ducts.

(b) No. The secretions of the adrenal cortex are controlled by blood-borne factors such as trophic hormones and not by neuronal activity.

(c) Yes. The secretions of the adrenal medulla depend on action potentials in the sympathetic nerves innervating the gland and the secretions cease if the gland is denervated.

(d) No. The nerve fibres innervating the adrenal medullary secretory cells are preganglionic sympathetic fibres and are thinly myelinated.

(e) Yes.

22.12
(a) Yes. Shivering depends on nerve impulses initiated in the hypothalamus and projecting down to the anterior horn cells of the spinal cord.

(b) No. Sweating may occur, for instance, below the level of the lesion in a person with a spinal transection of long-standing; such a subject has a functioning hypothalamus but it is disconnected from the spinal cord.

(c) Yes.

(d) Yes.

(e) No. 3 litres is mild dehydration, 6 litres is moderate, 9 litres is severe and about 12 litres is fatal.

22.13
(a) No. Cerebrospinal fluid is reabsorbed, not formed, by the arachnoid villi.

(b) Yes.

(c) No. Associated with its low concentration of protein, cerebrospinal fluid has less buffering capacity than blood.

(d) Yes.

(e) No. Cerebrospinal fluid drains into the arachnoid villi of the superior sagittal sinus; the brain has no lymphatic system.

22.14
(a) No. The endplate potential is a depolarization.

(b) No. The endplate potential is produced by acetylcholine released from the nerve endings.

(c) No. The endplate potential is due to an increase in the permeability of the muscle membrane at the endplate to all small inorganic ions.

(d) No. The endplate potential lasts typically for 3 msec.

(e) No. The endplate potential is a local phenomenon; it spreads passively, with decrement.

22.15
(a) Yes.

(b) Yes. The equilibrium potential depends on the ratio of the concentrations of that ion on the two sides of the membrane.

(c) No. The equilibrium potential of a given ion across a membrane depends on the ion's concentration gradient across the membrane and on its charge, not on the membrane potential.

(d) Yes.

(e) Yes.

22.16

(a)   No. It is an interesting general principle that all neurones with cell bodies in the central nervous system and with axons leaving the central nervous system are cholinergic. The principle holds for somatic neurones (motoneurones) and for both sympathetic and parasympathetic preganglionic neurones.

(b)   Yes. An IPSP in a mammalian motoneurone reduces the sensitivity of the motoneurone and so may prevent an EPSP from initiating an action potential.

(c)   No. An inhibitory postsynaptic potential in a mammalian motoneurone is blocked by strychnine.

(d)   No. An excitatory postsynaptic potential in a mammalian motoneurone is due to the opening of channels allowing all small inorganic ions to pass.

(e)   No. The neurotransmitter for excitatory postsynaptic potentials in mammalian motoneurones is glutamate. Glycine is an inhibitory neurotransmitter.

22.17

(a)   Yes. The subject uses 1 dioptre of his accommodation to view distant objects and so has another 1 dioptre for near vision; his near point is thus 1 m in front of his cornea.

(b)   Yes. With hypermetropia, his far point is virtual, 1 dioptre of hypermetropia indicating his far point to be 1 m behind his cornea.

(c)   Yes. Using 1 dioptre of accommodation, he can clearly see distant objects.

(d)   No. If the accommodation of a hypermetropic eye is paralysed by atropine, all images of objects in the visual field fall in front of the retina; in this situation, a hypermetrope cannot clearly see any objects in front of him.

(e)   No. If his accommodation is paralysed and a +2D spectacle lens placed in front of the eye, 1 dioptre will be required to counteract the hypermetropia and allow the subject to see distant objects clearly. This leaves 1 dioptre, which will allow him to see clearly an object 1 metre in front of him.

22.18

(a)   No. The sympathetic innervation to the pupil causes pupillary dilatation.

(b)   Yes.

(c)   Yes.

(d)   No. The sympathetic supply to the skin causes constriction of skin blood vessels.

(e)   Yes.

22.19

(a)   No, in alkalosis, the urinary pH can rise to 8.

(b)   No. In disorders of acid base status, the concentrations of potassium and hydrogen ions in the extracellular fluid tend to move in the same direction.

(c)   Yes. Acidaemia stimulates respiration, so the arterial PCO_2 falls.

(d)   Yes. In respiratory alkalosis, bicarbonate is excreted as part of the homeostatic mechanism for returning the blood pH towards normal and alkaline urine is excreted.

(e)   Yes. In this situation there is renal retention of bicarbonate so that, if corrected to a normal PCO_2, the blood is more alkaline than usual.

22.20

(a)   No. The main control of release of the secretions of the anterior pituitary gland is humoral, not neural.

(b)   No. Many of the secretions the anterior pituitary gland are controlled by releasing factors transported to it via a local portal system from the hypothalamus.

(c)   Yes. The anterior pituitary contains the cells that elaborate the anterior pituitary hormones.

(d)   Yes. The capillaries are fenestrated. This allows the hormones, which are relatively large molecules, to pass into the blood when released from the secretory cells.

(e)   Yes. The actions of anterior pituitary hormones are mainly on other endocrine glands.

22.21

(a)   No. Erythrocytes are biconcave discs.

(b)   No.

(c)   No. Erythrocytes respire anaerobically.

(d)   No. The life-span of an erythrocyte is typically 120 days.

(e)   No. When blood is centrifuged, the erythrocytes are thrown to the bottom of the tube, showing that they have a specific gravity higher than that of plasma.

22.22

(a)   No. Intracellular fluid has a lower pH than extracellular fluid.

(b)   No. Extracellular fluid constitutes about one-third of the total body water, intracellular fluid two-thirds.

(c)   Yes.

(d)   Yes. Chloride is quantitatively the principal anion in extracellular fluid. For intracellular fluid, organic anions and phosphate are quantitatively most important.

(e)   Yes. In extracellular fluid, the potassium concentration is typically 4 mmol and in intracellular fluid it is 150 mmol.

22.23

(a)   Yes. The lost fluid comes from the extracellular fluid, so there is a reduction in its volume.

(b)   No. There is no change of osmotic pressure of the extracellular fluid, so there is no reduction in the volume of intracellular fluid.

(c)   No. The loss of water is balanced by a loss of solute, so there is no change in the osmolarity of the extracellular fluid.

(d)   No. See (c).

(e)   Yes. Loss of electrolyte signifies a reduction in the total quantity of osmotically active material in the body.

22.24

(a)   Yes. This is because the ileum is the major site of absorption of necessary nutrients, and the terminal part is the only site of absorption of vitamin B12 (complexed with intrinsic factor).

(b)   Yes. As a general rule, parasympathetic stimulation enhances motility throughout the gut.

(c)   Yes. This fits in with the general rule that sympathetic activity inhibits gut activity – relaxation of the rectal wall and contraction of the internal sphincter (along with voluntary control of the external sphincter) postpone defaecation.

(d)   No. There is no evidence that constipation results in the absorption of toxic substances from the bowel.

(e)   Yes.

22.25

(a)   Yes. Inflation of the lungs involves work against surface tension in the alveolar lining, which is diminished by surfactant.

(b)   Yes. Blockage of capillaries causes alveolar dead space: air goes in and out of affected alveoli unchanged (CO_2 near zero) and mixes on the way out with gas from normally perfused alveoli (CO_2 over 5%); therefore the CO_2 partial pressure in end-expired gas is lower than the PCO_2 in blood leaving normal alveoli, and this latter determines the PCO_2 of arterial blood.

(c)   Yes. Collapse of alveoli causes shunting of some mixed venous blood.

(d)   Yes. Increased resistance to airflow results in incomplete emptying of alveoli during expiration and so causes an increase in functional residual capacity.

(e)   No. Increased resistance to airflow causes a decrease in FEV_1 but not in vital capacity.

22.26

(a)   No. The inspired PO_2 is three times normal – approximately 460 mmHg. Alveolar and arterial PO_2 are a little over 400 mmHg.

(b)   Yes. The usual control mechanisms keep arterial PCO_2 normal. (Note that a mole of carbon dioxide – as of any other gas – will take up only one-third of the volume at 3 atmospheres compared with sea-level; to excrete the necessary moles per min still requires the same alveolar ventilation: e.g. 4 litres per min, with 2% CO_2, would now carry away 80 ml of CO_2, as compared with 240 ml when it is 6% at sea-level; the 80 ml and the 240 ml would represent the same amount in moles).

(c)   Yes. Blood equilibrates with alveolar PN_2, and tissues in turn with blood. Although N_2 is very insoluble, approximately three times the amount becomes dissolved after sufficient time at this depth.

(d)   No. The partial pressure of water vapour, at body temperature, saturated, does not change with ambient pressure. The percentage in alveolar gas will be one-third.

(e)   No. The longer the period at depth the slower must decompression be to avoid nitrogen coming out of solution in the tissues. There is also a risk from rapid lung expansion and pulmonary barotrauma if breath is held on the way up.

22.27

(a)   No. Variation in ventilation controls the excretion of carbon dioxide. The urinary excretion of CO_2 cannot be controlled.

(b)   Yes. An increase in the urinary excretion of bicarbonate ions is a homeostatic mechanism for excreting alkali in alkalosis.

(c)   Yes. The synthesis of ammonia provides a vehicle for the excretion of acid in acidosis.

(d)   No. There is no renal mechanism for the synthesis of organic acids to buffer alkalosis.

(e)   No. There is no renal mechanism for the metabolism of organic acids to buffer acidosis.

22.28

(a)   Yes. This is a typical value for a normal subject.

(b)   Yes. (See (a).)

(c)   Yes. (See (a).)

(d)   Yes. (See (a).)

(e)   No. The maximum pressure drop across the mitral valve occurs at the height of ventricular contraction; the left ventricular pressure is then around 120 mmHg, while the left atrial pressure is close to zero, so the pressure drop is around 120 mmHg.

22.29

(a) No. At blood glucose concentrations below the renal Tm for glucose reabsorption, all filtered glucose is reabsorbed, so the amount of glucose reabsorbed is directly proportional to, and not independent of, the blood glucose concentration.

(b) No. At blood glucose concentrations above the renal Tm for glucose reabsorption, the amount of glucose reabsorbed is constant and the amount excreted in the urine equals the filtered load minus this constant amount that is reabsorbed; the amount of glucose excreted in the urine increases with increasing blood glucose concentration.

(c) No. In a subject with a high blood glucose concentration and glycosuria, lowering of the glomerular filtration rate results in a reduction in the filtered load of glucose and hence a reduction, not an increase, in the amount of glucose in the urine.

(d) Yes.

(e) No. Tubular reabsorption is reduced with damage to the renal tubules, so the glucose Tm is typically lower, not higher, than normal.

22.30

(a) No. The physically fit have a higher than average stroke volume at rest.

(b) Yes. The physically fit have a lower than average heart rate.

(c) Yes. Both water and solutes are lost, but the loss of water is the greater.

(d) No. Haemorrhage is followed by haemodilution.

(e) Yes. The fact that T and R waves are usually of the same polarity depends on rapid conduction through the ventricles.

22.31

(a) Yes. Water moves under osmotic forces across the tubule wall here.

(b) No. Electrolytes are pumped out here against a concentration gradient; if the wall were permeable to water, net movement of water would dissipate this gradient.

(c) Yes. The osmolarity of the plasma along with that of the interstitial fluid rises by at least a factor of 2 as the erythrocyte passes along one of the vasa recta.

(d) No. Except in the glomerulus, there is no net entry of water into the tubule along the nephron. So as tubular fluid flows along the several components of the nephron, there is no segment where the volume of the tubular fluid increases.

(e) Yes. As tubular fluid flows along the several components of the nephron, its osmolarity decreases as it flows along the ascending limb of the loop of Henle.

22.32

(a)   No. For an emmetrope, the relaxed eye is focused at infinity.

(b)   Yes. Since his near point is 1 metre and his far point is infinity, his power of accommodation is $1/1 = 1$ dioptre.

(c)   Yes. 25 cm = 0.25 m and $1/0.25 = 4$. So he needs a total of 4 dioptres of power to see clearly at 25 cm. His own accommodation provides 1 dioptre which, together with the spectacle lens of $+3$ dioptres, gives him the required optical power to see clearly at 25 cm.

(d)   No. If his accommodation is paralysed pharmacologically, he will be able to see clearly distant objects, not 100 cm ahead of him.

(e)   Yes. The lens is convex, so its removal reduces the optical power of the eye; removal of the lens results in the near point receding.

22.33

(a)   Yes.

(b)   No. The central nervous system infers the nature of the energy exciting a receptor from the sensory nerve fibre along which the information travels. So a receptor sensitive to cold and a receptor sensitive to touch must connect to different sensory nerve fibres.

(c)   Yes.

(d)   Yes. A rapidly adapting receptor responds when the intensity of the stimulus is changing, not when the intensity is constant. Hence it signals the rate of change of strength of a signal rather than its absolute intensity.

(e)   No. For somaesthetic receptors, the ending of the sensory nerve fibre is part of the receptor; for most of the special senses, there is a separate receptor cell which transduces the energy to which the receptor is sensitive and then relays it, via a chemical synapse, to the sensory nerve fibre.

22.34

(a)   Yes.

(b)   No. A lesion of the optic chiasma interrupts fibres from the nasal half of each eye, i.e. the temporal visual field of each eye. So the result is a bitemporal hemianopia.

(c)   No. The fovea is bilaterally represented; loss of one occipital pole gives the phenomenon of foveal sparing. This means that objects on and close to the visual axis are seen if the occipital pole of one hemisphere is damaged.

(d)   No. Light shone in the right eye will cause constriction of both pupils; the afferent pathway is the right optic nerve and the efferent pathway to the pupils runs with the 3rd cranial nerve.

(e)   No. The light reflex pathway is via the retinotectal projection, not via the cerebral cortex.

22.35

(a) Yes.

(b) No. The hormones that are released by the anterior pituitary gland are synthesized in the gland itself.

(c) No. The secretions of the posterior pituitary are elaborated in the hypothalamus.

(d) Yes. The capillaries are fenestrated. This allows the hormones, which are relatively large molecules, to pass into the blood when released.

(e) No. The posterior pituitary hormones act directly on target cells such as the cells of the collecting ducts of the kidney.

22.36

(a) Yes. Vomiting of gastric contents results in loss of hydrochloric acid from the body and hence an alkalosis.

(b) Yes.

(c) Yes. The kidney excretes an alkaline urine to rid the body of the unwanted alkali.

(d) No. The kidney excretes bicarbonate.

(e) No. Alkalosis depresses ventilation.

22.37

(a) No. There is a progressive rise in $[H^+]$ as the tubular fluid passes along the nephron.

(b) No. Reabsorption of water is by mechanisms which do not interact with mechanisms for the excretion of hydrogen ions.

(c) Yes. By removing water, the concentrations of all other chemicals in the tubular fluid, including hydrogen ions, are raised.

(d) No. A correct answer would be a pH of 4.5.

(e) No. They are being pumped against an ever-increasing concentration gradient.

22.38

(a) Yes. The peripheral apparatus functions normally; spinal shock is a phenomenon of the spinal cord itself.

(b) No. It has occasionally occurred that, after a first transection of the spinal cord, when sufficient time had elapsed for spinal shock to have disappeared, a second transection has occurred. The second transection is not followed by a phase of spinal shock. This shows that spinal shock is not due to release of toxins from the cord at the site of injury. Spinal shock is attributed to interruption of descending influences from higher centres.

(c)   Yes. As in (a).

(d)   No. Proprioceptive input still occurs.

(e)   No. Peripheral nerves below the segmental level of a spinal transection are not injured by the transection; they do not degenerate and therefore no regeneration occurs. In the period of time immediately following the transection the cessation of function in spinal centres is attributed to lack of descending influences and it is observed that, subsequently, these centres function autonomously. The mechanisms are poorly understood.

22.39

(a)   Yes.

(b)   No. Mathematical ability and logic are attributes of the left ('dominant') hemisphere in most subjects.

(c)   Yes.

(d)   Yes. Such an object projects to the hemisphere housing the speech areas.

(e)   No. The opposite. The right (non-speaking) hemisphere is better at recognition than the speaking hemisphere.

22.40

(a)   No. It is the principal excitatory transmitter for fast pathways.

(b)   Yes.

(c)   Yes. Glutamate, by attaching to the n-methyl D-aspartate (NMDA) sub-population of glutamate receptors, opens membrane channels permeable to calcium. There is therefore a net influx of calcium ions from the extracellular fluid.

(d)   Yes. By acting on the metabotropic glutamate receptors.

(e)   No. Hypoxia results in excessive release of glutamate.

22.41

(a)   Yes.

(b)   Yes.

(c)   Yes. In a patient with severe diarrhoea, the fluid lost is isosmotic with body fluids, so most of the loss is from the extracellular, not the intracellular compartment. Therefore the intracellular: extracellular volume ratio increases.

(d)   No. The total body water volume is controlled from centres in the hypothalamus.

(e)   No. Albumin injected intraveounsly remains in the plasma compartment and so can be used to estimate the plasma volume, not the total volume of water in the body.

22.42

(a)   Yes. The cell membrane is permeable to water, so to-and-fro move-
       ment of water will occur even if there is no concentration difference
       between the two solutions on either side of the membrane.

(b)   No. Simple diffusion is a physicochemical process and its rate is
       directly proportional to the absolute temperature. So a fall in
       temperature of 12°C from 37°C will result in a change in rate of
       diffusion of $12/(273+37) = 3\%$ approximately.

(c)   No. Simple diffusion is due to the thermal energy of particles and
       does not depend on chemical bonds.

(d)   Yes.

(e)   No. Simple diffusion occurs at a rate that decreases as the size of
       the molecule increases.

22.43

(a)   Yes. Local arteriolar constriction results in a reduction in pres-
       sure of blood in the capillaries and so results in less tissue fluid
       formation.

(b)   No. Most of the plasma colloid osmotic pressure is due to albumin,
       so halving of the plasma globulin concentration would reduce the
       plasma colloid osmotic pressure by much less than a half.

(c)   No. Fluid drainage in lymphatic channels is the mechanism of
       removing from the interstitial fluid protein that has filtered across
       the capillary wall.

(d)   Yes. Normally the capillary wall is almost impermeable to pro-
       tein, so when the capillary permeability is increased by histamine,
       the fluid formed contains a higher concentration of protein than
       normal.

(e)   Yes. When standing, the pressure of blood in the capillaries
       at the ankle is increased by the pressure of the column of blood
       between the heart and the ankle. So the rate of formation of tissue
       fluid at the ankle will be greater when standing still than when lying
       down.

22.44

(a)   Yes. In acute respiratory obstruction, the primary disturbance is a
       fall in arterial PO_2 and a rise in arterial PCO_2.

(b)   Yes. A rise in arterial PCO_2 is accompanied by a rise in arterial
       concentration of CO_2.

(c)   Yes. The reaction $H_2O + CO_2 = H^+ + HCO_3^-$ shows that a rise
       in concentration of CO_2 leads, by mass action, to a rise in arterial
       bicarbonate concentration.

(d)   No. There is a fall in arterial pH.

(e)   No. The pK in the Henderson–Hasselbalch equation is a constant, unaltered by changes in concentrations of the participating chemicals.

22.45

(a)   Yes. The glucose is reabsorbed unaltered.

(b)   No. Retrieval of filtered bicarbonate depends on its chemical reaction with hydrogen ions to yield CO_2, diffusion of CO_2 into the tubular cell cytoplasm and recombination with water to yield hydrogen ions and bicarbonate again.

(c)   Yes.

(d)   No. The opposite is the case.

(e)   No.

22.46

(a)   No. The high blood glucose concentration *per se* is not damaging; the coma is due to other factors such as ketoacidaemia.

(b)   Yes. Insulin is not required for glucose entry into brain cells; this is a point of contrast with skeletal muscle cells.

(c)   Yes. Hepatocytes are readily permeable to glucose and entry does not depend on insulin.

(d)   No. Due to mobilization of triglycerides from fat stores, the concentration of free fatty acids in the blood is high, often extremely high.

(e)   No. There is dehydration and haemoconcentration.

22.47

(a)   Yes.

(b)   No. Growth hormone is secreted by the anterior pituitary.

(c)   Yes.

(d)   No. It is the anterior pituitary that is connected with the hypothalamus via a portal blood system.

(e)   Yes.

22.48

(a)   No. Low extracellular $[K^+]$ results in K^+ moving from the renal tubular cell cytoplasm to the interstitial fluid. This transfer results in the movement of H^+ in the opposite direction, from interstitial fluid into the tubular cell cytoplasm as part of an electroneutrality balance. The rise in intracellular $[H^+]$ assists renal H^+ secretion.

(b)   Yes. A low extracellular [K⁺] is commonly associated with an extracellular alkalosis. There are several mechanisms: one is that, as a result of the low extracellular [K⁺], K⁺ moves from intra- to extracellular fluid. This transfer results in the movement of H⁺ in the opposite direction, from extra- to intracellular fluid to maintain electroneutrality. This movement of H⁺ lowers the extracellular [H⁺].

(c)   Yes. By the mechanism described in (b), a low extracellular [K⁺] leads to an intracellular acidosis.

(d)   Yes. Aldosteronism causes the renal retention of sodium and excretion of potassium.

(e)   Yes. Administration of insulin results in glucose and potassium entering cells.

22.49

(a)   No. In plasma, phosphate is a relatively unimportant buffer quantitatively because of its relatively low concentration.

(b)   Yes. In inflamed tissue, the capillary lining allows the passage of proteins, which act as good buffers.

(c)   No. The pK (6.1) is more than one pH unit from body pH (7.4).

(d)   Yes. This is because both PCO_2 and $[HCO_3^-]$ can be regulated.

(e)   No. They buffer most effectively at pH values close to their pK.

22.50

(a)   Yes. For extrafusal fibres, a threshold depolarization at any point initiates an action potential that travels away from that point in both directions to the end of the muscle fibre; the whole of the muscle fibre is involved.

(b)   No. Endplates are found at the poles of the intrafusal fibres.

(c)   No. The receptor is the terminal of the afferent nerve fibre. The initiation of impulses is by passive (electrotonic) conduction from the receptor to the first node of Ranvier of the nerve fibre.

(d)   No. This takes the stretch off the whole of the intrafusal muscle fibre.

(e)   Yes. The direct contribution of the intrafusal fibres to the tension developed by a muscle is insignificant.

22.51

(a)   Yes. There are only cones, no rods, in the fovea.

(b)   Yes. There are no photosensitive receptors at the centre of the optic disc, or blind spot.

(c) No. This is peripheral retina, where the density of rods exceeds that of cones.

(d) No. The photosensitive receptors are of epithelial origin. There is a chain of synapses between the receptor cells and the terminals of the optic nerve fibres.

(e) Yes. Rhodopsin is sensitive to blue light and rods are more sensitive than cones for light of this wavelength.

22.52

(a) No. The three speech areas lie in the frontal, parietal and temporal lobes of the left hemisphere.

(b) No. Disordered function of the speech areas results in difficulty with the structure of language, not with articulation.

(c) No. Just anterior.

(d) No. The motor speech area is released from control and characteristically subjects with such a lesion are verbose.

(e) No. This is true of young children but not of adults.

22.53

(a) No. The lungs, not the kidney, contribute to acid-base homeostasis by regulating the excretion of carbon dioxide.

(b) No. Ammonium excretion is a means of ridding the body of acid, not alkali.

(c) No. The titratable acid in the urine does not include the contribution made to urinary acid excretion by ammonium ions.

(d) No. In a healthy person excreting a concentrated urine, about 50% of the osmolarity of the urine is due to sodium chloride. The other 50% is due to urea.

(e) No. In a patient with renal failure, the urine osmolarity is close to that of plasma.

22.54

(a) Yes. This is a spinal reflex and does not depend on brain-stem function.

(b) No. The respiratory centres lie in the brain-stem and, with no brain-stem function, spontaneous respiratory movements do not occur.

(c) No. Grimacing involves activity in the nucleus of the facial nerve, which lies in the brain-stem.

(d) No. Vestibulo-ocular reflexes including caloric testing depend on the nuclei of cranial nerves III, IV and VI which lie in the brain-stem.

(e)   No. The subject cannot speak because he is unconscious due to lack of activity of the ascending reticular formation.

22.55

(a)   No. It is the proliferation of association areas that characterizes the human brain.

(b)   No. The sequence of myelination is the same as the sequence of phylogenetic development; the association areas are phylogenetically more recent than the primary receiving areas.

(c)   No. Myelination of association cortex, for instance proceeds until the late teens.

(d)   No. The primary motor area lies in precentral cortex; most primary sensory areas are post-central.

(e)   No. The specific somatosensory projection pathways, which are the most direct projections, traverse two synapses.

22.56

(a)   No. On tilting from the horizontal to the vertical position, arterial blood pressure is restored after a small initial fall.

(b)   Yes. Static exercise elicits reflex vasoconstriction, which raises the diastolic blood pressure as well as the systolic. This assists the flow of blood into the strongly contracted muscles, where it is mechanically impeded. In rhythmic exercise the diastolic pressure tends to fall because of the muscle vasodilatation, while systolic pressure rises.

(c)   Yes. This can happen to the extent of causing syncope – an unfortunate trick known as the 'fainting lark'.

(d)   Yes. Reduction of arterial PCO_2 by hyperventilation leads to cerebral vasoconstriction.

(e)   No. Heart rate increases during inspiration (sinus arrhythmia); this implies a decrease in the duration of diastole.

22.57

(a)   Yes.

(b)   No. In the spinal cord, the segments innervating the limbs are swelled because of the cell bodies associated with serving the motor and sensory innervation of the limbs; these segments are devoid of cell bodies of autonomic preganglionic fibres.

(c)   No. A motoneurone in the cord always supplies muscle fibres on the same side of the body.

(d)   Yes. This is the phenomenon of reciprocal innervation.

(e)   No. A reflex response never commands all the neurones in a motoneurone pool.

22.58

(a)   No. Portal venous blood provides the liver with oxygen, so the hepatic venous blood clearly has a lower oxygen saturation than does portal venous blood. Typical figures are: oxygen saturation of portal venous blood = 85%; hepatic venous blood = 75%.

(b)   Yes. Because of the high rate of blood flowing through the portal vein (blood flow 1200 ml per min), it provides the liver with more oxygen (about 43 ml oxygen per min) than does the hepatic artery (blood flow 300 ml per min), which provides the liver with about 17 ml oxygen per min.

(c)   No. During digestion, the portal blood flow markedly increases, reflecting increased metabolism in the gastro-intestinal tract.

(d)   Yes. Due to oxygen utilization in the processes of digestion and absorption during digestion, the oxygen saturation of the portal blood decreases.

(e)   Yes.

22.59

(a)   Yes. Sick cells swell and eventually burst; this is because of failure of the sodium extrusion mechanism.

(b)   Yes. Energy from metabolism is required for active pumping.

(c)   No. Active transport is required for net movement of a chemical against, but not down, its electrochemical gradient.

(d)   Yes. See (e).

(e)   Yes. Any mechanism yielding a fluid with a concentration of water high or lower than that of plasma requires energy. When a urine more dilute than plasma is being produced, this requires the active transport of solute from renal tubular fluid to renal interstitial fluid.

22.60

(a)   No. In the primary acinar secretion, the concentration of potassium is greater than in plasma.

(b)   Yes. As saliva passes along the ducts of the salivary glands, sodium ions are reabsorbed, thus reducing the concentration of sodium.

(c)   No. As saliva passes along the ducts of the salivary glands, despite the reabsorption of sodium, the salivary osmolarity is maintained by potassium secretion.

(d)   Yes.
(e)   Yes. The sodium reabsorption and potassium secretion are rate limited, so when the salivary flow rate is high, the saliva has a composition closer to that of plasma than when the flow rate is low; at low flow rates the salivary concentration of potassium is greater than at high flow rates.

Index

The numbers in this index refer to the questions and/or their answers